New Biomolecules and Drug Delivery Systems as Alternatives to Conventional Antibiotics

New Biomolecules and Drug Delivery Systems as Alternatives to Conventional Antibiotics

Editor

Helena P. Felgueiras

MDPI • Basel • Beijing • Wuhan • Barcelona • Belgrade • Manchester • Tokyo • Cluj • Tianjin

Editor
Helena P. Felgueiras
Centre for Textile Science and
Technology
University of Minho
Guimarães
Portugal

Editorial Office
MDPI
St. Alban-Anlage 66
4052 Basel, Switzerland

This is a reprint of articles from the Special Issue published online in the open access journal *Antibiotics* (ISSN 2079-6382) (available at: www.mdpi.com/journal/antibiotics/special_issues/Biomolecules_Antibiotics).

For citation purposes, cite each article independently as indicated on the article page online and as indicated below:

LastName, A.A.; LastName, B.B.; LastName, C.C. Article Title. *Journal Name* **Year**, *Volume Number*, Page Range.

ISBN 978-3-0365-4736-7 (Hbk)
ISBN 978-3-0365-4735-0 (PDF)

Contents

Helena P. Felgueiras
New Biomolecules and Drug Delivery Systems as Alternatives to Conventional Antibiotics
Reprinted from: *Antibiotics* **2022**, *11*, 318, doi:10.3390/antibiotics11030318 . . . . **1**

Marta O. Teixeira, Joana C. Antunes and Helena P. Felgueiras
Recent Advances in Fiber–Hydrogel Composites for Wound Healing and Drug Delivery Systems
Reprinted from: *Antibiotics* **2021**, *10*, 248, doi:10.3390/antibiotics10030248 . . . . **3**

Neveen M. Saleh, Yasmine S. Moemen, Sara H. Mohamed, Ghady Fathy, Abdullah A. S. Ahmed and Ahmed A. Al-Ghamdi et al.
Experimental and Molecular Docking Studies of Cyclic Diphenyl Phosphonates as DNA Gyrase Inhibitors for Fluoroquinolone-Resistant Pathogens
Reprinted from: *Antibiotics* **2022**, *11*, 53, doi:10.3390/antibiotics11010053 . . . . **37**

Jiaohong Li, Rongyu Li, Cheng Zhang, Zhenxiang Guo, Xiaomao Wu and Huaming An
Co-Application of Allicin and Chitosan Increases Resistance of *Rosa roxburghii* against Powdery Mildew and Enhances Its Yield and Quality
Reprinted from: *Antibiotics* **2021**, *10*, 1449, doi:10.3390/antibiotics10121449 . . . . **53**

Jaime Esteban, María Vallet-Regí and John J. Aguilera-Correa
Antibiotics- and Heavy Metals-Based Titanium Alloy Surface Modifications for Local Prosthetic Joint Infections
Reprinted from: *Antibiotics* **2021**, *10*, 1270, doi:10.3390/antibiotics10101270 . . . . **65**

Daphne T. Lianou, Efthymia Petinaki, Peter J. Cripps, Dimitris A. Gougoulis, Charalambia K. Michael and Katerina Tsilipounidaki et al.
Prevalence, Patterns, Association with Biofilm Formation, Effects on Milk Quality and Risk Factors for Antibiotic Resistance of Staphylococci from Bulk-Tank Milk of Goat Herds
Reprinted from: *Antibiotics* **2021**, *10*, 1225, doi:10.3390/antibiotics10101225 . . . . **89**

Arul Murugan Preethi and Jayesh R. Bellare
Concomitant Effect of Quercetin- and Magnesium-Doped Calcium Silicate on the Osteogenic and Antibacterial Activity of Scaffolds for Bone Regeneration
Reprinted from: *Antibiotics* **2021**, *10*, 1170, doi:10.3390/antibiotics10101170 . . . . **103**

Margarita N. Baranova, Polina A. Babikova, Arsen M. Kudzhaev, Yuliana A. Mokrushina, Olga A. Belozerova and Maxim A. Yunin et al.
Live Biosensors for Ultrahigh-Throughput Screening of Antimicrobial Activity against Gram-Negative Bacteria
Reprinted from: *Antibiotics* **2021**, *10*, 1161, doi:10.3390/antibiotics10101161 . . . . **119**

Hui-Ling Lin, Chen-En Chiang, Mei-Chun Lin, Mei-Lan Kau, Yun-Tzu Lin and Chi-Shuo Chen
Aerosolized Hypertonic Saline Hinders Biofilm Formation to Enhance Antibiotic Susceptibility of Multidrug-Resistant *Acinetobacter baumannii*
Reprinted from: *Antibiotics* **2021**, *10*, 1115, doi:10.3390/antibiotics10091115 . . . . **131**

Hani A. Alhadrami, Raha Orfali, Ahmed A. Hamed, Mohammed M Ghoneim, Hossam M. Hassan and Ahmed S. I. Hassane et al.
Flavonoid-Coated Gold Nanoparticles as Efficient Antibiotics against Gram-Negative Bacteria—Evidence from In Silico-Supported In Vitro Studies
Reprinted from: *Antibiotics* **2021**, *10*, 968, doi:10.3390/antibiotics10080968 . . . . **143**

Qiuping Wang, Cheng Zhang, Youhua Long, Xiaomao Wu, Yue Su and Yang Lei et al.
Bioactivity and Control Efficacy of the Novel Antibiotic Tetramycin against Various Kiwifruit Diseases
Reprinted from: *Antibiotics* **2021**, *10*, 289, doi:10.3390/antibiotics10030289 . . . . **161**

Hee-Won Han, Jin-Hwan Kwak, Tae-Su Jang, Jonathan Campbell Knowles, Hae-Won Kim and Hae-Hyoung Lee et al.
Grapefruit Seed Extract as a Natural Derived Antibacterial Substance against Multidrug-Resistant Bacteria
Reprinted from: *Antibiotics* **2021**, *10*, 85, doi:10.3390/antibiotics10010085 . . . . **173**

Vajravathi Lakkim, Madhava C. Reddy, Roja Rani Pallavali, Kakarla Raghava Reddy, Ch Venkata Reddy and Inamuddin et al.
Green Synthesis of Silver Nanoparticles and Evaluation of Their Antibacterial Activity against Multidrug-Resistant Bacteria and Wound Healing Efficacy Using a Murine Model
Reprinted from: *Antibiotics* **2020**, *9*, 902, doi:10.3390/antibiotics9120902 . . . . **187**

Vanessa Raquel Greatti, Fernando Oda, Rodrigo Sorrechia, Bárbara Regina Kapp, Carolina Manzato Seraphim and Ana Carolina Villas Bôas Weckwerth et al.
Poly-ε-caprolactone Nanoparticles Loaded with 4-Nerolidylcatechol (4-NC) for Growth Inhibition of *Microsporum canis*
Reprinted from: *Antibiotics* **2020**, *9*, 894, doi:10.3390/antibiotics9120894 . . . . **209**

antibiotics

MDPI

Editorial

New Biomolecules and Drug Delivery Systems as Alternatives to Conventional Antibiotics

Helena P. Felgueiras

Centre for Textile Science and Technology (2C2T), Campus de Azurém, University of Minho, 4800-058 Guimaraes, Portugal; helena.felgueiras@2c2t.uminho.pt

New approaches to deal with the growing concern associated with antibiotic-resistant bacteria are in high demand. For many years, antibiotics have been the gold standard for treating infections. However, their excessive consumption and misuse have contributed to the rise of microorganisms resistant to antibiotic action, leading to a global health crisis. Engineering new drug delivery platforms and uncovering alternative biomolecules with antimicrobial and regenerative potentials is becoming extremely urgent. This Special Issue aims at expanding our understanding of the antimicrobial action of specialized biomolecules, recently engineered or chemically modified from their ancient origins, and to introduce a broad audience to new systems of drug delivery.

In this collection of research, many important findings can be highlighted, namely the emergence of flavonoid-coated gold nanoparticles [1] and the concurrent effect of quercetin (also a bioflavonoid)- and magnesium-doped calcium silicates as highly effective antibacterial agents against Gram-negative bacteria [2], the engineering of silver nanoparticles via a new green synthesis methodology that improved the performance of these cues against multidrug-resistant bacteria [3], and the loading of poly-ε-caprolactone nanoparticles with 4-nerolidylcatechol that specifically inhibited the growth of *Microsporum canis* [4]. Another strategy against multidrug-resistant microbials was introduced by Han et al., whose findings demonstrated grapefruit seed extracts as effective antibacterial agents, even at low concentrations [5], while Lin et al. revealed the potentialities of aerosolized hypertonic saline against multidrug-resistant *Acinetobacter baumannii*, unveiling a new vehicle of delivery for conventional antibiotics capable of improving their effectiveness [6].

Discovering new pharmaceutical strategies to fight infection is a very challenging and time-consuming process. Considering DNA gyrase and topoisomerase IV are known targets for novel antibacterial drug design, Saleh et al. demonstrated the effectiveness of diphenylphosphonates as DNA gyrase inhibitors, with great potentially for new pharmaceutical formulations [7]. Furthermore, Baranova et al. followed a different route and resorted to live biosensors for ultra-high-throughput screening for deep profiling of antibacterial activity and antibiotic discovery [8].

Even though most of the focus of this Special Issue is on developing and unveiling new antimicrobial cues capable of mitigating or irradicating infection in humans, plants and animal products are also affected by similar issues, with pesticides and other chemical agents becoming highly ineffective against microbial plagues. Assessments of pathogenic resistance have been made by Lianou et al. on bulk-tank milk of goat herds, to identify potentially dangerous factors affecting the product quality [9]. These assessments are essential to better understand the mechanisms of action of microbial species, and hence, propose personalized solutions. Wang et al. investigated a novel polyene agriculture antibiotic, tetramycin, and determined that it could prevent several diseases in kiwi plants [10]. Allicin and chitosan were also found to increase the resistance of *Rosa roxburghii* against powdery mildew, being highlighted as a potential green, cost-effective and environmentally friendly strategy to raise production yields [11].

Citation: Felgueiras, H.P. New Biomolecules and Drug Delivery Systems as Alternatives to Conventional Antibiotics. *Antibiotics* **2022**, *11*, 318. https://doi.org/10.3390/antibiotics11030318

Received: 10 February 2022
Accepted: 11 February 2022
Published: 28 February 2022

Finally, recent advances in antibiotic- and heavy-metal-loaded titanium surfaces were examined as potential mechanisms for preventing local infection in bone-related applications [12], while for tissue engineering and wound healing, fiber–hydrogel composites were identified as prospective effective solutions [13]. Even though this Special Issue has provided significant evidence of the high level of research and dedication in finding potential options and solutions to the present antibiotic crisis, introducing readers to both techniques and molecules with an active profile against microbial agents, we anticipate that there are many antimicrobial cues and delivery systems with precise targets and mechanisms of action still to uncover.

Funding: This research was funded by the Portuguese Foundation for Science and Technology (FCT) grants PTDC/CTMTEX/28074/2017 and UID/CTM/00264/2020.

Conflicts of Interest: The authors declare no conflict of interest.

References

1. Alhadrami, H.A.; Orfali, R.; Hamed, A.A.; Ghoneim, M.M.; Hassan, H.M.; Hassane, A.S.I.; Rateb, M.E.; Sayed, A.M.; Gamaleldin, N.M. Flavonoid-Coated Gold Nanoparticles as Efficient Antibiotics against Gram-Negative Bacteria—Evidence from In Silico-Supported In Vitro Studies. *Antibiotics* **2021**, *10*, 968. [CrossRef] [PubMed]
2. Preethi, A.M.; Bellare, J.R. Concomitant Effect of Quercetin- and Magnesium-Doped Calcium Silicate on the Osteogenic and Antibacterial Activity of Scaffolds for Bone Regeneration. *Antibiotics* **2021**, *10*, 1170. [CrossRef] [PubMed]
3. Lakkim, V.; Reddy, M.C.; Pallavali, R.R.; Reddy, K.R.; Reddy, C.V.; Inamuddin; Bilgrami, A.L.; Lomada, D. Green Synthesis of Silver Nanoparticles and Evaluation of Their Antibacterial Activity against Multidrug-Resistant Bacteria and Wound Healing Efficacy Using a Murine Model. *Antibiotics* **2020**, *9*, 902. [CrossRef] [PubMed]
4. Greatti, V.R.; Oda, F.; Sorrechia, R.; Kapp, B.R.; Seraphim, C.M.; Weckwerth, A.C.V.B.; Chorilli, M.; Silva, P.B.D.; Eloy, J.O.; Kogan, M.J.; et al. Poly-ε-caprolactone Nanoparticles Loaded with 4-Nerolidylcatechol (4-NC) for Growth Inhibition of Microsporum canis. *Antibiotics* **2020**, *9*, 894. [CrossRef] [PubMed]
5. Han, H.-W.; Kwak, J.-H.; Jang, T.-S.; Knowles, J.C.; Kim, H.-W.; Lee, H.-H.; Lee, J.-H. Grapefruit Seed Extract as a Natural Derived Antibacterial Substance against Multidrug-Resistant Bacteria. *Antibiotics* **2021**, *10*, 85. [CrossRef] [PubMed]
6. Lin, H.-L.; Chiang, C.-E.; Lin, M.-C.; Kau, M.-L.; Lin, Y.-T.; Chen, C.-S. Aerosolized Hypertonic Saline Hinders Biofilm Formation to Enhance Antibiotic Susceptibility of Multidrug-Resistant Acinetobacter baumannii. *Antibiotics* **2021**, *10*, 1115. [CrossRef] [PubMed]
7. Saleh, N.M.; Moemen, Y.S.; Mohamed, S.H.; Fathy, G.; Ahmed, A.A.S.; Al-Ghamdi, A.A.; Ullah, S.; El Sayed, I.E.-T. Experimental and Molecular Docking Studies of Cyclic Diphenyl Phosphonates as DNA Gyrase Inhibitors for Fluoroquinolone-Resistant Pathogens. *Antibiotics* **2022**, *11*, 53. [CrossRef] [PubMed]
8. Baranova, M.N.; Babikova, P.A.; Kudzhaev, A.M.; Mokrushina, Y.A.; Belozerova, O.A.; Yunin, M.A.; Kovalchuk, S.; Gabibov, A.G.; Smirnov, I.V.; Terekhov, S.S. Live Biosensors for Ultrahigh-Throughput Screening of Antimicrobial Activity against Gram-Negative Bacteria. *Antibiotics* **2021**, *10*, 1161. [CrossRef] [PubMed]
9. Lianou, D.T.; Petinaki, E.; Cripps, P.J.; Gougoulis, D.A.; Michael, C.K.; Tsilipounidaki, K.; Skoulakis, A.; Katsafadou, A.I.; Vasileiou, N.G.C.; Giannoulis, T.; et al. Prevalence, Patterns, Association with Biofilm Formation, Effects on Milk Quality and Risk Factors for Antibiotic Resistance of Staphylococci from Bulk-Tank Milk of Goat Herds. *Antibiotics* **2021**, *10*, 1225. [CrossRef] [PubMed]
10. Wang, Q.; Zhang, C.; Long, Y.; Wu, X.; Su, Y.; Lei, Y.; Ai, Q. Bioactivity and Control Efficacy of the Novel Antibiotic Tetramycin against Various Kiwifruit Diseases. *Antibiotics* **2021**, *10*, 289. [CrossRef] [PubMed]
11. Li, J.; Li, R.; Zhang, C.; Guo, Z.; Wu, X.; An, H. Co-Application of Allicin and Chitosan Increases Resistance of Rosa roxburghii against Powdery Mildew and Enhances Its Yield and Quality. *Antibiotics* **2021**, *10*, 1449. [CrossRef] [PubMed]
12. Esteban, J.; Vallet-Regí, M.; Aguilera-Correa, J.J. Antibiotics- and Heavy Metals-Based Titanium Alloy Surface Modifications for Local Prosthetic Joint Infections. *Antibiotics* **2021**, *10*, 1270. [CrossRef] [PubMed]
13. Teixeira, M.O.; Antunes, J.C.; Felgueiras, H.P. Recent Advances in Fiber–Hydrogel Composites for Wound Healing and Drug Delivery Systems. *Antibiotics* **2021**, *10*, 248. [CrossRef] [PubMed]

antibiotics

Review

Recent Advances in Fiber–Hydrogel Composites for Wound Healing and Drug Delivery Systems

Marta O. Teixeira, Joana C. Antunes and Helena P. Felgueiras *

Centre for Textile Science and Technology (2C2T), Department of Textile Engineering, University of Minho, Campus of Azurém, 4800-058 Guimarães, Portugal; martasofia.teixeira@hotmail.com (M.O.T.); joana.antunes@2c2t.uminho.pt (J.C.A.)

* Correspondence: helena.felgueiras@2c2t.uminho.pt; Tel.: +351-253-510-283; Fax: +351-253-510-293

Abstract: In the last decades, much research has been done to fasten wound healing and target-direct drug delivery. Hydrogel-based scaffolds have been a recurrent solution in both cases, with some reaching already the market, even though their mechanical stability remains a challenge. To overcome this limitation, reinforcement of hydrogels with fibers has been explored. The structural resemblance of fiber–hydrogel composites to natural tissues has been a driving force for the optimization and exploration of these systems in biomedicine. Indeed, the combination of hydrogel-forming techniques and fiber spinning approaches has been crucial in the development of scaffolding systems with improved mechanical strength and medicinal properties. In this review, a comprehensive overview of the recently developed fiber–hydrogel composite strategies for wound healing and drug delivery is provided. The methodologies employed in fiber and hydrogel formation are also highlighted, together with the most compatible polymer combinations, as well as drug incorporation approaches creating stimuli-sensitive and triggered drug release towards an enhanced host response.

Keywords: fiber–hydrogel composite; biodegradable polymers; skin regeneration; drug delivery platforms; controlled release

Citation: Teixeira, M.O.; Antunes, J.C.; Felgueiras, H.P. Recent Advances in Fiber–Hydrogel Composites for Wound Healing and Drug Delivery Systems. *Antibiotics* **2021**, *10*, 248. https://doi.org/10.3390/antibiotics10030248

Academic Editor: Serena Riela

Received: 29 January 2021
Accepted: 25 February 2021
Published: 2 March 2021

1. Introduction

Biomaterials are defined as nonviable materials, with potential for applications in medical devices, that possess the ability to interact with biological systems to evaluate, treat, replace or enhance the performance of any tissue [1]. Biomaterials are classified in different ways; the most common refers to their chemical nature and is subdivided in metallic materials (ferrous and non244-ferrous) and non-metallic materials (organic: polymers, biological materials, and carbons; and inorganic: ceramics and glasses). Composites are considered another very important class of biomaterials and result from the combination of two classes of materials that work in synergy to improve the properties of the final product above those of the individual components [1,2].

The continued research in this field has raised the specificity level of the biomaterials developed and, therefore, has increased its impact in the healthcare global market [1]. Polymers represent a large portion of all biomaterials used in the biomedical field (about 45%) [2], and their application appears to have no end. They can be processed in the form of particles, foams, films, membranes, hydrogels and fibers, and combinations of these 3D structures can then be made to generated intricate, target-direct, specialized biomedical systems. Biomedicine has resorted to these constructs to understand specific biological processes and to engineer high-performance therapies to treat a variety of diseases. The need to match the desired functions/characteristics of a given tissue or cell has driven the combination of different classes of biomaterials in complex constructs (e.g., fiber–hydrogel composite) that can effectively respond to the local demands and provide the necessary tools to reach the desired goals. In recent years, fiber–hydrogel composites have been disclosed as one of those systems that combine different structures to improve individual features and enhance inherent advantages to achieve successful outcomes. In biomedical engineering, the importance of these constructs is particularly noticeable in wound healing and drug delivery. In both areas, fiber–hydrogel composites can be a good alternative to the use of antibiotics and/or their controlled administration.

The present review explores this subject further, starting with the introduction of basic concepts associated with polymer properties and processing in the form of fibers and hydrogels and then evolving towards the combination of these two structures in one to successfully respond to specific needs. The most recent studies highlighting fiber–hydrogel composites are here identified, giving particular attention to the engineering of wound dressings and drug delivery systems.

2. Polymers Natural/Synthetic

The word polymer is derived from the Greek *poly* and *meros*, meaning many and parts, respectively. Polymers are macromolecules that result from the repetition of smaller molecules, the monomers [3]. The nature of the monomers and the specific bonds generated between them, and their spatial rearrangement, determine the properties of the built polymer [4]. The process through which a polymer is formed is named polymerization and can be described as a chemical reaction in which the combination of one or more monomers occurs [3]. Polymers can also be biologically derived or synthetically produced [2]. Natural polymers are created in nature during the life cycles of biological systems, such as plants, microorganisms, and animals [5]. These polymers are widely used in scientific community, namely, in tissue engineering, wound dressing and drug delivery systems [6–8], due to their biocompatibility, non-toxicity, biodegradability and bioactivity, particularly their inherent anti-inflammatory and antibacterial properties [9]. These polymers include polysaccharides and polypeptides. Polysaccharides, the most abundant class of biopolymers, are polymeric carbohydrate molecules formed by glycosidic bonds with different structures and properties depending on molecular weight and chemical composition [8]. In particular, polysaccharides, compared to polypeptides, are generally more stable and usually do not denature on heating [10]. Regarding their chemical properties, they have polyfunctionality, high chemical reactivity, chirality, chelation and adsorption capacity, which allow them to be chemically and biochemically modified very easily. These modifications result in different polysaccharide derivatives, which increase the range of applications [6,8,11]. The alginate, hyaluronic acid (HA), cellulose and chitosan (CS) stand out between the polysaccharides for being the most used in biomedicine (Table 1). Just like polysaccharides, polypeptides are produced by microorganisms. Polypeptides are macromolecules composed of repeated units of amino acids linked by peptide bonds. Their versatility, flexibility, good performance in metabolic adaptation and imitation of the extracellular matrix makes them good candidates for tissue scaffolding and drug/gene delivery [12]. The most common polypeptides used in biomedicine are collagen and gelatin (Table 1). However, known limitations of natural polymers include their very low dimensional stability, susceptibility to immunogenic responses, possibility of pathogen transmission and high batch-to-batch variability [12,13]. For this reason, biodegradable synthetic polymers are frequently employed as alternatives.

Indeed, some of the key benefits of synthetic polymers are their reproducibility, which allows mass production, and their ability to be tuned according to specific requirements. Their degradation profile can also be easily manipulated via their hydrolytic groups [14], even though bulk degradation can occur [15]. Moreover, synthetic polymers are biologically inert, thus without a therapeutical impact, but may induce chronic inflammation [16]. In biomedicine, poly(ethylene oxide) (PEO), poly(ε-caprolactone) (PCL), polylactic acid (PLA), poly(lactic-co-glycolic acid) (PLGA), poly(vinylpyrrolidone)(PVP) and poly(vinyl alcohol) (PVA) [15,17] constitute the most studied polymers in the field (Table 1) [18]. They may additionally be combined with natural polymers. Hybrid polymers can result from the total or part combination of natural and synthetic polymers. As is the case of the combination of the PLGA (synthetic polymer) and the CS (natural polymer) that result in the PLGA-CS hybrid polymer that has been studied in several areas, namely in therapeutic delivery [19]. The choice of polymers for the formation of scaffolds, based on their characteristics, has proved to be crucial in the properties and applicability of the final scaffold. Currently, synergisms between synthetic and natural biomaterials in the form of 3D scaffolds, such as hydrogels and nanofibrous mats, are in high demand for biomedical applications, being frequently preferred over constructs made of polymers belonging to only one of these categories [7,15,20].

Table 1. Origins and main properties of natural and synthetic polymers commonly used in wound healing, tissue engineering and drug delivery applications.

	Polymer	Structural Formula	Origin/Synthesis Pathway	Main Characteristics	Known/Key/Main/Selected Applications	Reference
Natural	**Hyaluronic acid**	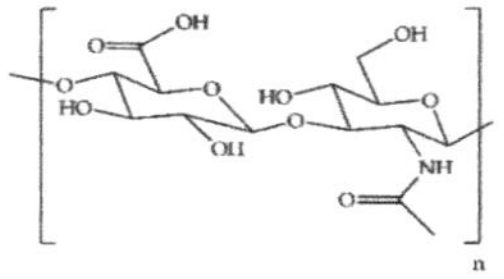	Connective tissues of any vertebrate	Non-sulfated anionic glycosaminoglycan; linear conformation; hydrophilic; water-soluble; highly viscoelastic; non-immunogenic; biodegradable	Wound healing; biomolecule (e.g., ocatdecyl acrylate) delivery; cartilage/bone regeneration; bioink in 3D printing	[11,21–24]
	Chitosan	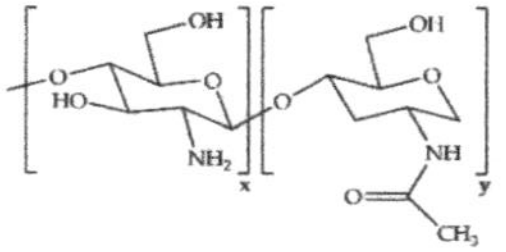	Chitin (mostly found in the exoskeleton of shrimps, crabs, lobster and squid pens; cuticles of insects; and in lesser amounts, in cell walls of fungi, yeast and plants)	Cationic linear polysaccharide; hydrophilic; pH-dependent charge density; physicochemical properties dependent on the degree of acetylation, crystallinity, molecular weight and degradation; non-toxic; biodegradable; non-antigenic; biologically adhesive; hemostatic effect; antimicrobial; anti-inflammatory	Wound healing; bone/cartilage regeneration; antibiotic/antibacterial agents/growth factors delivery	[20,22,25–27]
	Alginate	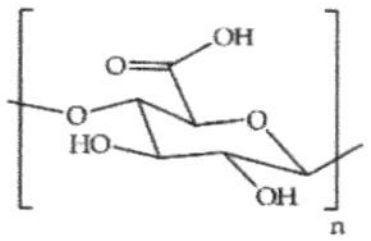	Brown seaweed or bacteria (*Azotobacter* and *Pseudomonas* specie)	Anionic linear polysaccharide; slow gelation time; hydrophilic; water soluble; low toxicity; low cost; water retaining capacity; biodegradable	Wound dressings; burn treatments; protein/small chemical drug delivery; bone/cartilage regeneration	[5,28–30]
	Cellulose	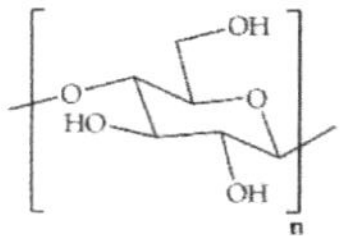	Plants (mainly derived from cotton fiber, dried hemp and wood), bacteria (e.g., *Acetobacter*, *Azotobacter*, *Rhizobium*, *Agrobacterium*, *Pseudomonas*, *Salmonella*, *Alcaligenes* and *Sarcina ventriculi* species)	Linear homopolysaccharide; hydrophilic; rigid; fibrous morphology; relatively easy extraction; non-toxicity; low cost; biodegradable	Bone/tendon tissue regeneration; wound healing; loading antimicrobial agents and antibiotics	[31–34]

Table 1. *Cont.*

	Polymer	Structural Formula	Origin/Synthesis Pathway	Main Characteristics	Known/Key/Main/Selected Applications	Reference
Natural	**Gelatin**	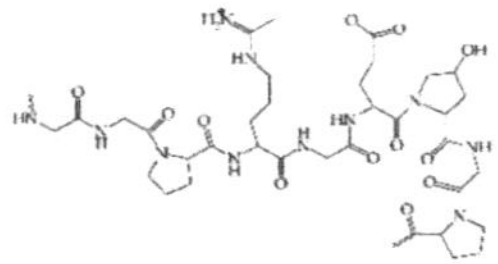	Skin and bone of bovine and porcine, fish and marine organisms (incomplete denaturalization of collagen)	Linear polypeptide; hydrophilic; water soluble (35 °C); soluble in polyhydric alcohols and several other organic solvents; cost efficient; easily available; biodegradable; non-antigenic; similarity to collagen	Wound healing; bone regeneration; articular cartilage repair; tendon tissue engineering	[26,35–37]
	Collagen	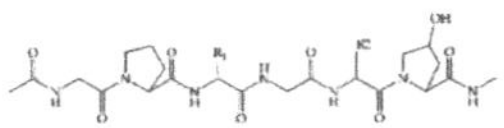 Collagen type I	Animals (e.g., Achilles tendon, bovine skin, porcine skin, and human cadaveric skin)	Polypeptide; good surface-active agent; enhanced water holding capacity; highly hydrophilic; twenty-eight different collagen types; low antigenic and cytotoxic responses; antioxidant; biodegradable; most abundant protein of animal origin	Wound healing; tissue replacement and regeneration (bone, cartilage, skin, blood vessels, trachea, esophagus); carriers for drug/protein delivery	[38–41]
Synthetic	**Poly(ethylene oxide)**	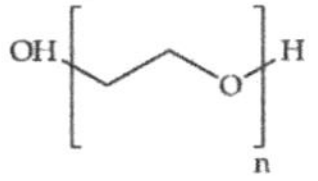	Anionic ring-opening polymerization of ethylene oxide (EO)	Neutral polymer; hydrophilic; water soluble; low toxic; biodegradable	Gene/drug delivery systems; biomedical implants; neocartilage tissue formation; transdermal delivery	[42–45]
	Poly(ε-caprolactone)	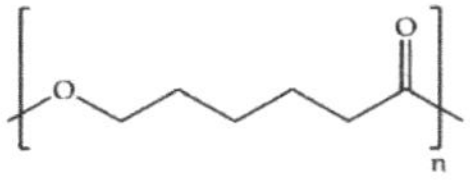	Ring-opening polymerization of ε-caprolactone monomer using a wide range of catalysts	Semicrystalline; hydrophobic; excellent mechanical strength; slow degradation rate; nontoxic; biodegradable	Tendon tissue engineering; skin regeneration; vascular scaffolds	[37,44,46,47]
	Polylactic acid	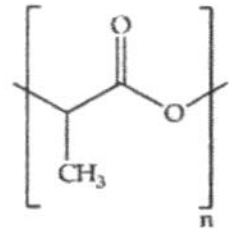	Polycondensation of lactic acid and ring opening polymerization of cyclic lactide	Thermoplastic aliphatic polyester; hydrophobic; poor ductility; low strength; bioabsorbable; biodegradable	Ligament and tendon repair; vascular stents; bone regeneration	[5,48–50]

Table 1. *Cont.*

	Polymer	Structural Formula	Origin/Synthesis Pathway	Main Characteristics	Known/Key/Main/Selected Applications	Reference
	Poly(lactic-co-glycolic acid)	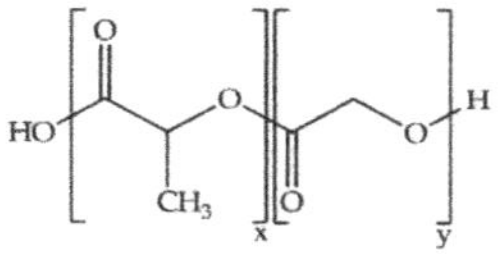	Ring-opening polymerization of lactide	Linear aliphatic copolymer; relatively hydrophobic; enhanced flexibility; thermal processibility; tunable degradation/biodegradation; minimal side effects	Wound healing; bone/cardiac/periodontal tissue regeneration; protein/growth facto/antibiotic/gene delivery	[51,52]
Synthetic	**Poly(vinylpyrrolidone)**	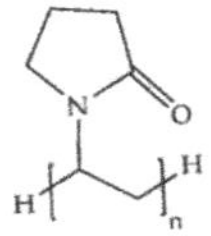	Free radical polymerization from the vinylpyrrolidone monomer	Neutral polymer; amorphous; hydrophilic; water soluble; stable; nontoxic; adhesive power; non-biodegradable	Wound healing; gene delivery; biomedical implants (orthopedic, dental, vaginal, breast); neural/cardiac/pancreatic tissue regeneration	[17,53–55]
	Poly(vinyl alcohol)	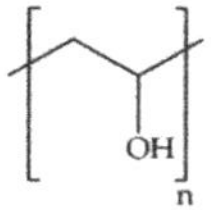	Vinyl acetate with base catalyzed transesterification with ethanol	Linear polymer; hydrophilic; semicrystalline; water soluble; pH sensitive; high swelling capability; excellent chemo-thermal stability; transparency; high tensile; strength; high elongation at break; flexibility; non-toxic; non-carcinogenic and bioadhesive properties; non-biodegradable	Drugs/protein/growth factor/nanoparticle/gene delivery; skin healing and reconstruction; kidney regeneration	[48,56,57]

3. Hydrogel

Hydrogels are 3D networks of hydrophilic polymers capable of absorbing and retaining significant amounts of fluids [58], which have also been widely applied in wound healing [30,59]; cartilage tissue engineering [36,60]; bone tissue engineering [61]; and delivery of proteins, growth factors and antibiotics [20,62].

Hydrogels can be classified based on their source, namely the composing polymers, in natural or synthetic (Table 2). Thus, nature-derived hydrogels may consist of natural polysaccharides or polypeptides [6,12], ergo carrying molecular recognition sites enabling cell/tissue communication pathways and modulation towards a therapeutical effect [63]. However, as hydrogels, they tend to present low stability in aqueous medium, poor mechanical properties and quick degradation rates [63]. On the other hand, hydrogels based on synthetic polymers are typically mechanically resilient and display superior elastic properties. Still, their biological inertness, blocking any chances of tuning cell behavior towards a healthier state, limits their use in biomedicine [63,64]. Hybrid hydrogels, combining natural and synthetic polymers [65], have been proven useful to create smart hydrogels (alginate-g-(PEO-poly(propylene oxide)-PEO) [66]), in biomedical materials (PVA/collagen [67]) and in tissue engineering applications (CS/PCL [47]), to name a few examples. Their polymer composition may also subdivide hydrogels in homopolymers, copolymers, multipolymers or interpenetrating polymer networks (IPN) [68]. Homopolymer hydrogels are made of crosslinked polymer networks derived from a single type of basic structural unit (monomers) [69]. Copolymer hydrogels are frequently crosslinked polymer networks made up of two co-monomer units with at least one hydrophilic component (not soluble in water). These networks can assume three types of configuration, arbitrary, block or may alternate between both along the chain [70,71]. Multipolymer hydrogels are the result of the reaction of three or more co-monomers [72]. In turn, IPNs are an important class made of two independent crosslinked synthetic and/or natural polymer components, in which a new hydrogel polymeric network is polymerized within a pre-existent [68,73]. In case only one polymer network from the two is crosslinked, the hydrogels are designated as semi-IPNs. [68].

Table 2. General classification of hydrogels considering their source, polymers charge, polymer composition, structural configuration, degradation, physical properties, response to stimuli, and type of crosslinking [68].

Hydrogels Classification	
Source	Natural, synthetic or hybrid
Charge of polymers	Ionic, non-ionic, amphoteric or zwitterionic
Polymeric composition	Homopolymer, copolymer, multipolymer, IPN or semi-IPN
Configuration	Amorphous, crystalline or semicrystalline
Degradability	Biodegradable or non-biodegradable
Physical properties	Conventional or smart
Response	Physical, chemical, or biochemical/biological
Type of crosslinking	Chemical or physical

Hydrogels may also be categorized as amorphous, crystalline or semi-crystalline, depending on their physical organization and chemical composition. Semicrystalline hydrogel networks are mixtures of crystalline as well as amorphous phases [74]. These properties may also affect the hydrogel degradation rate, sub-divided in degradable or non-degradable structures [68]. Most hydrogels used in tissue engineering and drug delivery systems are biodegradable and are developed to degrade into biologically acceptable molecules (non-toxic degradation biproducts) [75,76]. The degradation rate of biodegradable hydrogels may be manipulated via the polymers' molecular weight [77], by the action of oxidizing agents [78], or by the presence of enzymes [79]. Tanan et al. developed a semi-interpenetrating hydrogel (semi-IPN) consisting of a mixture of cassava starch-g-polyacrylic acid/natural rubber/PVA. This hydrogel exhibited an excellent water retention capacity and proved to be highly sensitive to salt concentration, type of cations, pH and swelling time. In addition, it demonstrated good biodegradation with a rate of 0.626 wt.%/day [80].

In terms of their physical properties, hydrogels can be categorized as conventional or smart. Conventional hydrogels are characterized by low response rates, in general. They have a very low swelling rate due to their small matrix size. This limitation has triggered a greater interest in macroscopic hydrogels, where the size of the pores allows a higher swelling rate. Smart hydrogels are hydrogels that react to changes in environmental conditions (external stimuli) by swelling or reversibly collapsing [81,82]. Hydrogels can be physical, chemical or biochemical/biological in relation to the type of response/stimulus [68]. Physical stimuli like temperature, electric field, magnetic field, light and pressure and chemical stimuli like pH, solvent composition and ionic strength can change the swelling state of the hydrogel. Hydrogels with biochemical/biological responses are capable of interacting with the surrounding environment [81,83]. In terms of production, hydrogels can be formed by physical [30] and/or chemical [21] crosslinking of polymers, which will be discussed in the following sections. Hydrogels can also be classified based on their charge in non-ionic (neutral), ionic (anionic or cationic), amphoteric (acidic and basic groups) or zwitterionic (anionic and cationic groups in each structural unit) [68].

Hydrogels benefit from a high degree of flexibility, adjustable viscoelasticity, biocompatibility, high permeability to oxygen and essential nutrients, high water content and low interfacial tension with aqueous medium [7,22]. The hydrogel biocompatibility, that is, its ability to perform its intended function without inducing side effects in the host, is one of its most crucial characteristics. Further, in case of wounds, for instance, their limited adhesion may allow removal from the wound bed without causing additional trauma or destroying the newly formed tissues [84,85].

Certain hydrogels even have capacity to alter their swelling state in response to environmental variations; these function as triggers to change the physical and/or chemical properties of the hydrogel. For example, in the case of pH-sensitive hydrogels, the polymers that make up the hydrogel contain hydrophobic moieties that swell in water according to the pH of the external environment. Thus, in the absence of this stimulus, the hydrogel maintains its initial swelling state [81]. This property makes them good candidates for drug delivery systems. In this case, altering the swelling state in response to a change in pH opens opportunities for controlling the timing of drug release. Kwon et al. described the synthesis via chemical crosslinking of pH-sensitive hydrogels based on hydroxyethyl cellulose and HA for transdermal delivery of the drug isoliquiritigenin. At pH 7, the electrostatic repulsions between the carboxylate groups of HA lead to the enlargement of mesh and, consequently, to an increase in the amount of isoliquiritigenin released. The authors observed an efficacy greater than 70% of the release of the drug due to the pH and excellent adhesive properties of the hydrogel, which makes it a good candidate for treating skin lesions [86].

Hydrogel Formation: Techniques

Considering that many hydrogels degrade very easily in biological systems or in contact with water-based fluids, the purpose of the crosslinking process is to improve the insolubility, mechanical strength, and rigidity of the polymer network. Hydrogels can be physically or chemically crosslinked (Table 3) [87]. Physical hydrogels are networks with transient junctions (reversible connections), traditionally disordered and fragile. They result from interactions such as ionic bonding [88], hydrogen bonding [89], hydrophobic interactions [90], and crystallization [91]. The physical properties of the polymers and the gelation conditions determine the internal structure of the hydrogel, by modulating properties such as gel density, porosity and mechanical performance (e.g., rigidity) [92].

Physical hydrogels tend to exhibit low mechanical strength and are often unstable [93]. The dissolution of physically crosslinked hydrogels can occur in response to changes in temperature, application of stress, ionic strength, pH and solvent composition. Because of their reversible character, the polymer solution resulting from the dissolution process may undergo again gelation and restore the original hydrogel features [65,94].

Unlike physical, chemical hydrogels are polymer networks with permanent junctions, formed via covalent bonds, which are capable of maintaining the structure integrity for longer (increased degradation time) [95]. Chemically crosslinked hydrogels are known to be mechanically strong. However, although they present a permanently fixed shape, they have low fracture resistance and extensibility [93]. Further, certain chemical crosslinking agents are toxic and can cause adverse reactions; thus, they must be extracted from the gels before use [96]. Photopolymerization, enzymatic crosslinking, crosslinking molecules and polymer–polymer crosslinking are the four major chemical crosslinking methods that can be employed to form crosslinked hydrogels.

Table 3. Properties and limitations of different types of physical and chemical crosslinking.

Hydrogels	Crosslinking Engine	Concept	Advantages	Disadvantages	Reference
Physical	**Ionic/Electrostatic Interaction**	Interaction between a polyanion and a multivalent cation or a polycation, and vice versa (interaction between opposite charges)	Simple method; self-healing ability	Low stability in physiological environments and limited mechanical strength	[29,94,97,98]
	Hydrogen Bonding	Hydrogen bond between polymer chains (electron-deficient hydrogen atom and a high electronegativity functional group)	Absence of chemical crosslinkers	High dilution and dispersion rate over a few hours in vivo	[85,99]
	Hydrophobic Interaction	Polymers with hydrophobic domains are capable of crosslinking in aqueous environments by means of reverse thermal gelation ("sol-gel") (increased temperature leads to the aggregation of these domains)	Shape memory; autonomously self-healing properties; high degree of toughness	Poor mechanical properties	[99–101]
	Crystallization	The principle of freezing polymers at low temperatures, followed by thawing at room temperature causes the formation of crystals which leads to the formation of hydrogels	Stability and mechanical properties can be increased with increasing the freezing time and freeze–thaw cycles; simple method; not require additional chemicals and high temperature	Freeze/thaw processes applied for long periods of time can alter the behavior of the hydrogel	[96,102–104]
Chemical	**Photo-crosslinked**	The crosslinking of monomers or oligomers is initiated in the presence of an irradiation of UV/visible light and a photoinitiator that, when absorbing photons, is cleaved and forms free radicals that trigger polymerization	No toxic crosslinking agents are required; excellent spatial and temporal selectivity; low processing cost and energy requirements	The photoinitiator can produce free radicals with effects on immunogenicity and cytotoxicity responses	[105,106]
	Enzymatic Reaction	Certain enzymes (e.g., transglutaminases, horseradish peroxidase and tyrosinase) help to catalyze crosslinked reactions between two or more polymers	Mildness of the enzymatic reactions at normal physiological conditions; high efficiency; selectivity; non-toxicity; good biocompatibility; fast gelation process; tunable mechanical properties	Instability and poor availability of some of the enzymes	[107–109]

Table 3. *Cont.*

Hydrogels	Crosslinking Engine	Concept	Advantages	Disadvantages	Reference
Chemical	Crosslinking Molecules	Crosslinkers (e.g., glutaraldehyde, carbodiimide agents, genipin and citric acid) are small molecules with two or more reactive functional groups responsible for the formation of bridges between polymers chains	Easiness and versatility method	Possible cytotoxicity of the crosslinking agent (e.g., glutaraldehyde)	[110–112]
	Polymer-Polymer	Crosslinking reaction occurs between pre-functionalized polymer chains with reactive functional groups under favorable conditions. Polymer–polymer bonds can be formed by Schiff bases and by Michael addition reactions	Not using crosslinking molecules	Requires the modification of the polymer chains before their conjugation	[113,114]

Hybrid hydrogels result from the combination of physical and chemical crosslinking of polymers. These double crosslinked hydrogels combine the advantages of both strategies, namely, low surface tension, remarkable thermodynamic stability and elevated capacity of solubilization [65,93].

Various chemical and physical hydrogels have been prepared from natural and/or synthetic polymers for a variety of biomedical purposes. Chitosan hydrogels formed with the crosslinking agent trisodium salt 6-phosphogluconic (6-PG-Na^+) loaded with the drug piroxicam were developed by Martinez-Martinez et al. The interaction between ionic polymer cationic groups and anionic groups of the 6-PG-Na^+ crosslinker led to the formation of ionic hydrogels. The authors observed that the hydrogel had potential as a drug vehicle for topical administration since at pH close to neutrality there was less degradation than at lower pH, with a release of 90% of piroxicam during 7 h (release controlled by pH). This hydrogel proved to be a good candidate as a wound dressing given its good adhesion properties, non-toxicity and ability to induce healing and regeneration [115]. In another study, Wang et al. developed a hydrogel based on gelatin methacrylamine/poly(ethylene glycol)diacrylate (GelMA/PEGDA) via photo-crosslinking (with photoinitiator I2959). The engineered hydrogel was shown to have stronger mechanical properties than pure GelMA hydrogels and a degradation rate that lasted 4 weeks. Here, osteoblasts were able to adhere and proliferate along the surface, showing great cell viability and biocompatibility. Such characteristics make this hydrogel a good candidate for guided bone regeneration [116]. Table 4 lists some of the most recent examples physical, chemical and hybrid hydrogels employed in biomedicine and their respective production techniques.

Table 4. Examples of hydrogel crosslinking systems employed in wound dressing, tissue engineering and drug delivery.

Hydrogels	Crosslinking Engine	Hydrogel Composition	Applications	Reference
Physical	Ionic Interaction	6-PG-Na^+-crosslinked CS	Drug delivery; wound dressing	[115]
		$CaCl_2$-crosslinked alginate-pectin	Wound dressing	[30]
		Poloxamer-heparin/gellan gum	Bone marrow stem cells delivery	[117]
		$Al_3{}^+$-crosslinked cellulose	Drug delivery	[118]
	Hydrogen Bonding	PVA/poly(acrylic acid)	Surgical sutures and load-bearing fields	[119]
		1,6-hexamethylenediamine (HMDA)-crosslinked cytosine and guanosine modified HA	Injectable drug delivery; soft tissue engineering; regenerative medicine	[120]
	Crystallization	PVA/poly(ethylene glycol)	Wound dressing	[121]
		CS/PVA	Anti-inflammatory drug loading and release	[102]
		PVA/cellulose	2-layered skin model	[122]
Chemical	Photo-crosslinked	PEGDA	Tissue engineered heart valves	[123]
		GelMA	Tissue engineering; drug delivery; regenerative medicine	[124]
		GelMA/PEGDA	Bone regeneration	[116]
		GelMA/CS	Tissue engineering	[60]

Table 4. *Cont.*

Hydrogels	Crosslinking Engine	Hydrogel Composition	Applications	Reference
Chemical	Enzymatic Reaction	Horseradish peroxidase -crosslinked HA/silk fibroin	Tissue engineering	[21]
		Horseradish peroxidase -crosslinked Silk fibroin-tyramine-substituted silk fibroin or gelatin	Cell delivery	[125]
		Transglutaminase-crosslinked gelatin–laminin	Neuromuscular tissue engineering	[126]
	Crosslinking Molecules	Genipin-crosslinked CS	Drug delivery systems in oral administration applications	[111]
		Genipin-crosslinked CS/gelatin	Drug delivery	[127]
		Glutaraldehyde-crosslinked CS	Tissue engineering	[128]
	Polymer–Polymer	CS/Alginate	Neuronal tissue engineering	[129]
Hybrid	Chemical Crosslinking followed by Crystallization	Ethylene glycol diglycidyl ether-crosslinked microcrystalline Cellulose/PVA	Drug delivery	[130]

4. Fiber

The use and production of polymer-based fibers by humans has been described since pre-historic times. The earliest account of the biomedical use of fibers is suggested in decorations of the Tassili caves, engraved between 5000–2500 BC [131]. Ancient records, date the beginning of the use of cotton to the first half of the 6th millennium BC and the cultivation of silkworms to produce silk fibers to the 4th millennium BC [132,133]. With the industrial revolution, there was a need to create more efficient fiber production strategies. In the 14th century, the spindle to manufacture wool and cotton fibers emerged. The evolution in this field did not stagnate and the production of fibers continue evolving until the 19th century, dramatically increasing the use of natural fibers in the 1940s [11,134]. Years later, in the middle of the 20th century, the production of synthetic fibers began [11]. Nowadays, this area is constantly evolving, being already available several high precision methods of fiber production [133,135]. The application of fibers in biomedicine occurs in several areas, namely in wound dressings [136], bone tissue engineering [137], drug-controlled release [138], among others.

Fibers can be divided in two classes, natural and synthetic. Natural fibers can be extracted from plants, animals or minerals. Synthetic or man-made fibers usually arise from chemical processing [135]. In general, all plant-derived fibers are composed of cellulose, while animal-derived fibers contain proteins [139]. Natural fibers are made of millions of macrofibrils, which in turn are formed by microfibrils [140], composed mainly of crystalline cellulose (30–90%, that varies depending on the part of the plant concerned) surrounded by an amorphous matrix of lignin and hemicellulose [141]. These three fiber components are linked together by covalent bonds [140], with the fiber properties being defined by their composition, microfibril angle, crystallinity and internal structure. The stiffness of the fibers depends essentially on the angle of the cellulose microfibrils, the smaller the angle the greater the stiffness. Other properties, such as water absorption, moisture resistance, swelling and integration of the fiber bundle are determined by the other components, like hemicellulose [141]. In general, vegetable fibers are characterized by their biodegradable nature, lightweight, renewable capacity, abundance, improved mechanical properties, low cost and low density [142,143]. Because of these characteristics, natural fibers can be processed in various forms, including rope, yarn and reinforcing agents for biocomposites [144]. However, as reinforcements, the quality and efficiency of the final product are dependent on environment conditions which may be unpredictable from batch to batch, generating heterogeneity between fibers with the same origin [142]. Cellulose nanofibers have been applied in areas such as drug delivery [145] and tissue engineering [146]. Doench et al. reported the development of non-cellularized injectable suspensions of viscous CS solutions, filled with cellulose nanofibers as a strategy for visco-supplementation of the intervertebral disc nucleus pulposus tissue [146]. Natural fibers derived from animal sources can be collected from wool, silk and hair, for instance [139]. In the case of wool, depending on the animal it is collected from, be it sheep, lama or rabbit, there are properties that vary, namely, the color and the weight of the fibers [147]. Keratin is the main component of wool and hair [148]. This protein has excellent biocompatibility, biodegradability and is capable of increasing scaffolds elasticity and mechanical resilience by self-assembly and polymerization [149]. Silk fibers, on the other hand, are mainly made up of two structural proteins, fibroin (mechanical strength) and sericin (coating) that can be organized in a linear structure [150]. Silk fibers are characterized by being biodegradable and biocompatible. Although in the past their use was limited to clothing, today, silk is used in surgical knits, sutures, and wound healing. In addition, several researches are now in course to examine their use in films, scaffolds, electroplated materials and hydrogels [133,151]. In fact, the increase in research on polymeric composites reinforced with natural fibers has emerged side by side with the use of synthetic fibers in polymeric composites [143].

Synthetic fibers can be classified in inorganic or organic. Inorganic fibers are those that are not made of organic compounds [152]. As such, organic fibers can be manufactured either from natural or synthetic polymers. Most of the fibers used are of polymeric origin. Thus, the molecular weight of the polymer fiber plays a crucial role in influencing the tensile strength and the physical properties of the final construct [153]. Synthetic polymer fibers can be prepared from various polymers, as can be seen in Table 5 [153]. However, in biomedicine, those endowed with biodegradable features attract much more attention, namely, the PLA and the PCL polyesters [154]. PLA has the potential to replace fossil-based polymers [139]. It is biocompatible and its degradation biproducts are non-toxic, which favors its application in health-related fields [155]. On its turn, PCL is a biocompatible, linear polyester with improved elastic properties (despite having low tensile strength, it is capable of very high elongation) [154] that make it highly desirable for tissue engineering systems [156].

Table 5. Examples of natural and synthetic fibers [135,153].

Type of Fibers		
Natural	**Plant**	Bast fibers (e.g., jute and flax); seed fibers (e.g., cotton and coir); leaf fibers (e.g., banana and abaca); grass fibers (e.g., sugarcane bagasse and bamboo); straw fibers (e.g., rice, corn and wheat); wood fibers (e.g., softwood and hardwood)
	Animal-Based	Wool; silk; hair
Synthetic	**Inorganic**	Metals and alloys (e.g., metals fiber); metal or semi-metal compounds (e.g., glass and ceramics fibers); carbon-based fibers (e.g., carbon and graphene fibers)
	Organic	Synthetic polymers (e.g., polyamide nylon, polyethylene terephthalate, phenol-formaldehyde, PVA, polycarbonate, polyvinyl chloride and polyolefins (polypropylene and polyethylene)); natural polymer (e.g., chitosan and alginate)

Numerous researches describe the combination of synthetic polymers and natural polymers as the key for a successful fiber production [157–159]. For instance, Hu et al., reported the production of alginate/PCL composite nanofibers by co-electrospinning to enrich cancer stem cells (CSCs) constructs. The author studied the impact of the separated PCL and alginate fibers and the alginate/PCL composite having observed that the application of composite fibers is more effective in selecting cells than pure fibers. The fact that these scaffolds can be adjusted (composition proportion) to isolate CSCs from different tissues may potentially facilitate cancer research [157]. Levengood et al. developed CS/PCL nanofiber structures that combined the biological properties of CS and the stability and mechanical integrity of PCL for prospective applications in skin tissue engineering. Throughout the study, it was found that the nanofiber structure increased the wound healing rate, promoted general closure, re-epithelialization, maturity of the neoepidermis and collagen deposition when compared to the control. Such facts strengthen the potential of CS/PCL nanofiber structures for skin repair [158]. The other section of synthetic fibers, the inorganic fibers, can be subdivided in three main groups, which are the metals and alloys, the metal or semi-metal compounds and the carbon-based fibers (Table 5).

Many of the inorganic fibers generally exhibit high strength, high thermal and chemical stability and stability against any kind of organic solvent [152]. Regarding fiber glass, they have a relatively low cost, high tensile strength, high chemical resistance and good insulation properties. In case of carbon fibers, these have numerous advantages, such as high stiffness and tensile strength, high chemical resistance, high temperature tolerance, present low cost and low thermal expansion. Because of these characteristics, both glass fibers and carbon fibers are often used as reinforcement in polymeric composites [143]. These fibers can be combined with other components. Naskar et al. described a composite of regenerated silk protein fibroin reinforced with functionalized carbon nanofibers, loaded with growth factors (BMP-2 and TGF-β1) essential to bone regeneration. The matrices formed were porous, immune-compatible and bioactive when incubated in simulated body fluid. Here, it was seen that the reinforcement of the nanofibers influenced the mechanical property of the matrices, increasing the compression module up to 46.54 MPa [160].

Fibers can be classified according to their internal structure (uniform fibers or core-shell) or orientation (aligned or arranged randomly). They can also be formed of continuous monofilament yarns or multifilament yarns. Both natural and synthetic fibers can be characterized physically (diameter, length, density and moisture gain) and mechanically (tensile strength, specific strength young's modulus, specific young's modulus and failure strain) [161]. Natural fibers have moderate mechanical properties, high thermal sensitivity, low density, acceptable modulus-weight ratio, low cost, can be extracted from unlimited sources, and display good recyclability and biodegradability. However, the high sensitivity to humidity, higher variability of physical and mechanical properties and low durability are some of the disadvantages of natural fibers. In turn, synthetic fibers have high mechanical properties, low sensitivity to moisture and low thermal sensitivity. Limited sources and moderate recyclability are some disadvantages of synthetic fibers. [162,163]. Even though their mechanical resilience is highly attractive, the energy necessary to produce synthetic fibers tends to be more than that required for natural [140].

Fiber Production: Techniques

As explained earlier, the fiber final properties depend on the polymer composition. However, they are also dependent on the processing conditions. The four most used fiber production methods include electrospinning, melt-spinning, wet-spinning and dry-spinning (Table 6). The electrospinning is a technique that allows the generation of polymeric fibers with submicron or nanometric diameters while conventional techniques such as melt-spinning, wet-spinning and dry-spinning can produce polymer fibers with diameters up to the micrometer range.

Table 6. Set up, concept, advantages and disadvantages of the most common fiber manufacturing techniques, namely, electrospinning, wet-spinning, melt-spinning and dry-spinning.

	Electrospinning	Wet-Spinning	Melt-Spinning	Dry-Spinning
Set Up	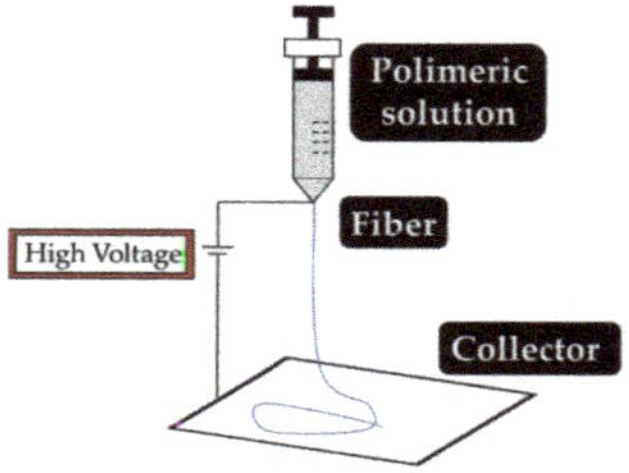	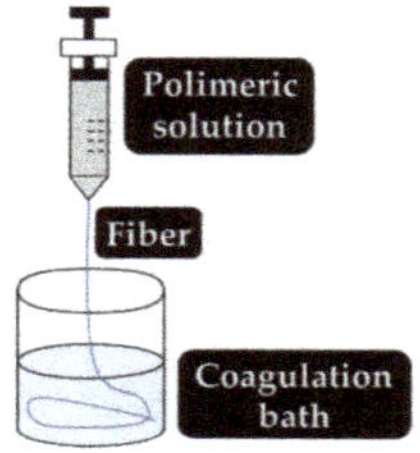	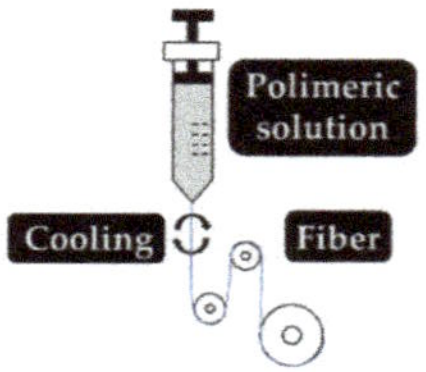	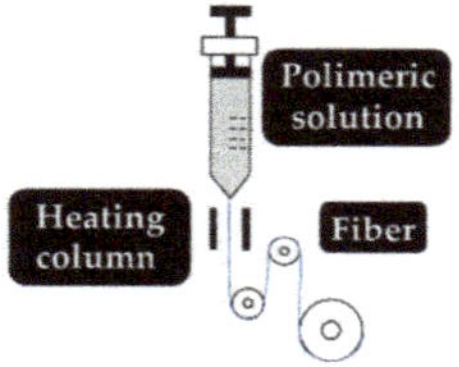
Concept	The polymer dissolved in an appropriate solvent is injected by a needle towards a collection plate. Due to the high applied electric field, potential difference generated between the syringe (acts as an electrode) and the plate (acts as an electrode count), the polymer is attracted by the collecting plate, and the polymer solution is converted into nanofibers	The polymer is dissolved in an appropriate solvent and later injected through a fiery into a coagulation bath containing a non-solvent liquid. In the coagulation bath, continuous polymerization of the filaments occurs. After the formation of the fibers, they are extracted from the coagulation bath by means of rollers-induced capture	The solid polymer is heated above its melting point within the extruder and is then expelled through a die, solidifying on cooling. In a pick-up, the fibers are then recovered and mechanically stretched	The polymer is dissolved in a suitable solvent (must be highly volatile). The initial solution is injected through the spinneret and through a heating column that causes the solvent to evaporate. Consequently, the polymer solidifies, and dry fibers are attained
Advantages	Fibers with a large surface area, high porosity, great flexibility, and excellent mechanical properties; simple and straightforward process; cost efficiency	Wet-spun structures have greater intrinsic porosity and larger interconnected pores; versatile technique in terms of material selection	Fabrication process is quick; Not require added solvents	Enables spinning of polymers vulnerable to thermal degradation
Disadvantages	Fiber thickness increases density and reduces pore size in 3D structures that can limited the interaction of cells with the fibers; toxicity of the solvents and the instability of the jets; slow process	Long exposure to chemicals during the processing and coagulation may impact negatively on the cells' microenvironments	Limited to thermically-resistant polymers; unstable in the production of fine fibers	Requires high temperatures which can affect the properties/characteristics of the fibers/fiber surface
Ref.	[164–170]	[171–174]	[175]	[176,177]

Depending on the fiber production method employed, several precautions must be taken into consideration, such is the case with the processing of CS fibers via wet-spinning. CS fibers have a very low tensile strength (due to their increased hydrophilicity) and, therefore, chemical crosslinking must be induced by Epichlorohydrin (ECH) to improve its wet tenacity [178]. According to the chemical (e.g., composition and rate of degradation) and physical (e.g., diameter, strength and porosity) characteristics, the electrospun nanofibers can guide and interact with the injured tissue to improve wound healing [179].

5. Fiber–Hydrogel Composites

As seen in the previous sections, both hydrogels and fibers display great potential in biomedicine, particularly in the wound healing and drug delivery areas [88,156,157,180]. Despite the many advantages that make these scaffolding systems promising, there are still aspects that often limit their application. For instance, the low mechanical stability of natural hydrogels and the not-so-great biocompatibility of synthetic hydrogels tend to constrain their uses [63]. In the case of fibers, there is a limitation associated with the lack of 3D network formations which can restrict cell migration/infiltration [181]. Given these limitations, a number of researches are now dedicated in combining the advantages of fibers and hydrogels to produce an optimal, highly functional composite system [182–184]. In this sense, the objective of these investigations is to optimize the mechanical/biological functionalities of composites by promoting the combination of beneficial properties of both components (fiber/hydrogel) and reducing the impact of their undesirable features in the final application. The mechanical properties of hydrogels, in this case fiber–hydrogel composites, are significantly influenced by the addition of fibers [185], as they serve as a structural support for the hydrogel to surround, for instance [184]. Regev et al. reported that the incorporation of bovine serum albumin fibers in dextran/gelatin hydrogels increases the elasticity modulus of the hydrogel and decreases its gelation time [186]. Gelatin nanofibers aligned and infiltrated in alginate hydrogels may also increase the tensile modulus and rigidity of the overall hydrogel construct [187].

The fibers used in fiber–hydrogel composite can have different origins, natural or synthetic, and, at a morphological level, they can also differ depending on the desired application. Generally, the fibers used in these composites can be classified as long or short, and within the composite, they can exhibit a continuous or discontinuous pattern. Specifically, long and continuous fibers produced by electrospinning tend to possess small pores that limit cellular penetration and growth [188]. Based on the potential application of the scaffold, the organization of the fibers is a crucial element for the performance of the intended function, which can be oriented uniformly or randomly [185]. Although the available literature is still limited, several methods of combining fibers with hydrogels for the creation of composites with different structures have been reported. Of all, the most common arrangements of composite fiber–hydrogel structures are the stacked, with hydrogels and fibers forming layers (laminated composites) [189], the encapsulated, with fibers being enclosed within the hydrogel matrix [190], the injectable composites [191] and the electrospinning and electrospraying combination [192] (Figure 1). In fiber production, electrospinning is one the most used techniques due to its simplicity, cost efficiency, flexibility, scalability the advantage of mimicking the natural extracellular matrix (ECM) [16,166,193,194], so its combination with hydrogel fabrication methodologies is very frequent.

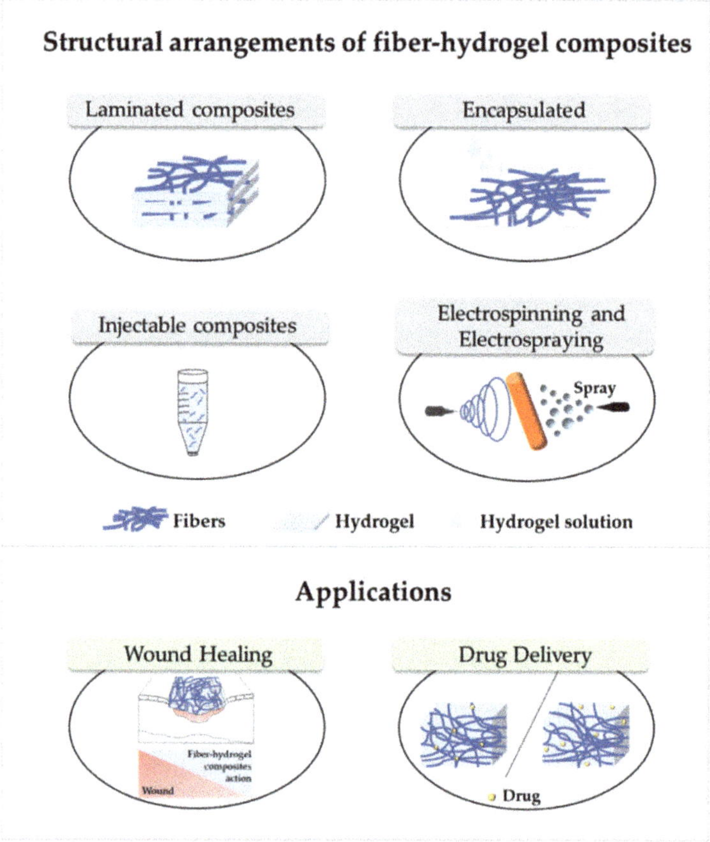

Figure 1. Structural arrangements of fiber–hydrogel composites and their applications in wound healing and drug delivery. Fiber–hydrogel composites with laminated structure result from the junction of individually manufactured fibers and hydrogels that can be organized in layers with different orientations. The encapsulation of fibers in hydrogels can result from crosslinking of the hydrogel solution directly into the fibers. In case of injectable composites, small individual fiber fragments are added to the hydrogel solution, resulting in an encapsulated and injectable composite structure. These composites can also be formed by the simultaneous combination of electrospinning and electrospraying applied directly towards a single collecting system (shown in orange).

Laminating is the simplest method to yield a fiber–hydrogel composite scaffold. Laminated composites consist of the junction of individually manufactured hydrogels and fibers in different layers. The number of fiber layers influences the mechanical properties of the composite. These composites can be formed by a single layer of fibers or by multilayers, with different orientations (e.g., 0°, 45° and 90°). The orientation of the fibers within the composite allows to control the toughness and strength of the final structure. These constructs exhibit significantly improved tensile properties compared to hydrogels alone [195]. However, they can undergo delamination very easily after water absorption due to the weak interactions between layers [196]. Additionally, the 2D structure of the fibers becomes a limitation for applications where it is essential to mimic the ECM, since this structure makes cell migration very challenging [197]. Encapsulating fibers in hydrogels can be accomplished by crosslinking the hydrogel directly into fibers with a pre-determined architecture or by immersing the fibers in a hydrogel precursor solution. In this process, the gaps between the fibers are occupied by the hydrogel precursor solution that later crosslinks.

Based on encapsulation fibers in hydrogel, McMahon et al. hypothesized a composite with a tubular structure with circumferential mechanical properties similar to coronary artery vessels [187,190]. Papaparaskeva et al. projected prefabricated fibrous mats of PVP/silver nanocomposites incorporated within semi-IPN hydrogels in two unique forms of laminated dispersion (a prefabricated electrospun fibrous mat was placed in the circumference of the fiber/hydrogel composite) and homogeneous (a 2D circular fibrous mat was homogeneously encapsulated within a 3D hydrogel matrix). They noted that the dispersion mode of electrically spun fibrous mats within the hydrogel significantly influences the mechanical performance of the resulting composite [198]. Injectable composites have been considered an alternative to produce fiber–hydrogel constructs with homogeneous qualities. In this type of composite, small individual fiber fragments (smaller sizes facilitate injectability) are added to a hydrogel precursor solution. Subsequently, these fibers are incorporated into the crosslinked hydrogel matrix (in the desired environment), playing a reinforcing role. This production strategy is minimally invasive; however, the absence of connections between fibers can become a restriction for certain applications [188,199]. The electrospraying process has been used to form fiber–hydrogel composites. Here, the hydrogel solution is sprayed in fine droplets on fibers produced by electrospinning. These drops, which are deposited on the fibers, can have different sizes, from nanometers to several micrometers. The electrospinning–electrospraying has therefore low cost and is easy to operate. Furthermore, it allows to obtain a composite fiber–hydrogel with different structures and with adjustable size and morphology [200–202]. Despite the formation processes of fiber–hydrogel composites mentioned above, which are already used in investigations, a less positive aspect can be highlighted. This focuses on the differences in hydrophilicity between the fibers and the hydrogels that can cause some incompatibility, which then may result in a separation of the compound. In this sense, the modification of the fiber surface is considered a potential solution to improve this limitation [203–205].

There are several approaches that have been used to improve the properties of fibrous scaffolds and hydrogels, namely the development of fiber–hydrogels composites (Figure 1). As seen, these composites continue to conform to the same guidelines applied for the fabrication of the individual parts, with peculiarities related to their fabrication being, as expected, associated to polymer and solvent selection and combination of compatible processing methodologies. In general, the applications of scaffolds depend on their mechanical and biological properties and, as such, many possibilities have emerged in recent years.

6. Applications of Fiber–Hydrogel Composites

Recently, research on fiber–hydrogel composites has increased significantly. These scaffolding systems have been investigated for a range of applications, including wound healing [206], regeneration of corneal stroma [184], nucleus pulposus regeneration [201], bone tissue engineering [207], antibiotic delivery [208] and heart valve tissue engineering [209]. Scaffolds with an architecture that mimics native ECM and allows cell infiltration and differentiation has emerged as a prospective solution for the treatment of various health complications. For instance, the fibrous structure in fiber–hydrogel composites is considered of enormous importance for a greater efficiency of the scaffold. This is because tissues have biological fibers with specific composition and architecture that contribute to the normal function of the tissues. Thus, with this, it is possible to simulate biological fibers, approximating the foreign scaffold to living tissue and, thus, enhance cellular growth and maturation (e.g., cell differentiation) [184]. In the following sections, we will contextualize and list in more detail some recent examples of fiber–hydrogel composites applied in wound healing and drug delivery.

6.1. Wound Healing

Wound healing is a complex physiological response that involves a cascade of cells, matrix components and other biological factors [16]. In healthy people, wound healing includes four important phases: hemostasis, inflammation, proliferation, and remodeling. This complex process allows skin functions to be restored. Wounds that fail the normal healing process in a predictable amount of time are considered chronic wounds (CW) [210,211]. Currently, wound care is based on the application of a wide variety of wound dressings (gauzes, absorbent cotton and bandages), debridement, vacuum assisted closure and grafts. Even though they are considered the therapy of choice, wound dressing have some limitations, they are incapable of maintaining the moist environment necessary for wound healing and tend to adhere to the wound, which may cause discomfort to the patient when the dressing is removed [212]. CW treatments are often associated to high economic costs, an increase in surgical procedures and the greater susceptibility of the patient to infection. Microorganisms such as *Acinetobacter baumannii, Enterococcus faecalis, Pseudomonas aeruginosa* and *Staphylococcus aureus* have the ability to colonize and infect wounds, which complicate the healing process [6,210]. In the most severe cases, patients with infected wounds, such as diabetic foot infections, include mainly antibiotics in their therapy [213]. The impact of excess and inappropriate use of antibiotics has been explored in relation to the various adverse effects, such as bacterial resistance, which has been highlighted as a serious global concern [135]. Several alternatives have been developed for a more efficient wound healing in order to prevent infection to evolve and, in the case of CW, to try and shorten the treatment period [212,214–217]. There are some properties that ideally a modern wound dressing should have, specifically, the capacity for mechanical protection and adaptation to the shape of the wound, without adhering to wound tissue per se, so as not to cause pain to the patient when removed. Absorption capacity, cytocompatibility, flexibility, ability to ensure a balanced moist environment, induce wound healing, facilitate ECM regeneration, protect the wound from external contaminants and promote debridement are also important features in the development of an effective wound dressing [6,33,166,212]. Wound dressings can be classified based on the affinity of the dressing with the wound into four distinct groups: passive, interactive, advanced and smart dressings [211]. Modern dressings take the most varied forms, including hydrogels, films, sponges, foams, nanofiber mats and, more recently, fiber–hydrogel composites [33,206]. The hydrogel has the ability to absorb exudates and maintain a balance of moisture at the wounded site. In turn, the fiber mimics the fibrous structure of ECM. Since both structures present limitations, the fibers do not facilitate cell migration and hydrogels have low mechanical stability, scaffolds combining both have been the research target of many investigations in order to uncover alternatives for the treatment of wounds [206,217,218]. The combination of the two structure in one scaffold is expected to facilitate healing by generating an environment conducive with cell recognition and attachment (ECM mimicking) with a moist and breathable atmosphere required for a healthy tissue formation. It is known that a large part of mammalian ECM has an aqueous matrix (gel) containing diverse fibrous proteins, essentially collagen, elastin and fibronectin. These proteins surround and guide cells in vivo and act as an anchoring matrix [219,220]. In humans, fibrillar collagen provides tensile strength for ECM, which limits tissue/organ distensibility as is the case of the skin [221]. The ECM is mainly responsible for cell adhesion, migration, proliferation, and regulation of their action. For a complete and effective skin regeneration, it is important that a scaffold is created that mimics the structure and normal skin conditions. Studies have shown that the reinforcement of hydrogels with fibers improves cell function, differentiation and proliferation, as well as structural stability [182,183,195]. Indeed, Schulte et al. described the manufacture of an artificial ECM scaffold consisting of biofunctionalized fibers incorporated in a semi-synthetic hydrogel of HA that allowed the control of cell adhesion [220].

There are several polymers used in fiber–hydrogel composites, namely gelatin [206,217,222]. The combination of two separate scaffolds (bilayer scaffold) was studied by Franco et al. for a possible application in skin regeneration. The formulation consisted of a first layer based on a PCL/PLGA membrane (80:20) formed by electrospinning and a second layer of CS/gelatin hydrogel (50:50) crosslinked with glutaraldehyde. The first layer showed excellent mechanical properties and biocompatibility. In the case of the second layer, they obtained a porous structure, capable of swelling more than 500% of its dry size (excellent absorbent properties). The junction of the fibrous membranes provided better mechanical support to the scaffold and, at the same time, reduced the rate of degradation of the layer formed by the hydrogel [222]. In the same light, Zhao et al. through a chemical reaction of the methacrylamide groups with gelatin formed a prepolymer to produce fibers by electrospinning (GelMA). The electrospun GelMA nanofibers were crosslinked by photo-crosslinking, with UV radiation. By manipulating the degree of modification of the gelatin with the methacrylamide groups and the photo-crosslinking time, it is possible to adjust the physical and biological properties. Characteristics such as water vapor permeability, water retention, mechanical resistance and kinetic degradation can be adapted by adjusting the time of UV light radiation. These GelMA scaffolds, which mimic the structure of the native ECM, demonstrated a better orientation of the cellular processes (e.g., cell migration of fibroblasts) and biocompatibility compared to the controls (gelatin and PLGA). The in vivo tests reinforce the potential of this scaffold since it was visible that they accelerated wound repair [217]. Sun et al. went a step further and reported the ability of the GelMA to improve the elastic biodegradable mechanical properties of the construct and its ability to improve cell adhesion, proliferation and vascularization [223]. In turn, Li et al. reports the use of gelatin for the development of a hydrogel fibers. Initially the gelatin-based compound hydrogel fibers were prepared by gel-spinning with PEG6000. Subsequently, the crosslinking agent dialdehyde carboxymethyl cellulose (DCMC) was incorporated in order to improve the thermal and mechanical properties of the hydrogel fibers composed of gelatin-PEG. This scaffold showed a strong capacity to absorb free water due to its 3D structure and porous network. The higher the DCMC content in hydrogel fibers, the more slowly they degrade. In addition, DCMC increased the compatibility of the hydrogel fibers with blood [206]. HA nanofibers are reported to promote wound healing. Due to their high solubility in water, crosslinking is required to increase their water stability. Chen et al. developed an electrospun a mixture of maleicated hyaluronate/poly(vinyl alcohol) methacrylate (MHA/MaPVA) that allowed the formation of mats with the capacity to swell and form fibrous hydrogels. The weight ratio of the nanofiber components influenced the morphology and diameter of the nanofibers. This structure was cytocompatible, promoted cell fixation and displayed high water absorption capacities [218]. PVA has also been combined with PCL to form double layer structures resultant from the combination of PCL nanofibers (hydrophobic) and PVA hydrogel (hydrophilic). After exposure to water, the PVA fiber layer was completely dissolved, and a hydrogel-like structure was formed. Despite this change, the defined shape of the scaffold was maintained due to the stability of the PCL layer in water-based environments. Several aspects were tested in this scaffold, namely, its morphology, wettability, and adhesion and proliferation of mouse fibroblasts. Here, it was seen that fibroblasts exhibited greater proliferative activity on the PCL side of the double layer. In the case of the PVA layer, the same was not seen, which may be a consequence of the greater hydrophilicity of the layer. Based on the behavior and characteristics of the double layer scaffold, the authors concluded that the scaffold had the potential to be used as a dressing or in the prevention of abdominal adhesions [194].

The rapid dissolution of fibers in an aqueous medium becomes a limitation for their application in active wound dressings. In the case of PVP fibers, their rapid solubility remains a problem despite their self-adhesive properties and their ability to incorporate molecules. Recently, to overcome this limitation Contardi et al. proposed to develop PVP-based fiber hydrogels containing hydroxycinnamic acid derivatives. A controlled release of p-cumaric and ferulic acids (derived from hydroxycinnamic acid) from the fibers was observed due to the incorporation of these in the hydrogel. The author also observed in burned skin a reduction in the levels of enzymes known to be positively regulated by reactive oxidative species in burned skin [224]. By electrospinning/electrospraying methods, Azarniya et al. reported the production of a hybrid fiber–hydrogel by combining fibrous mats and hydrogel particles. Through electrospinning, keratin/bacterial cellulose (BC) fibers were produced and simultaneously sprayed with thermosensitive hydrogel particles. The chemically crosslinked hydrogel was composed of non-ionic triblock copolymers (PEO99-PPO65-PEO99; Pluronic F127) conjugated with Tragacanto gum (TG). Due to the low spinning power of keratin, poly(oxide of ethylene) (PEO) was added to the formulation forming the keratin/BC/PEO fibers. Reductions in the diameter of keratin/PEO fibers from 243 $\pm$ 57 nm to 150 $\pm$ 43 nm and hydrophobicity were observed with the addition of 1% or more of BC. However, despite the reduction of pores, TG and BC modified mats promoted cell fixation and proliferation in fibrous structures. It was seen that the hydrogel particles were uniformly incorporated into the junction of the fibrous network. This modification improved several features of the scaffolds, including hydrophilicity, modulus of elasticity (31%), tensile strength (35%) and ductility (23%) [225]. More recently, Loo et al. developed "intelligent" peptide hydrogels, in which the short aliphatic peptides had the tendency to self-assemble into helical fibers, forming nanofiber hydrogels. These nanofibrous hydrogels were found to possess regenerative properties and to display potential to accelerate the healing of burn wounds [226].

6.2. Drug Delivery

In conventional therapies, rapid degradation and excretion of drugs during the circulation process in the body is frequently detected. Consequently, only a small amount of medication will have therapeutic effects in places of interest [227]. Several research groups have focused on the development of new controlled drug delivery systems to allow an effective distribution of drugs in the intended locations at a controlled release rate [193,228]. A drug delivery system is used to transport therapeutic substances in the body more effectively and safely, having the ability to control the amount, the time and the targeted place for drug release [229]. Several scaffolds have been used to encapsulate and deliver therapeutic drugs, namely, fibers and hydrogels [102,230–232].

Electrospinning systems allow drugs to be incorporated into the fibers, giving them a high drug loading capacity, increased initial burst, sustained release, and prolonged circulation. Methods of incorporation include blend (or co-, the drug is mixed in the polymer solution), side-by-side (vehicle/polymer solution and the biomolecules are loaded in a separate spinneret), multi-jet (use of multiple nozzles with one or more jets, or a nozzle with different jets), co-axial (two concentric aligned capillaries connected to a high voltage source) and emulsion electrospinning (the drug is encapsulated in an appropriate solvent to be protected from the fiber/solvent system) [48]. Just as there are different ways to incorporate drugs into fibers, drugs may also be released via three distinct mechanisms: desorption of the fiber surface, diffusion in the solid state through the fibers, and fiber degradation [233]. The fiber morphology and its high therapeutic load capacity are beneficial properties that make them potential candidates for drug delivery systems. Electrospun fibers have several advantages especially due to their large surface area and their absorption/release properties [234]. However, large-burst drug release, uncontrolled duration of drug release, and incomplete drug release are recurring problems. The possible agglomeration of bioactive agents on the surface of the fibers becomes a disadvantage of the electrospinning method since it can trigger an initial burst release, which may cause toxicity of the release site [48,224,235]. Such limitations may have implications in the scaffold biomedical goals.

To incorporate drugs into hydrogels, they can be loaded into the precursor solutions before crosslinking or can be absorbed after gelation [236]. Regarding drug release, swelling is an important property in some stimulus-sensitive drug delivery system. Certain changes in the environment may trigger swelling that allows the release of the drug due to the alterations in mesh size of the polymeric network [237]. Features like hydrophilicity, biocompatibility and tunable mechanical properties are the reason why hydrogels have been used extensively for the controlled release of drugs [193]. Although hydrogels are widely used in controlled release systems, there are some limitations that must be overcome. These scaffolds suffer from low mechanical resistance, which may be responsible for inhomogeneous release [236]. In most hydrogels, their ability to absorb large amounts of water and the presence of large pore sizes may trigger a rapid drug release [208]. In accordance, some investigations have developed/obtained better kinetic release profiles when there is a combination of hydrogels with other structures, namely fibers [193]. The effectiveness of fiber–hydrogel composites for drug administration has been demonstrated [208,227,228]. Nanofiber–hydrogel scaffolds as biofunctionalized platforms appear as attractive alternatives to the ineffective treatments related to direct drug administration.

Persistent neurological dysfunctions are usually triggered by spinal cord injuries due to failure in axon regeneration. Nguyen et al. synthesized lined mats of poly(ε-caprolactone-co-ethyl ethylene phosphate) (PCLEEP) by electrospinning and distributed them in a collagen hydrogel matrix. Both the fibers and the hydrogel contained neurotrophin-3 (model protein) known for promoting neuronal survival, axonal sprouting and regeneration. Additionally, the hydrogel contained miR-222 (model microRNA) known to contribute to the control of local protein synthesis at distal axons. Overtime, it was seen that degradation occurred within the collagen hydrogel, but the PCLEEP fibers maintained their morphology and alignment after 3 months. The composite framework allowed localized and sustained drug/gene delivery, while aligned nanofibers acted to direct remyelination of the injured area. Furthermore, they observed the regeneration of the animal model axon [227]. In a similar study, small fragmented nanofibers of poly(3-caprolactone-$_{co}$-D,L-lactide) (PCL:DLLA) and collagen were individually dispersed in a hyaluronane-methylcellulose hydrogel (HAMC). These fiber–hydrogel composites were used as a cell-transport system multipotent neural/progenitor stem cells (NSPCs) for the treatment of spinal cord injuries. The results showed that the incorporation of fibers in the HAMC hydrogel influenced the behavior of the NSPC cells, highlighting a better neuronal and oligodendrocytic differentiation in the scaffold PCL:DLLA/HAMC compared to collagen/HAMC [199]. In both studies, the complex generated from the combination of fibers and hydrogels allowed for a faster cell development and consequent regeneration.

A laminated fiber–hydrogel composite based on PCL electrospun fiber mats coupled with poly(ethylene glycol)-poly(ε-caprolactone) diacrylate (PEGPCL) hydrogels processed by UV polymerization was developed to control the release of a model hydrophilic protein (e.g., bovine albumin serum, BSA). To study the release of the hydrophilic protein, BSA was added to the system before crosslinking. The results reported by Han et al. suggested the relevant role of PLC fibers (diameter of approximately 0.45 μm) in the release of the drug in a uniform and delayed manner, by reducing swelling of hydrogels and water penetration rates and by increasing the length of the diffusion path and the diffusivity of the drug. In addition, the bioactivity of proteins after release was proven since extension of PC12 cell neuritis was detected. In general, the PCL fibers in the PEGPCL hydrogel demonstrated an important role in three main areas: control of the release kinetics of the hydrophilic protein, reduction of burst release (initial) and increased duration of drug release (more than two months) [193].

Osteomyelitis is a bone disease caused mainly by methicillin-resistant *Staphylococcus aureus* (MRSA). Various antibiotics are administered to reduce this infection, namely the glycopeptide vancomycin hydrochloride (vanco-HCl). The bacterial plaque that forms around the infected area limits treatment by preventing the diffusion of the antibiotic vanco-HCL to the infected site, which then requires the administration of high doses. This overuse of antibiotics in addition to their impropriate function can lead to systemic toxicity. To try and solve this problem, Ahadi et al. developed a scaffold made of poly(L-lactide) (PLLA) fibers produced by electrospinning followed by aminolysed, encased in a hydrogel of silk fibroin/oxidized pectin. PLLA fibers were loaded with vanco-HCl to promote a more sustainable release of the antibiotic at the affected site, resulting in a 61% reduction in drug release. This scaffold revealed better mechanical properties compared to the single hydrogel (without fibers), namely, a higher crosslinking density (52%), a higher compression module (30%) and a lower expansion rate (15%). Biologically, the fiber–hydrogel composite was seen to have activity against MRSA and to be cytocompatible with cells, largely due to the presence of fibers aminolized with drugs [208]. Ekaputra et al. developed by electrospinning/electrospraying a hybrid mesh of PCL/collagen and HA hydrogel, Heprasil^{TM}, loaded with vascular endothelial growth factors (VEGF) and platelet-derived growth factors (PDGF). It was seen that the fiber–hydrogel composite PCL/collagen-Heprasil was successful in allowing a double simultaneous loading of the growth factors VEGF165 and PDGF-BB and to promote their controlled release over a period of five weeks, in vitro [192]. Recently, biocompatible vehicles for the release of the crystal violet drug (CV) have also been described, in which polydopamine microfibers (PDA) were incorporated in a pullulan (PHG) hydrogel crosslinked by poly(ethylene glycol) diglicidyl ether (chemical crosslinker). PDA fibers attributed the pH-responsive drug release behavior to the PHG hydrogel. This happens in response to the acidic conditions, which increase the electrostatic repulsion force between the PDA (protonated and positively charged) and the drug CV (positive charge). This repulsion promotes the release of the drug, with a detectable a cumulative release of 60.3% (pH 7.4), which increased to 87% with a decrease in pH to 5. In addition, the incorporation of PDA fibers and the adjustment of their content allowed to regulate several properties of the composite PHG-PDAs, namely, its viscoelastic characteristics, mechanical performance, mesh size and swelling/disintegration properties of the PHG hydrogel. The developed scaffold proved to have great potential to be used in drug delivery systems, given its good cytocompatibility, non-toxicity and easily adjustable properties for a controlled release of CV [238]. Overall, data demonstrated the ability of the engineered systems to promote a controlled drug delivery, in which the fibrous mesh guaranteed the mechanical stability of the construct while the hydrogel released the loaded active compounds.

A new physical approach based on hydrogel and nanofibers (or NEEDs) for cell encapsulation has been described in the work of An et al. Here, tubular constructs with different compartments were developed, consisting of Nylon 6,6 nanofibers, manufactured by electrospinning, being subsequently impregnated in different hydrogel precursor solutions (alginate, chitosan or collagen) and crosslinked. Fibers had an average diameter of 200 nm with 1 μm interconnected pores. Compartmentation proved to be an asset for co-encapsulation, co-culture and co-distribution of different individual cells and cellular aggregates (islets), with cell viability being observed. Finally, the potential application of NEEDs for cell therapies using a type 1 diabetic model was tested, and the disease was corrected (in 8 weeks), which proved the therapeutic potential of NEEDs within primary rat islets (without the disease) [228].

In wound healing, it is important to pay attention to the biomaterials used to produce wound dressing. To achieve the desired objectives, the properties of each biomaterial are optimally combined. Studies have shown that local administration of therapeutic agents through wound dressings can improve the wound healing process [16]. In fact, a bioactive dressing of fibers of silk fibroin (SF) produced via electrospinning was developed and then combined with the alginate hydrogel (ALG) capable of supplying amniotic fluid (AF). This dressing had the ability to release AF, highly enriched with various therapeutic agents, at the wound site. The AF release profile was related to the concentration of ALG (greater release of AF in lower amounts of ALG). The increase in cell proliferation and collagen dissemination and secretion due to AF in fibroblast cultures strengthens the potential of the SF/ALG fiber–hydrogel composite to accelerate the healing process in severe wounds [239]. In a similar study, a bi-layer dressing of gelatin nanofiber mats loaded with epigallocatechin gallate (EGCG)/PVA hydrogel was produced for the treatment of acute wounds. The hydrogel was used as a protective and hydrating outer layer of the bi-layer dressing. Jaiswal el al. observed that the decrease in crosslinking time led to a slower EGCG release profile. This increased in the 2-4 days release period demonstrating the ability of this scaffold to guarantee a gradual drug release. Faster wound contraction, improvement in angiogenesis, reepithelization and less inflammatory response compared to control were also observed [240]. More recently, Chen et al. developed CS/gelatin hydrogels with polydopamine-intercalated silicate nanoflakes (PDA-Silicate). These were electrospun in the form of nanofibers loaded with the antibiotic tetracycline hydrochloride

(TH). In this sandwich-like nanofiber/hydrogel composite (NF-HG) the incorporation of the fibers in the hydrogel resulted in a restriction in the release of antibiotic TH. However, it allowed a sustained release rate of TH in NF-HG for long-term protection. In addition, this structure reduced the toxicity of the drug associated to the rapid release. Furthermore, the excellent adhesiveness and anti-infectious properties demonstrated by the NF-HG, turned this formulation particularly attractive to be used as a wound dressing [241].

7. Conclusions

The world of biomaterials, specifically polymers, continues to significantly impact on the field of biomedicine. The diversity of polymers and the different ways of using them in scaffolds have evolved considerably in the last years, proposing active solutions for daily problems. In recent decades, combinations of different scaffolding systems in one solution have been researched, demonstrating great potential in wound healing and drug delivery systems, particularly in the fight against antibiotic-resistant pathogens. Indeed, hydrogel and fiber composites have been engineered as effective therapies, overcoming many of the mechanical, physical, and biological limitations of fibers and hydrogels when used in individual systems. Although research in this field is still very limited and is basically taking the first steps, the potential is clear. In the next years, it is expected the research on these composites to continue evolving and growing, as the need for more adaptable and specialized biomedical devices grows as well.

Author Contributions: Conceptualization, M.O.T., J.C.A. and H.P.F.; writing original draft, M.O.T.; supervision, J.C.A. and H.P.F.; funding acquisition, H.P.F. All authors have read and agreed to the published version of the manuscript.

Funding: This research received funding from the Portuguese Foundation for Science and Technology (FCT) under the scope of the projects PTDC/CTM-TEX/28074/2017 (POCI-01-0145-FEDER-028074) and UID/CTM/00264/2021.

Institutional Review Board Statement: Not applicable.

Informed Consent Statement: Not applicable.

Data Availability Statement: Not available.

Acknowledgments: Authors acknowledge the Portuguese Foundation for Science and Technology (FCT), FEDER funds by means of Portugal 2020 Competitive Factors Operational Program (POCI), and the Portuguese Government (OE) for funding the project PEPTEX with reference PTDC/CTM-TEX/28074/2017 (POCI-01-0145-FEDER-028074). The authors also acknowledge project UID/CTM/00264/2021 of the Centre for Textile Science and Technology (2C2T), funded by national funds through FCT/MCTES.

Conflicts of Interest: The authors declare no conflict of interest.

References

1. Ratner, B.D.; Hoffman, A.S.; Schoen, F.J.; Lemons, J.E.; Wagner, W.R.; Sakiyama-Elbert, S.E.; Zhang, G.; Yaszemski, M.J. Introduction to Biomaterials Science: An Evolving, Multidisciplinary Endeavor. In *Biomaterials Science: An Introduction to Materials in Medicine*; Wagner, W., Sakiyama-Elbert, S., Zhang, G., Yaszemski, M., Eds.; Academic Press: Cambridge, MA, USA, 2020; pp. 3–19.
2. Mariani, E.; Lisignoli, G.; Borzì, R.M.; Pulsatelli, L. Biomaterials: Foreign Bodies or Tuners for the Immune Response? *Int. J. Mol. Sci.* **2019**, *20*, 636. [CrossRef]
3. Asim, M.; Jawaid, M.; Saba, N.; Ramengmawii; Nasir, M.; Sultan, M.T.H. Processing of hybrid polymer composites-a review. In *Hybrid Polymer Composite Materials*; Thakur, V.K., Thakur, M.K., Gupta, R.K., Eds.; Elsevier: Amsterdam, The Netherlands, 2017; pp. 1–22.
4. Ivanova, E.P.; Bazaka, K.; Crawford, R.J. Advanced synthetic polymer biomaterials derived from organic sources. In *New Functional Biomaterials for Medicine and Healthcare*; Ivanova, E.P., Bazaka, K., Crawford, R.J., Eds.; Woodhead Publishing: Cambridge, UK, 2014; pp. 71–99.
5. Asghari, F.; Samiei, M.; Adibkia, K.; Akbarzadeh, A.; Davaran, S. Biodegradable and biocompatible polymers for tissue engineering application: A review. *Artif. Cells Nanomed. Biotechnol.* **2016**, *45*, 185–192. [CrossRef]

6. Ribeiro, D.M.L.; Júnior, A.R.C.; de Macedo, G.H.R.V.; Chagas, V.L.; Silva, L.D.S.; da Silva Cutrim, B.; Santos, D.M.; Soares, B.L.L.; Zagmignan, A.; de Càssia Mendonça de Miranda , R.; et al. Polysaccharide-Based Formulations for Healing of Skin-Related Wound Infections: Lessons from Animal Models and Clinical Trials. *Biomolecules* **2020**, *10*, 1–16.
7. Singh, M.R.; Patel, S.; Singh, D. Natural polymer-based hydrogels as scaffolds for tissue engineering. In *Nanobiomaterials in Soft Tissue Engineering*; Grumezescu, A.M., Ed.; William Andrew Publishing: Norwich, NY, USA, 2016; pp. 231–260.
8. Liu, Z.; Jiao, Y.; Wang, Y.; Zhou, C.; Zhang, Z. Polysaccharides-based nanoparticles as drug delivery systems. *Adv. Drug Deliv. Rev.* **2008**, *60*, 1650–1662. [CrossRef]
9. Mele, E. Electrospinning of natural polymers for advanced wound care: Towards responsive and adaptive dressings. *J. Mater. Chem. B* **2016**, *4*, 4801–4812. [CrossRef] [PubMed]
10. Bealer, E.J.; Onissema-Karimu, S.; Rivera-Galletti, A.; Francis, M.; Wilkowski, J.; la Cruz, D.S.; Hu, X. Protein–Polysaccharide Composite Materials: Fabrication and Applications. *Polymer* **2020**, *12*, 464. [CrossRef] [PubMed]
11. Miranda, C.S.; Ribeiro, A.R.M.; Homem, N.C.; Felgueiras, H.P. Spun Biotextiles in Tissue Engineering and Biomolecules Delivery Systems. *Antibiotics* **2020**, *9*, 174. [CrossRef] [PubMed]
12. Vandghanooni, S.; Eskandani, M. Natural polypeptides-based electrically conductive biomaterials for tissue engineering. *Int. J. Biol. Macromol.* **2020**, *147*, 706–733. [CrossRef] [PubMed]
13. Poole-Warren, L.A.; Patton, A.J. Introduction to biomedical polymers and biocompatibility. In *Biosynthetic Polymers for Medical Applications*; Poole-Warren, L., Martens, P., Green, R., Eds.; Woodhead Publishing: Cambridge, UK, 2016; pp. 3–31.
14. Nair, L.S.; Laurencin, C.T. Biodegradable polymers as biomaterials. *Prog. Polym. Sci.* **2007**, *32*, 762–798. [CrossRef]
15. Manavitehrani, I.; Fathi, A.; Badr, H.; Daly, S.; Shirazi, A.N.; Dehghani, F. Biomedical applications of biodegradable polyesters. *Polymers* **2016**, *8*, 20. [CrossRef] [PubMed]
16. Negut, I.; Dorcioman, G.; Grumezescu, V. Scaffolds for Wound Healing Applications. *Polymers* **2020**, *12*, 2010. [CrossRef]
17. Mondal, D.; Mollick, M.M.R.; Bhowmick, B.; Maity, D.; Bain, M.K.; Rana, D.; Mukhopadhyay, A.; Dana, K.; Chattopadhyay, D. Effect of poly(vinyl pyrrolidone) on the morphology and physical properties of poly(vinyl alcohol)/sodium montmorillonite nanocomposite films. *Prog. Nat. Sci. Mater. Int.* **2013**, *23*, 579–587. [CrossRef]
18. Salehi-Nik, N.; Rezai Rad, M.; Nazeman, P.; Khojasteh, A. Polymers for oral and dental tissue engineering. In *Biomaterials for Oral and Dental Tissue Engineering*; Tayebi, L., Moharamzadeh, K., Eds.; Woodhead Publishing: Cambridge, UK, 2017; pp. 25–46.
19. Duskey, J.T.; Baraldi, C.; Gamberini, M.C.; Ottonelli, I.; Da Ros, F.; Tosi, G.; Forni, F.; Vandelli, M.A.; Ruozi, B. Investigating Novel Syntheses of a Series of Unique Hybrid PLGA-Chitosan Polymers for Potential Therapeutic Delivery Applications. *Polymers* **2020**, *12*, 823. [CrossRef]
20. Liu, H.; Wang, C.; Li, C.; Qin, Y.; Wang, Z.; Yang, F.; Li, Z.; Wang, J. A functional chitosan-based hydrogel as a wound dressing and drug delivery system in the treatment of wound healing. *RSC Adv.* **2018**, *8*, 7533–7549. [CrossRef]
21. Raia, N.R.; Partlow, B.P.; McGill, M.; Kimmerling, E.P.; Ghezzi, C.E.; Kaplan, D.L. Enzymatically crosslinked silk-hyaluronic acid hydrogels. *Biomaterials* **2017**, *131*, 58–67. [CrossRef] [PubMed]
22. Tran, H.D.N.; Park, K.D.; Ching, Y.C.; Huynh, C.; Nguyen, D.H. A Comprehensive Review on Polymeric Hydrogel and Its Composite: Matrices of Choice for Bone and Cartilage Tissue Engineering. *J. Ind. Eng. Chem.* **2020**, *89*, 58–82. [CrossRef]
23. Felgueiras, H.P.P.; Wang, L.-M.; Ren, K.-F.; Querido, M.M.; Jin, Q.; Barbosa, M.; Ji, J.; Martins, M.C.L. Octadecyl chains immobilized onto hyaluronic acid coatings by thiolene "click chemistry" increase the surface antimicrobial properties and prevent platelet adhesion and activation to polyurethane. *ACS Appl. Mater. Interfaces* **2017**, *9*, 7979–7989. [CrossRef]
24. Shi, W.; Hass, B.; Kuss, M.A.; Zhang, H.; Ryu, S.; Zhang, D.; Li, T.; Li, Y.; Duan, B. Fabrication of versatile dynamic hyaluronic acid-based hydrogels. *Carbohydr. Polym.* **2020**, *233*, 115803. [CrossRef]
25. Dave, P.N.; Gor, A. Natural Polysaccharide-Based Hydrogels and Nanomaterials: Recent Trends and Their Applications. In *Handbook of Nanomaterials for Industrial Applications*; Hussain, C.M., Ed.; Elsevier: Amsterdam, The Netherlands, 2018; pp. 36–66.
26. Ranganathan, S.; Balagangadharan, K.; Selvamurugan, N. Chitosan and gelatin-based electrospun fibers for bone tissue engineering. *Int. J. Biol. Macromol.* **2019**, *133*, 354–364. [CrossRef]
27. Antunes, J.C.; Conçalves, R.M.; Barbosa, M.A. Chitosan/Poly(γ-glutamic acid) Polyelectrolyte Complexes: From Self-Assembly to Application in Biomolecules Delivery and Regenerative Medicine. *Res. Rev. J. Mater. Sci.* **2016**, *4*, 12–36. [CrossRef]
28. Goh, C.H.; Heng, P.W.S.; Chan, L.W. Alginates as a useful natural polymer for microencapsulation and therapeutic applications. *Carbohydr. Polym.* **2012**, *88*, 1–12. [CrossRef]
29. Lee, K.Y.; Mooney, D.J. Alginate: Properties and biomedical and applications. *Prog. Polym. Sci.* **2012**, *37*, 106–126. [CrossRef] [PubMed]
30. Rezvanain, M.; Ahmad, N.; Amin, M.C.I.M.; Ng, S.-F. Optimization, characterization, and in vitro assessment of alginate-pectin ionic cross-linked hydrogel film for wound dressing applications. *Int. J. Biol. Macromol.* **2017**, *97*, 131–140. [CrossRef] [PubMed]
31. Yan, G.; Chen, B.; Zeng, X.; Sun, Y.; Tang, X.; Lin, L. Recent advances on sustainable cellulosic materials for pharmaceutical carrier applications. *Carbohydr. Polym.* **2020**, *244*, 116492. [CrossRef]
32. Wang, J.; Tavakoli, J.; Tang, Y. Bacterial cellulose production, properties and applications with different culture methods–A review. *Carbohydr. Polym.* **2019**, *219*, 63–76. [CrossRef]
33. Teixeira, M.A.; Paiva, M.C.; Amorim, M.T.P.; Felgueiras, H.P. Electrospun Nanocomposites Containing Cellulose and Its Derivatives Modified with Specialized Biomolecules for an Enhanced Wound Healing. *Nanomaterials* **2020**, *10*, 557. [CrossRef] [PubMed]

34. Fu, L.-H.; Qi, C.; Ma, M.-G.; Wan, P. Multifunctional cellulose-based hydrogels for biomedical applications. *J. Mater. Chem. B* **2019**, *7*, 1541–1562. [CrossRef]
35. Gaspar-Pintiliescu, A.; Stanciuc, A.-M.; Craciunescu, O. Natural composite dressings based on collagen, gelatin and plant bioactive compounds for wound healing: A review. *Int. J. Biol. Macromol.* **2019**, *138*, 854–865. [CrossRef]
36. Lin, H.; Cheng, A.W.-M.; Alexander, P.G.; Beck, A.M.; Tuan, R.S. Cartilage Tissue Engineering Application of Injectable Gelatin Hydrogel with *In Situ* Visible-Light-Activated Gelation Capability in both Air and Aqueous Solution. *Tissue Eng. Part A* **2014**, *20*, 2402–2411. [CrossRef]
37. Yang, G.; Lin, H.; Rothrauff, B.B.; Yu, S.; Tuan, R.S. Multilayered Polycaprolactone/Gelatin Fiber-Hydrogel Composite for Tendon Tissue Engineering. *Acta Biomater.* **2016**, *35*, 68–76. [CrossRef] [PubMed]
38. Gurumurthy, B.; Janorkar, A.V. Improvements in Mechanical Properties of Collagen-Based Scaffolds for Tissue Engineering. *Curr. Opin. Biomed. Eng.* **2021**, *17*, 100253. [CrossRef]
39. Nuñez, S.M.; Guzmán, F.; Valencia, P.; Almonacid, S.; Cárdenas, C. Collagen as a source of bioactive peptides: A bioinformatics approach. *Electron. J. Biotechnol.* **2020**, *48*, 101–108. [CrossRef]
40. Hashim, P.; Mohd Ridzwan, M.S.; Bakar, J.; Mat Hashim, D. Collagen in food and beverage industries. *Int. Food Res. J.* **2015**, *22*, 1–8.
41. Ferreira, A.M.; Gentile, P.; Chiono, V.; Ciardelli, G. Collagen for bone tissue regeneration. *Acta Biomater.* **2012**, *8*, 3191–3200. [CrossRef]
42. Yu, F.; Prashantha, K.; Soulestin, J.; Lacrampe, M.-F.; Krawczak, P. Plasticized-starch/poly(ethylene oxide) blends prepared by extrusion. *Carbohydr. Polym.* **2013**, *91*, 253–261. [CrossRef]
43. Theodosopoulos, G.V.; Zisis, C.; Charalambidis, G.; Nikolaou, V.; Coutsolelos, A.G.; Pitsikalis, M. Synthesis, Characterization and Thermal Properties of Poly(ethylene oxide), PEO, Polymacromonomers via Anionic and Ring Opening Metathesis Polymerization. *Polymers* **2017**, *9*, 145. [CrossRef] [PubMed]
44. Kundu, J.; Pati, F.; Jeong, Y.H.; Cho, D.-W. Biomaterials for Biofabrication of 3D Tissue Scaffolds. In *Biofabrication*; Forgacs, G., Sun, W., Eds.; William Andrew Publishing: Norwich, NY, USA, 2013; pp. 23–46.
45. Wong, R.S.H.; Dodou, K. Effect of Drug Loading Method and Drug Physicochemical Properties on the Material and Drug Release Properties of Poly (Ethylene Oxide) Hydrogels for Transdermal Delivery. *Polymer* **2017**, *9*, 286. [CrossRef] [PubMed]
46. Venugopal, J.; Ramakrishna, S. Biocompatible nanofiber matrices for the engineering of a dermal substitute for skin regeneration. *Tissue Eng.* **2005**, *11*, 847–854. [CrossRef] [PubMed]
47. Zhong, X.; Ji, C.; Chan, A.K.L.; Kazarian, S.G.; Ruys, A.; Dehghani, F. Fabrication of chitosan/poly(ε-caprolactone) composite hydrogels for tissue engineering applications. *J. Mater. Sci. Mater. Med.* **2011**, *22*, 279–288. [CrossRef] [PubMed]
48. Teixeira, M.A.; Amorim, M.T.P.; Felgueiras, H.P. Poly(Vinyl Alcohol)-Based Nanofibrous Electrospun Scaffolds for Tissue Engineering Applications. *Polymers* **2020**, *12*, 7. [CrossRef]
49. Manavitehrani, I.; Fathi, A.; Wang, Y.; Maitz, P.; Dehghani, F. Reinforced Poly(Propylene Carbonate) Composite with Enhanced and Tunable Characteristics, an Alternative for Poly(lactic Acid). *ACS Appl. Mater. Interfaces* **2015**, *7*, 22421–22430. [CrossRef] [PubMed]
50. Maitz, M.F. Applications of synthetic polymers in clinical medicine. *Biosurface Biotribol.* **2015**, *1*, 161–176. [CrossRef]
51. Virlan, M.J.R.; Miricescu, D.; Totan, A.; Greabu, M.; Tanase, C.; Sabliov, C.M.; Caruntu, C.; Calenic, B. Current Uses of Poly(lactic-co-glycolic acid) in the Dental Field: A Comprehensive Review. *J. Chem.* **2015**, *2015*, 1–12. [CrossRef]
52. Sun, X.; Xu, C.; Wu, G.; Ye, Q.; Wang, C. Poly(Lactic-co-Glycolic Acid): Applications and Future Prospects for Periodontal Tissue Regeneration. *Polymer* **2017**, *9*, 189. [CrossRef]
53. Del Prado, A.; Civantos, A.; Martínez-Campos, E.; Levkin, P.A.; Reinecke, H.; Gallardo, A.; Elvira, C. Efficient and Low Cytotoxicity Gene Carriers Based on Amine-Functionalized Polyvinylpyrrolidone. *Polymers* **2020**, *12*, 2724. [CrossRef]
54. Voronova, M.; Rubleva, N.; Kochkina, N.; Afineevskii, A.; Zakharov, A.; Surov, O. Preparation and Characterization of Polyvinylpyrrolidone/Cellulose Nanocrystals Composites. *Nanomaterials* **2018**, *8*, 1011. [CrossRef] [PubMed]
55. Kurakula, M.; Rao, G.K. Moving polyvinyl pyrrolidone electrospun nanofibers and bioprinted scaffolds toward multidisciplinary biomedical applications. *Eur. Polym. J.* **2020**, *136*, 109919. [CrossRef]
56. Mc Gann, M.J.; Higginbotham, C.L.; Geever, L.M.; Nugent, M.J.D. The synthesis of novel pH-sensitive poly(vinyl alcohol) composite hydrogels using a freeze/thaw process for biomedical applications. *Int. J. Pharm.* **2009**, *372*, 154–161. [CrossRef]
57. Costa-Júnior, E.S.; Barbosa-Stancioli, E.F.; Mansur, A.A.P.; Vasconcelos, W.L.; Mansur, H.S. Preparation and characterization of chitosan/poly(vinyl alcohol) chemically crosslinked blends for biomedical applications. *Carbohydr. Polym.* **2009**, *76*, 472–481. [CrossRef]
58. Kopeček, J. Hydrogel biomaterials: A smart future? *Biomaterials* **2007**, *28*, 5185–5192. [CrossRef]
59. Hwang, M.-R.; Kim, J.O.; Lee, J.H.; Kim, I.Y.; Kim, J.H.; Chang, S.W.; Jin, S.G.; Kim, J.A.; Lyoo, W.S.; Han, S.S.; et al. Gentamicin-loaded wound dressing with polyvinyl alcohol/dextran hydrogel: Gel characterization and *in vivo* healing evaluation. *AAPS PharmSciTech* **2010**, *11*, 1092–1103. [CrossRef]
60. Suo, H.; Zhang, D.; Yin, J.; Qian, J.; Wu, Z.L.; Fu, J. Interpenetrating polymer network hydrogels composed of chitosan and photocrosslinkable gelatin with enhanced mechanical properties for tissue engineering. *Mater. Sci. Eng. C* **2018**, *92*, 612–620. [CrossRef]
61. Hernández-González, A.C.; Téllez-Jurado, L.; Rodríguez-Lorenzo, L.M. Alginate hydrogels for bone tissue engineering, from injectables to bioprinting: A Review. *Carbohydr. Polym.* **2019**, *229*, 115514. [CrossRef] [PubMed]

62. Li, S.; Dong, S.; Xu, W.; Tu, S.; Yan, L.; Zhao, C.; Ding, J.; Chen, X. Antibacterial Hydrogels. *Adv. Sci.* **2018**, *5*, 1700527. [CrossRef] [PubMed]
63. Tsou, Y.-H.; Khoneisser, J.; Huang, P.-C.; Xu, X. Hydrogel as a bioactive material to regulate stem cell fate. *Bioact. Mater.* **2016**, *1*, 39–55. [CrossRef] [PubMed]
64. Abbasian, M.; Massoumi, B.; Mohammad-Rezaei, R.; Samadian, H.; Jaymand, M. Scaffolding polymeric biomaterials: Are naturally occurring biological macromolecules more appropriate for tissue engineering? *Int. J. Biol. Macromol.* **2019**, *134*, 673–694. [CrossRef] [PubMed]
65. Vasile, C.; Pamfil, D.; Stoleru, E.; Baican, M. New Developments in Medical Applications of Hybrid Hydrogels Containing Natural Polymers. *Molecules* **2020**, *25*, 1539. [CrossRef]
66. White, J.C.; Saffe, E.M.; Bhatia, S.R. Alginate/PEO-PPO-PEO Composite Hydrogels with Thermally-Active Plasticity. *Biomacromolecules* **2013**, *14*, 4456–4464. [CrossRef]
67. Bai, Z.; Wang, T.; Zheng, X.; Huang, Y.; Chen, Y.; Dan, W. High strength and bioactivity polyvinyl alcohol/collagen composite hydrogel with tannic acid as cross-linker. *Polym. Eng. Sci.* **2020**, 1–10.
68. Ahmed, E.M. Hydrogel: Preparation, characterization, and applications: A review. *J. Adv. Res.* **2015**, *6*, 105–121. [CrossRef]
69. Burkert, S.; Schmidt, T.; Gohs, U.; Dorschner, H.; Arndt, K.-F. Cross-linking of poly (N-vinyl pyrrolidone) films by electron beam irradiation. *Radiat. Phys. Chem.* **2007**, *76*, 1324–1328. [CrossRef]
70. Yang, L.; Chu, J.S.; Fix, J.A. Colon-specific drug delivery: New approaches and in *vitro/in vivo* evaluation. *Int. J. Pharm.* **2002**, *235*, 1–15. [CrossRef]
71. Teijón, C.; Guerrero, S.; Olmo, R.; Teijón, J.M.; Blanco, M.D. Swelling Properties of Copolymeric Hydrogels of Poly(ethylene glycol) Monomethacrylate and Monoesters of Itaconic Acid for Use in Drug Delivery. *J. Biomed. Mater. Res. Part B Appl. Biomater.* **2009**, *91*, 716–726. [CrossRef]
72. Lowman, A.M.; Peppas, N.A. Analysis of the Complexation/Decomplexation Phenomena in Graft Copolymer Networks. *Macromolecular* **1997**, *30*, 4959–4965. [CrossRef]
73. Jana, S.; Saha, A.; Nayak, A.K.; Sen, K.K.; Basu, S.K. Aceclofenac-loaded chitosan-tamarind seed polysaccharide interpenetrating polymeric network microparticles. *Colloids Surf. B Biointerfaces* **2013**, *105*, 303–309. [CrossRef] [PubMed]
74. Okay, O. Semicrystalline physical hydrogels with shape-memory and self-healing properties. *J. Mater. Chem. B* **2019**, *7*, 1581–1596. [CrossRef]
75. BaoLin, G.; MA, P.X. Synthetic biodegradable functional polymers for tissue engineering: A brief review. *Sci. China Chem.* **2014**, *57*, 490–500.
76. Iglesias, N.; Galbis, E.; Valencia, C.; Díaz-Blanco, M.J.; Lacroix, B.; De-Paz, M.-V. Biodegradable double cross-linked chitosan hydrogels for drug delivery: Impact of chemistry on rheological and pharmacological performance. *Int. J. Biol. Macromol.* **2020**, *165*, 2205–2218. [CrossRef]
77. Kong, H.J.; Kaigler, D.; Kim, K.; Mooney, D.J. Controlling Rigidity and Degradation of Alginate Hydrogels via Molecular Weight Distribution. *Biomacromolecules* **2004**, *5*, 1720–1727. [CrossRef]
78. Bouhadir, K.H.; Lee, K.Y.; Alsberg, E.; Damm, K.L.; Anderson, K.W.; Mooney, D.J. Degradation of partially oxidized alginate and its potential application for tissue engineering. *Biotechnol. Prog.* **2001**, *17*, 945–950. [CrossRef]
79. West, J.L.; Hubbell, J.A. Polymeric biomaterials with degradation sites for proteases involved in cell migration. *Macromolecules* **1999**, *32*, 241–244. [CrossRef]
80. Tanan, W.; Panichpakdee, J.; Saengsuwan, S. Novel Biodegradable Hydrogel Based on Natural Polymers: Synthesis, Characterization, Swelling/Reswelling and Biodegradability. *Eur. Polym. J.* **2018**, *112*, 678–687. [CrossRef]
81. Mantha, S.; Pillai, S.; Khayambashi, P.; Upadhyay, A.; Zhang, Y.; Tao, O.; Pham, H.M.; Tran, S.D. Smart Hydrogels in Tissue Engineering and Regenerative Medicine. *Materials* **2019**, *12*, 3323. [CrossRef] [PubMed]
82. Fänger, C.; Wack, H.; Ulbricht, M. Macroporous Poly(N-isopropylacrylamide) Hydrogels with Adjustable size "Cut-off" for the Efficient and Reversible Immobilization of Biomacromolecules. *Macromol. Biosci.* **2006**, *6*, 393–402. [CrossRef]
83. Sood, N.; Bhardwaj, A.; Mehta, S.; Mehta, A. Stimuli-responsive hydrogels in drug delivery and tissue engineering. *Drug Deliv.* **2014**, *7544*, 1–23. [CrossRef] [PubMed]
84. Bag, M.A.; Valenzuela, L.M. Impact of the Hydration States of Polymers on Their Hemocompatibility for Medical Applications: A review. *Int. J. Mol. Sci.* **2017**, *18*, 1422. [CrossRef]
85. Gupta, A.; Kowalczuk, M.; Heaselgrave, W.; Britland, S.T.; Martin, C.; Radecka, I. The production and application of hydrogels for wound management: A review. *Eur. Polym. J.* **2019**, *111*, 134–151. [CrossRef]
86. Kwon, S.S.; Kong, B.J.; Park, S.N. Physicochemical properties of pH-sensitive hydrogels based on hydroxyethyl cellulose–hyaluronic acid and for applications as transdermal delivery systems for skin lesions. *Eur. J. Pharm. Biopharm.* **2015**, *92*, 146–154. [CrossRef]
87. Salleh, K.M.; Zakaria, S.; Sajab, M.S.; Gan, S.; Chia, C.H.; Jaafar, S.N.S.; Amran, U.A. Chemically crosslinked hydrogel and its driving force towards superabsorbent behaviour. *Int. J. Biol. Macromol.* **2018**, *118*, 1422–1430. [CrossRef]
88. Zhao, Q.S.; Ji, Q.X.; Xing, K.; Li, X.Y.; Liu, C.S.; Chen, X.G. Preparation and characteristics of novel porous hydrogel films based on chitosan and glycerophosphate. *Carbohydr. Polym.* **2009**, *76*, 410–416. [CrossRef]
89. Kimura, M.; Fukumoto, K.; Watanabe, J.; Ishihara, K. Hydrogen-bonding-driven spontaneous gelation of water-soluble phospholipid polymers in aqueous medium. *J. Biomater. Sci. Polym. Ed.* **2004**, *15*, 631–644. [CrossRef]

90. Tuncaboylu, D.C.; Sari, M.; Oppermann, W.; Okay, O. Tough and Self-healing Hydrogels Formed via Hydrophobic Interactions. *Macromolecules* **2011**, *44*, 4997–5005. [CrossRef]
91. Stenekes, R.J.H.; Talsma, H.; Hennink, W.E. Formation of dextran hydrogels by crystallization. *Biomaterials* **2001**, *22*, 1891–1898. [CrossRef]
92. George, J.; Hsu, C.-C.; Nguyen, L.T.B.; Ye, H.; Cui, Z. Neural tissue engineering with structured hydrogels in CNS models and therapies. *Biotechnol. Adv.* **2019**, *42*, 1–17. [CrossRef]
93. Czarnecki, S.; Rossow, T.; Seiffert, S. Hybrid Polymer-Network Hydrogels with Tunable Mechanical Response. *Polymers* **2016**, *8*, 82. [CrossRef]
94. Hoffman, A.S. Hydrogels for biomedical applications. *Adv. Drug Deliv. Rev.* **2002**, *43*, 3–12. [CrossRef]
95. Rosiak, J.M.; Yoshii, F. Hydrogels and their medical applications. *Nucl. Instrum. Methods Phys. Res. Sect. B Beam Interact. Mater. Atoms* **1999**, *151*, 56–64. [CrossRef]
96. Zhang, H.; Zhang, F.; Wu, J. Physically crosslinked hydrogels from polysaccharides prepared by freeze-thaw technique. *React. Funct. Polym.* **2013**, *73*, 923–928. [CrossRef]
97. Zhong, M.; Liu, Y.-T.; Xie, X.-M. Self-healable, super tough graphene oxide/poly(acrylic acid) nanocomposite hydrogels facilitated by dual cross-linking effects through dynamic ionic interactions. *J. Mater. Chem. B* **2015**, *3*, 4001–4008. [CrossRef] [PubMed]
98. Hu, W.; Wang, Z.; Xiao, Y.; Zhanga, S.; Wang, J. Advances in crosslinking strategies of biomedical hydrogels. *Biomater. Sci.* **2019**, *7*, 843–855. [CrossRef] [PubMed]
99. Hoare, T.R.; Kohane, D.S. Hydrogels in drug delivery: Progress and challenges. *Polymers* **2008**, *49*, 1993–2007. [CrossRef]
100. Abdurrahmanoglu, S.; Can, V.; Okay, O. Design of high-toughness polyacrylamide hydrogels by hydrophobic modification. *Polymer* **2009**, *50*, 5449–5455. [CrossRef]
101. Zhang, Y.; Zhao, X.; Yang, W.; Jiang, W.; Chen, F.; Fu, Q. Enhancement of mechanical property and absorption capability of hydrophobically associated polyacrylamide hydrogels by adding cellulose nanofiber. *Mater. Res. Express* **2020**, *7*, 015319. [CrossRef]
102. Figueroa-Pizano, M.D.; Vélaz, I.; Peñas, F.J.; Zavala-Rivera, P.; Rosas-Durazo, A.J.; Maldonado-Arce, A.D.; Martínez-Barbosa, M.E. Effect of freeze-thawing conditions for preparation of chitosan-poly (vinyl alcohol) hydrogels and drug release studies. *Carbohydr. Polym.* **2018**, *195*, 476–485. [CrossRef] [PubMed]
103. Ricciardi, R.; Auriemma, F.; De Rosa, C.; Lauprêtre, F. X-ray Diffraction Analysis of Poly (vinyl alcohol) Hydrogels, Obtained by Freezing and Thawing Techniques. *Macromolecules* **2004**, *37*, 1921–1927. [CrossRef]
104. Lotfipour, F.; Alami-Milani, M.; Salatin, S.; Hadavi, A.; Jelvehgari, M. Freeze-thaw- induced cross-linked PVA/chitosan for oxytetracycline-loaded wound dressing: The experimental design and optimization. *Res. Pharm. Sci.* **2019**, *14*, 175–189.
105. Sabnis, A.; Rahimi, M.; Chapman, C.; Nguyen, K.T. Cytocompatibility studies of an in situ photopolymerized thermoresponsive hydrogel nanoparticle system using human aortic smooth muscle cells. *J. Biomed. Mater. Res. Part A* **2008**, *91*, 52–59.
106. Han, W.T.; Jang, T.; Chen, S.; Chong, L.S.H.; Jung, H.; Song, J. Improved cell viability for large-scale biofabrication with photo-crosslinkable hydrogel systems through a dual-photoinitiator approach. *Biomater. Sci.* **2020**, *8*, 450–461. [CrossRef]
107. Zhao, L.; Li, X.; Zhao, J.; Ma, S.; Ma, X.; Fan, D.; Zhu, C.; Liu, Y. A novel smart injectable hydrogel prepared by microbial transglutaminase and human-like collagen: Its characterization and biocompatibility. *Mater. Sci. Eng. C* **2016**, *68*, 317–326. [CrossRef]
108. Ren, K.; He, C.; Cheng, Y.; Li, G.; Chen, X. Injectable enzymatically crosslinked hydrogels based on a poly(L-glutamic acid) graft copolymer. *Polym. Chem.* **2014**, *5*, 5069–5076. [CrossRef]
109. Teixeira, L.S.M.; Feijen, J.; Van Blitterswijk, C.A.; Dijkstra, P.J.; Karperien, M. Enzyme-catalyzed crosslinkable hydrogels: Emerging strategies for tissue engineering. *Biomaterials* **2012**, *33*, 1281–1290. [CrossRef] [PubMed]
110. Kanafi, N.M.; Rahman, N.A.; Rosdi, N.H. Citric acid cross-linking of highly porous carboxymethyl cellulose poly(ethylene oxide) composite hydrogel films for controlled release applications. *Mater. Today Proc.* **2019**, *7*, 721–731. [CrossRef]
111. Dimida, S.; Demitri, C.; De Benedictis, V.M.; Scalera, F.; Gervaso, F.; Sannino, A. Genipin-cross-linked chitosan-based hydrogels: Reaction kinetics and structure-related characteristics. *J. Appl. Polym. Sci.* **2015**, *132*, 1–8. [CrossRef]
112. Lai, J.-Y. Solvent Composition is Critical for Carbodiimide Cross-Linking of Hyaluronic Acid as an Ophthalmic Biomaterial. *Materials* **2012**, *5*, 1986–2002. [CrossRef]
113. Jin, R.; Teixeira, L.S.M.; Krouwels, A.; Dijkstra, P.J.; Van Blitterswijk, C.A.; Karperien, M.; Feijen, J. Synthesis and characterization of hyaluronic acid-poly(ethylene glycol) hydrogels via Michael addition: An injectable biomaterial for cartilage repair. *Acta Biomater.* **2010**, *6*, 1968–1977. [CrossRef] [PubMed]
114. Parhi, R. Cross-Linked Hydrogel for Pharmaceutical Applications: A Review. *Adv. Pharm. Bull.* **2017**, *7*, 515–530. [CrossRef] [PubMed]
115. Martinez-Martinez, M.; Rodriguez-Berna, G.; Gonzalez-Alvarez, I.; Hernández, M.J.; Corma, A.; Bermejo, M.; Merino, V.; Gonzalez-Alvarez, M. Ionic hydrogel based on chitosan crosslinked with 6-Phosphogluconic Trisodium salt as a drug delivery system. *Biomacromolecules* **2018**, *19*, 1294–1304. [CrossRef] [PubMed]
116. Wang, Y.; Ma, M.; Wang, J.; Zhang, W.; Lu, W.; Gao, Y.; Zhang, B.; Guo, Y. Development of a Photo-Crosslinking, Biodegradable GelMA/PEGDA Hydrogel for Guided Bone Regeneration Materials. *Materials* **2018**, *11*, 1345. [CrossRef] [PubMed]

117. Choi, J.H.; Choi, O.K.; Lee, J.; Noh, J.; Lee, S.; Park, A.; Rim, M.A.; Reis, R.L.; Khang, G. Evaluation of double network hydrogel of poloxamer-heparin/gellan gum for bone marrow stem cells delivery carrier. *Colloids Surfaces B Biointerfaces* **2019**, *181*, 879–889. [CrossRef]
118. Masruchin, N.; Park, B.-D.; Causin, V. Influence of sonication treatment on supramolecular cellulose microfibril-based hydrogels induced by ionic interaction. *J. Ind. Eng. Chem.* **2015**, *29*, 265–272. [CrossRef]
119. Liu, T.; Jiao, C.; Peng, X.; Chen, Y.-N.; Chen, Y.; He, C.; Liu, R.; Wang, H. Super-strong and tough poly(vinyl alcohol)/poly(acrylic acid) hydrogels reinforced by hydrogen bonding. *J. Mater. Chem. B* **2018**, *6*, 8105–8114. [CrossRef]
120. Ye, X.; Li, X.; Shen, Y.; Chang, G.; Yang, J.; Gu, Z. Self-healing pH-sensitive cytosine- and guanosine-modified hyaluronic acid hydrogels via hydrogen bonding. *Polymer* **2017**, *108*, 348–360. [CrossRef]
121. Ahmed, A.S.; Mandal, U.K.; Taher, M.; Susanti, D.; Jaffri, J.M. PVA-PEG physically cross-linked hydrogel film as a wound dressing: Experimental design and optimization. *Pharm. Dev. Technol.* **2018**, *23*, 751–760. [CrossRef]
122. Hurtado, M.M.; de Vries, E.G.; Zeng, X.; van der Heide, E. A tribo-mechanical analysis of PVA-based building-blocks for implementation in a 2-layered skin model. *J. Mech. Behav. Biomed. Mater.* **2016**, *62*, 319–332. [CrossRef]
123. Nachlas, A.L.Y.; Li, S.; Jha, R.; Singh, M.; Xu, C.; Davis, M.E. Human iPSC-derived mesenchymal stem cells matured into valve interstitial- like cells using PEGDA hydrogels. *Acta Biomater.* **2018**, *71*, 235–246. [CrossRef]
124. Yoon, H.J.; Shin, S.R.; Cha, J.M.; Lee, S.H.; Kim, J.H.; Do, J.T.; Song, H.; Bae, H. Cold Water Fish Gelatin Methacryloyl Hydrogel for Tissue Engineering Application. *PLoS ONE* **2016**, *11*, 1–18. [CrossRef] [PubMed]
125. Hasturk, O.; Jordan, K.E.; Choi, J.; Kaplan, D.L. Enzymatically crosslinked silk and silk-gelatin hydrogels with tunable gelation kinetics, mechanical properties and bioactivity for cell culture and encapsulation. *Biomaterials* **2020**, *232*, 119720. [CrossRef]
126. Besser, R.R.; Bowles, A.C.; Alassaf, A.; Carbonero, D.; Claure, I.; Jones, E.; Reda, J.; Wubker, L.; Batchelor, W.; Ziebarth, N.; et al. Enzymatically crosslinked gelatin-laminin hydrogels for applications in neuromuscular tissue engineering. *Biomater. Sci.* **2020**, *8*, 591–606. [CrossRef] [PubMed]
127. Ubaid, M.; Murtaza, G. Fabrication and characterization of genipin cross-linked chitosan/gelatin hydrogel for pH-sensitive, oral delivery of metformin with an application of response surface methodology. *Int. J. Biol. Macromol.* **2018**, *114*, 1174–1185. [CrossRef] [PubMed]
128. Martínez-Mejía, G.; Vázquez-Torres, N.A.; Castell-Rodríguez, A.; del Río, J.M.; Corea, M.; Jiménez-Juárez, R. Synthesis of new chitosan-glutaraldehyde scaffolds for tissue engineering using schiff reactions. *Colloids Surfaces A Physicochem. Eng. Asp.* **2019**, *579*, 123658. [CrossRef]
129. Wang, G.; Wang, X.; Huang, L. Feasibility of chitosan-alginate (Chi-Alg) hydrogel used as scaffold for neural tissue engineering: A pilot study in vitro. *Biotechnol. Biotechnol. Equip.* **2017**, *31*, 766–773. [CrossRef]
130. Seera, S.D.K.; Kundu, D.; Banerjee, T. Physical and chemical crosslinked microcrystalline cellulose-polyvinyl alcohol hydrogel: Freeze–thaw mediated synthesis, characterization and in vitro delivery of 5- fluorouracil. *Cellulose* **2020**, *27*, 6521–6535. [CrossRef]
131. Marin, E.; Boschetto, F.; Pezzotti, G. Biomaterials and biocompatibility: An historical overview. *J. Biomed. Mater. Res. Part A* **2020**, *108*, 1617–1633. [CrossRef]
132. Moulherat, C.; Tengberg, M.; Haquet, J.F.; Mille, B. First evidence of cotton at Neolithic Mehrgarh, Pakistan: Analysis of Mineralized Fibres from a Copper Bead. *J. Archaeol. Sci.* **2002**, *29*, 1393–1401. [CrossRef]
133. Holland, C.; Numata, K.; Rnjak-Kovacina, J.; Seib, F.P. The Biomedical Use of Silk: Past, Present, Future. *Adv. Healthc. Mater.* **2018**, *8*, 1800465. [CrossRef]
134. Bari, E.; Morrell, J.J.; Sistani, A. Durability of natural/synthetic/biomass fiber-based polymeric composites: Laboratory and field tests. In *Durability and Life Prediction in Biocomposites, Fibre-Reinforced Composites and Hybrid Composites*; Jawaid, M., Thariq, M., Saba, N., Eds.; Woodhead Publishing: Cambridge, UK, 2019; pp. 15–26.
135. Tavares, T.D.; Antunes, J.C.; Ferreira, F.; Felgueiras, H.P. Biofunctionalization of natural Fiber-Reinforced Biocomposites for Biomedical Applications. *Biomolecules* **2020**, *10*, 148. [CrossRef]
136. Pankongadisak, P.; Sangklin, S.; Chuysinuan, P.; Suwantong, O.; Supaphol, P. The use of electrospun curcumin-loaded poly(L-lactic acid) fiber mats as wound dressing materials. *J. Drug Deliv. Sci. Technol.* **2019**, *53*, 101121. [CrossRef]
137. Heydari, Z.; Mohebbi-Kalhori, D.; Afarani, M.S. Engineered electrospun polycaprolactone (PCL)/octacalcium phosphate (OCP) scaffold for bone tissue engineering. *Mater. Sci. Eng. C* **2017**, *81*, 127–132. [CrossRef] [PubMed]
138. Wang, J.; Windbergs, M. Controlled dual drug release by coaxial electrospun fibers–Impact of the core fluid on drug encapsulation and release. *Int. J. Pharm.* **2018**, *556*, 363–371. [CrossRef] [PubMed]
139. Gurunathan, T.; Mohanty, S.; Nayak, S.K. A review of the Recent Developments in Biocomposites Based on Natural Fibres and Their Application Perspectives. *Compos. Part A Appl. Sci. Manuf.* **2015**, *77*, 1–25. [CrossRef]
140. Hao, L.C.; Sapuan, S.M.; Hassan, M.R.; Sheltami, R.M. Natural fiber reinforced vinyl polymer composites. In *Natural Fibre Reinforced Vinyl Ester and Vinyl Polymer Composites*; Sapuan, S.M., Ismail, H., Zainudin, E.S., Eds.; Woodhead Publishing: Cambridge, UK, 2018; pp. 27–70.
141. Balla, V.K.; Kate, K.H.; Satyavolu, J.; Singh, P.; Tadimeti, J.G.D. Additive manufacturing of natural fiber reinforced polymer composites: Processing and prospects. *Compos. Part B Eng.* **2019**, *174*, 106956. [CrossRef]
142. Fidelis, M.E.A.; Pereira, T.V.C.; Gomes, O.D.F.M.; de Andrade Silva, F.; Filho, R.D.T. The effect of fiber morphology on the tensile strength of natural fibers. *Integr. Med. Res.* **2013**, *2*, 149–157.

143. Rahman, R.; Putra, S.Z.F.S. Tensile properties of natural and synthetic fiber-reinforced polymer composites. In *Mechanical and Physical Testing of Biocomposites, Fibre-Reinforced Composites and Hybrid Composites*; Jawaid, M., Thariq, M., Saba, N., Eds.; Woodhead Publishing: Cambridge, UK, 2019; pp. 81–102.
144. Sanjay, M.R.; Madhu, P.; Jawaid, M.; Senthamaraikannan, P.; Senthil, S.; Pradeep, S. Characterization and Properties of Natural Fiber Polymer Composites: A Comprehensive Review. *J. Clean. Prod.* **2017**, *172*, 566–581. [CrossRef]
145. Bannow, J.; Benjamins, J.-W.; Wohlert, J.; Löbmann, K.; Svagan, A.J. Solid nanofoams based on cellulose nanofibers and indomethacin–the effect of processing parameters and drug content on material structure. *Int. J. Pharm.* **2017**, *526*, 291–299. [CrossRef]
146. Doench, I.; Torres-Ramos, M.E.W.; Montembault, A.; de Oliveira, P.N.; Halimi, C.; Viguier, E.; Heux, L.; Siadous, R.; Thiré, R.M.S.M.; Osorio-Madrazo, A. Injectable and Gellable Chitosan Formulations Filled with Cellulose Nanofibers for Intervertebral Disc Tissue Engineering. *Polymers* **2018**, *10*, 1202. [CrossRef]
147. Ramamoorthy, S.K.; Skrifvars, M.; Persson, A. A Review of Natural Fibers Used in Biocomposites: Plant, Animal and Regenerated Cellulose Fibers. *Polym. Rev.* **2015**, *55*, 107–161. [CrossRef]
148. Costa, F.; Silva, R.; Boccaccini, A.R. Fibrous protein-based biomaterials (silk, keratin, elastin, and resilin proteins) for tissue regeneration and repair. In *Peptides and Proteins as Biomaterials for Tissue Regeneration and Repair*; Barbosa, M.A., Martins, M.C.L., Eds.; Woodhead Publishing: Cambridge, UK, 2018; pp. 175–204.
149. McLellan, J.; Thornhill, S.G.; Shelton, S.; Kumar, M. Keratin-Based Biofilms, Hydrogels, and Biofibers. In *Keratin as a Protein Biopolymer*; Sharma, S., Kumar, A., Eds.; Springer: Cham, Switzerland, 2019; pp. 187–200.
150. Koh, L.-D.; Cheng, Y.; Teng, C.-P.; Khin, Y.-W.; Loh, X.-J.; Tee, S.-Y.; Low, M.; Ye, E.; Yu, H.-D.; Zhang, Y.-W.; et al. Structures, mechanical properties and applications of silk fibroin materials. *Prog. Polym. Sci.* **2015**, *46*, 86–110. [CrossRef]
151. Babu, K.M. Natural Textile Fibres: Animal and Silk Fibres. In *Textiles and Fashion*; Sinclair, R., Ed.; Woodhead Publishing: Cambridge, UK, 2015; pp. 57–78.
152. Mahltig, B. Introduction to inorganic fibers. In *Inorganic and Composite Fibers: Production, Properties, and Applications*; Mahltig, B., Kyosev, Y., Eds.; Woodhead Publishing: Cambridge, UK, 2018; pp. 1–29.
153. Bhat, G.; Kandagor, V. Synthetic polymer fibers and their processing requirements. In *Advances in Filament Yarn Spinning of Textiles and Polymers*; Zhang, D., Ed.; Woodhead Publishing: Cambridge, UK, 2014; pp. 3–30.
154. Ivorra-Martinez, J.; Verdu, I.; Fenollar, O.; Sanchez-Nacher, L.; Balart, R.; Quiles-Carrillo, L. Manufacturing and Properties of Binary Blend from Bacterial Polyester Poly(3-hydroxybutyrate-co-3-hydroxyhexanoate) and Poly(caprolactone) with Improved Toughness. *Polymers* **2020**, *12*, 1118. [CrossRef]
155. Gupta, B.; Revagade, N.; Hilborn, J. Poly(lactic acid) fiber: An overview. *Prog. Polym. Sci.* **2007**, *32*, 455–482. [CrossRef]
156. McNeil, S.E.; Griffiths, H.R.; Perrie, Y. Polycaprolactone Fibres as a Potential Delivery System for Collagen to Support Bone Regeneration. *Curr. Drug Deliv.* **2011**, *8*, 448–455. [CrossRef]
157. Hu, W.-W.; Lin, C.-H.; Hong, Z.-J. The enrichment of cancer stem cells using composite alginate/polycaprolactone nanofibers. *Carbohydr. Polym.* **2018**, *206*, 70–79. [CrossRef] [PubMed]
158. Levengood, S.L.; Erickson, A.E.; Chang, F.; Zhang, M. Chitosan-poly(caprolactone) nanofibers for skin repair. *J. Mater. Chem. B* **2017**, *5*, 1822–1833. [CrossRef] [PubMed]
159. Kan, Y.; Salimon, A.I.; Korsunsky, A.M. On the electrospinning of nanostructured collagen-PVA fiber mats. *Mater. Today Proc.* **2020**, *33*, 2013–2019. [CrossRef]
160. Naskar, D.; Ghosh, A.K.; Mandal, M.; Das, P.; Nandi, S.K.; Kundu, S.C. Dual growth factor loaded nonmulberry silk fibroin/carbon nanofiber composite 3D scaffolds for in vitro and in vivo bone regeneration. *Biomaterials* **2017**, *136*, 67–85. [CrossRef]
161. Latif, R.; Wakeel, S.; Khan, N.Z.; Siddiquee, A.N.; Verma, S.L.; Khan, Z.A. Surface treatments of plant fibers and their effects on mechanical properties of fiber-reinforced composites: A review. *J. Reinf. Plast. Compos.* **2018**, *38*, 15–30. [CrossRef]
162. Sanjay, M.R.; Arpitha, G.R.; Naik, L.L.; Gopalakrisha, K.; Yogesha, B. Applications of Natural Fibers and Its Composites: An Overview. *Nat. Resour.* **2016**, *7*, 108–114. [CrossRef]
163. Peças, P.; Carvalho, H.; Salman, H.; Leite, M. Natural Fibre Composites and Their Applications: A Review. *J. Compos. Sci.* **2018**, *2*, 66. [CrossRef]
164. Padil, V.V.T.; Cheong, J.Y.; KP, A.; Makvandi, P.; Zare, E.N.; Torres-Mendieta, R.; Wacławek, S.; Černík, M.; Kim, I.D.; Varma, R.S. Electrospun fibers based on carbohydrate gum polymers and their multifaceted applications. *Carbohydr. Polym.* **2020**, *247*, 116705. [CrossRef] [PubMed]
165. Liang, D.; Hsiao, B.S.; Chu, B. Functional electrospun nanofibrous scaffolds for biomedical applications. *Adv. Drug Deliv. Rev.* **2007**, *59*, 1392–1412. [CrossRef] [PubMed]
166. Felgueiras, H.P.; Amorim, M.T.P. Functionalization of electrospun polymeric wound dressings with antimicrobial peptides. *Colloids Surfaces B Biointerfaces* **2017**, *156*, 133–148. [CrossRef]
167. Shabani, I.; Haddadi-Asl, V.; Seyedjafari, E.; Soleimani, M. Cellular infiltration on nanofibrous scaffolds using a modified electrospinning technique. *Biochem. Biophys. Res. Commun.* **2012**, *423*, 50–54. [CrossRef] [PubMed]
168. Kumbar, S.G.; James, R.; Nukavarapu, S.P.; Laurencin, C.T. Electrospun nanofiber scaffolds: Engineering soft tissues. *Biomed. Mater.* **2008**, *3*, 034002. [CrossRef] [PubMed]
169. Al-Hazeem, N.Z.A. Nanofibers and Electrospinning Method. In Novel Nanomaterials-Synthesis and Applications. Kyzas, G., Mitropoulos, A.C., Eds.; IntechOpen: London, UK, 2018; pp. 191–210.

170. Greiner, A.; Wendorff, J.H. Electrospinning: A fascinating Method for the Preparation of Ultrathin Fibers. *Angew. Chemie Int. Ed.* **2007**, *46*, 5670–5703. [CrossRef] [PubMed]
171. Puppi, D.; Chiellini, F. Wet-spinning of Biomedical Polymers: From Single Fibers Production to Additive Manufacturing of 3D Scaffolds. *Polym. Int.* **2017**, *66*, 1690–1696. [CrossRef]
172. Ozipek, B.; Karakas, H. Wet spinning of synthetic polymer fibers. In *Advances in Filament Yarn Spinning of Textiles and Polymers*; Zhang, D., Ed.; Woodhead Publishing: Cambridge, UK, 2014; pp. 174–186.
173. Tronci, G.; Kanuparti, R.S.; Arafat, M.T.; Yin, J.; Wood, D.J.; Russell, S.J. Wet-spinnability and crosslinked fibre properties of two collagen polypeptides with varied molecular weight. *Int. J. Biol. Macromol.* **2015**, *81*, 112–120. [CrossRef] [PubMed]
174. Bonhomme, O.; Leng, J.; Colin, A. Microfluidic wet-spinning of alginate microfibers: A theoretical analysis of fiber formation. *Soft Matter* **2012**, *8*, 10641–10649. [CrossRef]
175. Jia, J.; Yao, D.; Wang, Y. Melt spinning of continuous fibers by cold air attenuation I: Experimental studies. *Text. Res. J.* **2014**, *84*, 593–603. [CrossRef]
176. Gajjar, C.R.; King, M.W. *Resorbable Fiber-Forming Polymers for Biotextile Applications*; Springer International Publishing: New York, NY, USA, 2014.
177. Imura, Y.; Hogan, R.M.C.; Jaffe, M. Dry spinning of synthetic polymer fibers. In *Advances in Filament Yarn Spinning of Textiles and Polymers*; Zhang, D., Ed.; Woodhead Publishing: Cambridge, UK, 2014; pp. 187–202.
178. Lee, S.-H.; Park, S.-Y.; Choi, J.-H. Fiber Formation and Physical Properties of Chitosan Fiber Crosslinked by Epichlorohydrin in a Wet Spinning System: The effect of the Concentration of the Crosslinking Agent Epichlorohydrin. *J. Appl. Polym. Sci.* **2004**, *92*, 2054–2062. [CrossRef]
179. Azimi, B.; Maleki, H.; Zavagna, L.; la Ossa, J.G.D.; Linari, S.; Lazzeri, A.; Danti, S. Bio-Based Electrospun Fibers for Wound Healing. *J. Funct. Biomater.* **2020**, *11*, 67. [CrossRef]
180. Mirzaei, B.E.; Ramazani, S.A.A.; Shafiee, M.; Danaei, M. Studies on Glutaraldehyde Crosslinked Chitosan Hydrogel Properties for Drug Delivery Systems. *Int. J. Polym. Mater. Polym. Biomater.* **2013**, *62*, 605–611. [CrossRef]
181. Blakeney, B.A.; Tambralli, A.; Anderson, J.M.; Andukuri, A.; Lim, D.-J.; Dean, D.R.; Jun, H.-W. Cell Infiltration and Growth in a Low Density, Uncompressed Three-Dimensional Electrospun Nanofibrous Scaffold. *Biomaterials* **2012**, *32*, 1583–1590. [CrossRef] [PubMed]
182. Kim, J.H.; Choi, Y.-J.; Yi, H.-G.; Wang, J.H.; Cho, D.-W.; Jeong, Y.H. A cell-laden hybrid fiber/hydrogel composite for ligament regeneration with improved cell delivery and infiltration. *Biomed. Mater.* **2017**, *12*, 055010. [CrossRef] [PubMed]
183. Jordan, A.M.; Kim, S.-E.; Van de Voorde, K.; Pokorski, J.K.; Korley, L.T.J. In Situ Fabrication of Fiber Reinforced Three-Dimensional Hydrogel Tissue Engineering Scaffolds. *ACS Biomater. Sci. Eng.* **2017**, *3*, 1869–1879. [CrossRef]
184. Kong, B.; Chen, Y.; Liu, R.; Liu, X.; Liu, C.; Shao, Z.; Xiong, L.; Liu, X.; Sun, W.; Mi, S. Fiber reinforced GelMA hydrogel to induce the regeneration of corneal stroma. *Nat. Commun.* **2020**, *11*, 1435. [CrossRef]
185. Sheffield, C.; Meyers, K.; Johnson, E.; Rajachar, R.M. Application of Composite Hydrogels to Control Physical Properties in Tissue Engineering and Regenerative Medicine. *Gels* **2018**, *4*, 51. [CrossRef]
186. Regev, O.; Reddy, C.S.; Nseir, N.; Zussman, E. Hydrogel Reinforced by Short Albumin Fibers: Mechanical Characterization and Assessment of Biocompatibility. *Macromol. Mater. Eng.* **2012**, *298*, 283–291. [CrossRef]
187. Tonsomboon, K.; Oyen, M.L. Composite electrospun gelatin fiber-alginate gel scaffolds for mechanically robust tissue engineered cornea. *J. Mech. Behav. Biomed. Mater.* **2013**, *21*, 185–194. [CrossRef]
188. Mohabatpour, F.; Karkhaneh, A.; Sharifi, A.M. A hydrogel/fiber composite scaffold for chondrocyte encapsulation in cartilage tissue regeneration. *RSC Adv.* **2016**, *6*, 83135–83145. [CrossRef]
189. Xu, W.; Ma, J.; Jabbari, E. Material properties and osteogenic differentiation of marrow stromal cells on fiber-reinforced laminated hydrogel nanocomposites. *Acta Biomater.* **2010**, *6*, 1992–2002. [CrossRef] [PubMed]
190. McMahon, R.E.; Qu, X.; Jimenez-Vergara, A.C.; Bashur, C.A.; Guelcher, S.A.; Goldstein, A.S.; Hahn, M.S. Hydrogel–Electrospun Mesh Composites for Coronary Artery Bypass Grafts. *Tissue Eng. Part C* **2011**, *17*, 451–461. [CrossRef] [PubMed]
191. Li, X.; Cho, B.; Martin, R.; Seu, M.; Zhang, C.; Zhou, Z.; Choi, J.S.; Jiang, X.; Chen, L.; Walia, G.; et al. Nanofiber-hydrogel composite–mediated angiogenesis for soft tissue reconstruction. *Sci. Transl. Med.* **2019**, *11*, eaau6210. [CrossRef] [PubMed]
192. Ekaputra, A.K.; Prestwich, G.D.; Cool, S.M.; Hutmacher, D.W. The three-dimensional vascularization of growth factor-releasing hybrid scaffold of poly (ε-caprolactone)/collagen fibers and hyaluronic acid hydrogel. *Biomaterials* **2011**, *32*, 8108–8117. [CrossRef] [PubMed]
193. Han, N.; Johnson, J.; Lannutti, J.J.; Winter, J.O. Hydrogel–electrospun fiber composite materials for hydrophilic protein release. *J. Control. Release* **2012**, *158*, 165–170. [CrossRef] [PubMed]
194. Klicova, M.; Klapstova, A.; Chvojka, J.; Koprivova, B.; Jencova, V.; Horakova, J. Novel double-layered planar scaffold combining electrospun PCL fibers and PVA hydrogels with high shape integrity and water stability. *Mater. Lett.* **2020**, *263*, 127281. [CrossRef]
195. Tonsomboon, K.; Butcher, A.L.; Oyen, M.L. Strong and tough nanofibrous hydrogel composites based on biomimetic principles. *Mater. Sci. Eng. C* **2016**, *72*, 220–227. [CrossRef] [PubMed]
196. Jang, J.; Lee, J.; Seol, Y.-J.; Jeong, Y.H.; Cho, D.-W. Improving mechanical properties of alginate hydrogel by reinforcement with ethanol treated polycaprolactone nanofibers. *Compos. Part B* **2013**, *45*, 1216–1221. [CrossRef]
197. Khorshidi, S.; Solouk, A.; Mirzadeh, H.; Mazinani, S.; Lagaron, J.M.; Shari, S.; Ramakrishna, S. A review of key challenges of electrospun scaffolds for tissue-engineering applications. *J. Tissue Eng. Regen. Med.* **2015**, *10*, 715–738. [CrossRef] [PubMed]

198. Papaparaskeva, G.; Louca, M.; Voutouri, C.; Tanasă, E.; Stylianopoulos, T.; Krasia-Christoforou, T. Amalgamated Fiber/Hydrogel Composites Based on Semi-Interpenetrating Polymer Networks and Electrospun Nanocomposite Fibrous Mats. *Eur. Polym. J.* **2020**, *140*, 110041. [CrossRef]
199. Hsieh, A.; Zahir, T.; Lapitsky, Y.; Amsden, B.; Wan, W.; Shoichet, M.S. Hydrogel/electrospun fiber composites influence neural stem/progenitor cell fate. *Soft Matter* **2010**, *6*, 2227–2237. [CrossRef]
200. Ekaputra, A.K.; Prestwich, G.D.; Cool, S.M.; Hutmacher, D.W. Combining Electrospun Scaffolds with Electrosprayed Hydrogels Leads to Three-Dimensional Cellularization of Hybrid Constructs. *Biomacromolecules* **2008**, *9*, 2097–2103. [CrossRef] [PubMed]
201. Thorvaldsson, A.; Silva-Correia, J.; Oliveira, J.M.; Reis, R.L.; Gatenholm, P.; Walkenström, P. Development of Nanofiber-Reinforced Hydrogel Scaffolds for Nucleus Pulposus Regeneration by a Combination of Electrospinning and Spraying Technique. *J. Appl. Polym. Sci.* **2013**, *128*, 1158–1163. [CrossRef]
202. Li, J.; Pan, K.; Tian, H.; Yin, L. The Potential of Electrospinning/Electrospraying Technology in the Rational Design of Hydrogel Structures. *Macromol. Mater. Eng.* **2020**, *2000285*, 1–26. [CrossRef]
203. Wang, J.-Y.; Wang, K.; Gu, X.; Luo, Y. Polymerization of Hydrogel Network on Microfiber Surface: Synthesis of Hybrid Water-Absorbing Matrices for Biomedical Applications. *ACS Biomater. Sci. Eng.* **2016**, *6*, 887–892. [CrossRef]
204. Huang, Y.; Li, X.; Lu, Z.; Zhang, H.; Huang, J.; Yan, K.; Wang, D. Nanofiber-reinforced bulk hydrogel: Preparation and structural, mechanical and biological properties. *J. Mater. Chem. B* **2020**, *8*, 9794–9803. [CrossRef]
205. Lin, S.; Cao, C.; Wang, Q.; Gonzalez, M.; Dolbow, J.E.; Zhao, X. Design of stiff, tough and stretchy hydrogel composites via nanoscale hybrid crosslinking and macroscale fiber reinforcement. *Soft Matter* **2014**, *10*, 7519–7527. [CrossRef] [PubMed]
206. Li, D.; Ye, Y.; Li, D.; Li, X.; Mu, C. Biological properties of dialdehyde carboxymethyl cellulose crosslinked gelatin-PEG composite hydrogel fibers for wound dressings. *Carbohydr. Polym.* **2015**, *137*, 508–514. [CrossRef] [PubMed]
207. Patel, M.; Koh, W.-G. Composite Hydrogel of Methacrylated Hyaluronic Acid and Fragmented Polycaprolactone Nanofiber for Osteogenic Differentiation of Adipose-Derived Stem Cells. *Pharmaceutics* **2020**, *12*, 902. [CrossRef] [PubMed]
208. Ahadi, F.; Khorshidi, S.; Karkhaneh, A. A hydrogel/fiber scaffold based on silk fibroin/oxidized pectin with sustainable release of vancomycin hydrochloride. *Eur. Polym. J.* **2019**, *118*, 265–274. [CrossRef]
209. Eslami, M.; Vrana, N.E.; Zorlutuna, P.; Sant, S.; Jung, S.; Masoumi, N.; Ramazan Ali, Khavari-Nejad; Javadi, G.; Khademhosseini, A. Fiber-reinforced hydrogel scaffolds for heart valve tissue engineering. *J. Biomater. Appl.* **2014**, *29*, 399–410. [CrossRef] [PubMed]
210. Goldberg, S.R.; Diegelmann, R.F. What Makes Wounds Chronic. *Surg. Clin. N. Am.* **2020**, *100*, 681–693. [CrossRef] [PubMed]
211. Ambekar, R.S.; Kandasubramanian, B. Advancements in nanofibers for wound dressing: A review. *Eur. Polym. J.* **2019**, *117*, 304–336. [CrossRef]
212. Radhakumary, C.; Antonty, M.; Sreenivasan, K. Drug loaded thermoresponsive and cytocompatible chitosan based hydrogel as a potential wound dressing. *Carbohydr. Polym.* **2011**, *83*, 705–713. [CrossRef]
213. Abbas, M.; Uçkay, I.; Lipsky, B.A. In diabetic foot infections antibiotics are to treat infection, not to heal wounds. *Expert Opin. Pharmacother.* **2015**, *16*, 821–832. [CrossRef]
214. Rubio-Elizalde, I.; Bernáldez-Sarabia, J.; Moreno-Ulloa, A.; Vilanova, C.; Juárez, P.; Licea-Navarro, A.; Castro-Cesenã, A.B. Scaffolds based on alginate-PEG methyl ether methacrylate-Moringa oleifera-Aloe vera for wound healing applications. *Carbohydr. Polym.* **2018**, *206*, 455–467. [CrossRef]
215. Joseph, B.; Augustine, R.; Kalarikkal, N.; Thomas, S.; Seantier, B.; Grohens, Y. Recent advances in electrospun polycaprolactone based scaffolds for wound healing and skin bioengineering applications. *Mater. Today Commun.* **2019**, *19*, 319–335. [CrossRef]
216. Felgueiras, H.P.; Teixeira, M.A.; Tavares, T.D.; Homem, N.C.; Zille, A.; Amorim, M.T.P. Antimicrobial action and clotting time of thin, hydrated poly(vinyl alcohol)/cellulose acetate fi lms functionalized with LL37 for prospective wound-healing applications. *J. Appl. Polym. Sci.* **2019**, *138*, 48626.
217. Zhao, X.; Sun, X.; Yildirimer, L.; Lang, Q.; Lin, Z.Y.; Zheng, R.; Zhang, Y.; Cui, W.; Annabi, N.; Khademhosseini, A. Cell infiltrative hydrogel fibrous scaffolds for accelerated wound healing. *Acta Biomater.* **2016**, *49*, 66–77. [CrossRef] [PubMed]
218. Chen, X.; Lu, B.; Zhou, D.; Shao, M.; Xu, W.; Zhou, Y. Photocrosslinking maleilated hyaluronate/methacrylated poly(vinyl alcohol) nanofibrous mats for hydrogel wound dressings. *Int. J. Biol. Macromol.* **2019**, *155*, 903–910. [CrossRef] [PubMed]
219. Lutolf, M.P.; Hubbell, J.A. Synthetic biomaterials as instructive extracellular microenvironments for morphogenesis in tissue engineering. *Nat. Biotechonol.* **2005**, *23*, 47–55. [CrossRef] [PubMed]
220. Schulte, V.A.; Hahn, K.; Dhanasingh, A.; Heffels, K.-H.; Groll, J. Hydrogel–fibre composites with independent control over cell adhesion to gel and fibres as an integral approach towards a biomimetic artificial ECM. *Biofabrication* **2014**, *6*, 024106. [CrossRef]
221. Bonnans, C.; Chou, J.; Werb, Z. Remodelling the extracellular matrix in development and disease. *Nat. Rev. Mol. Cell Biol.* **2014**, *15*, 786–801. [CrossRef] [PubMed]
222. Franco, R.A.; Nguyen, T.H.; Lee, B.-T. Preparation and characterization of electrospun PCL/PLGA membranes and chitosan/gelatin hydrogels for skin bioengineering applications. *J. Mater. Sci. Mater. Med.* **2011**, *22*, 2207–2218. [CrossRef]
223. Sun, X.; Lang, Q.; Zhang, H.; Cheng, L.; Zhang, Y.; Pan, G. Electrospun Photocrosslinkable Hydrogel Fibrous Scaffolds for Rapid In Vivo Vascularized Skin Flap Regeneration. *Adv. Funct. Mater.* **2016**, *27*, 1604617. [CrossRef]
224. Contardi, M.; Kossyvaki, D.; Picone, P.; Summa, M.; Guo, X.; Heredia-Guerrero, J.A.; Giacomazza, D.; Carzino, R.; Goldoni, L.; Scoponi, G.; et al. Electrospun Polyvinylpyrrolidone (PVP) hydrogels containing hydroxycinnamic acid derivatives as potential wound dressings. *Chem. Eng. J.* **2020**, *409*, 128144. [CrossRef]

225. Azarniya, A.; Tamjid, E.; Eslahi, N.; Simchi, A. Modification of bacterial cellulose/keratin nanofibrous mats by a tragacanth gum-conjugated hydrogel for wound healing. *Int. J. Biol. Macromol.* **2019**, *134*, 280–289. [CrossRef]
226. Loo, Y.; Wong, Y.-C.; Cai, E.Z.; Ang, C.-H.; Raju, A.; Lakshmanan, A.; Koh, A.G.; Zhou, H.J.; Lim, T.-C.; Moochhala, S.M.; et al. Ultrashort peptide nanofibrous hydrogels for the acceleration of healing of burn wounds. *Biomaterials* **2014**, *35*, 4805–4814. [CrossRef]
227. Nguyen, L.H.; Gao, M.; Lin, J.; Wu, W.; Wang, J.; Chew, S.Y. Three-dimensional aligned nanofibers-hydrogel scaffold for controlled non-viral drug/gene delivery to direct axon regeneration in spinal cord injury treatment. *Sci. Rep.* **2017**, *7*, 42212. [CrossRef]
228. An, D.; Ji, Y.; Chiu, A.; Lu, Y.-C.; Song, W.; Zhai, L.; Qi, L.; Luo, D.; Ma, M. Developing robust, hydrogel-based, nano fiber-enabled encapsulation devices (NEEDs) for cell therapies. *Biomaterials* **2015**, *37*, 40–48. [CrossRef]
229. Jain, K.K. An Overview of Drug Delivery Systems. In *Methods in Molecular Biology*; Jain, K.K., Ed.; Humana Press: New York, NY, USA, 2020; Volume 2059, pp. 1–54.
230. Norouzi, M.; Shabani, I.; Ahvaz, H.H.; Soleimani, M. PLGA/gelatin hybrid nanofibrous scaffolds encapsulating EGF for skin regeneration. *J. Biomed. Mater. Res. Part A* **2015**, *103*, 2225–2235. [CrossRef]
231. Sun, Y.; Cheng, S.; Lu, W.; Wang, Y.; Zhang, P.; Yao, Q. Electrospun fibers and their application in drug controlled release, biological dressings, tissue repair, and enzyme immobilization. *RSC Adv.* **2019**, *9*, 25712–25729. [CrossRef]
232. Gao, Q.; Liu, L.; Lu, X.; Zhou, H. In situ forming hydrogels based on chitosan for drug delivery and tissue regeneration. *Asian J. Pharm. Sci.* **2016**, *11*, 673–683.
233. Sill, T.J.; von Recum, H.A. Electrospinning: Applications in drug delivery and tissue engineering. *Biomaterials* **2008**, *29*, 1989–2006. [CrossRef]
234. Torres-Martinez, E.J.; Bravo, J.M.C.; Medina, A.S.; González, G.L.P.; Gómez, L.J.V. A Summary of Electrospun Nanofibers as Drug Delivery System: Drugs Loaded and Biopolymers Used as Matrices. *Curr. Drug Deliv.* **2018**, *15*, 1360–1374. [CrossRef]
235. Chou, S.-F.; Carson, D.; Woodrow, K.A. Current strategies for sustaining drug release from electrospun nanofibers. *J. Control. Release* **2015**, *220*, 584–591. [CrossRef] [PubMed]
236. Bas, O.; De-Juan-Pardo, E.M.; Catelas, I.; Hutmacher, D.W. The quest for mechanically and biologically functional soft biomaterials via soft network composites. *Adv. Drug Deliv. Rev.* **2018**, *132*, 214–234. [CrossRef] [PubMed]
237. Lee, K.Y.; Rowley, J.A.; Eiselt, P.; Moy, E.M.; Bouhadir, K.H.; Mooney, D.J. Controlling mechanical and Swelling Properties of Alginate Hydrogels Independently by Cross-Linker Type and Cross-Linking Density. *Macromolecules* **2000**, *33*, 4291–4294. [CrossRef]
238. Su, T.; Zhao, W.; Wu, L.; Dong, W.; Qi, X. Facile fabrication of functional hydrogels consisting of pullulan and polydopamine fibers for drug delivery. *Int. J. Biol. Macromol.* **2020**, *163*, 366–374. [CrossRef] [PubMed]
239. Ghalei, S.; Nourmohammadi, J.; Solouk, A.; Mirzadeh, H. Enhanced Cellular Response Elicited by Addition of Amniotic fluid to Alginate Hydrogel-Electrospun Silk Fibroin Fibers for Potential Wound Dressing Application. *Colloids Surfaces B Biointerfaces* **2018**, *172*, 82–89. [CrossRef]
240. Jaiswal, M.; Gupta, A.; Agrawal, A.K.; Jassal, M.; Dinda, A.K.; Koul, V. Bi-Layer Composite Dressing of Gelatin Nanofibrous Mat and Poly Vinyl Alcohol Hydrogel for Drug Delivery and Wound Healing Application: In-Vitro and In-Vivo Studies. *J. Biomed. Nanotechnol.* **2013**, *9*, 1495–1508. [CrossRef]
241. Chen, Y.; Qiu, Y.; Wang, Q.; Li, D.; Hussain, T.; Ke, H.; Wei, Q. Mussel-inspired sandwich-like nanofibers/hydrogel composite with super adhesive, sustained drug release and anti-infection capacity. *Chem. Eng. J.* **2020**, *399*, 125668. [CrossRef]

antibiotics

MDPI

Article

Experimental and Molecular Docking Studies of Cyclic Diphenyl Phosphonates as DNA Gyrase Inhibitors for Fluoroquinolone-Resistant Pathogens

Neveen M. Saleh [1,*], Yasmine S. Moemen [2], Sara H. Mohamed [1], Ghady Fathy [3], Abdullah A. S. Ahmed [3], Ahmed A. Al-Ghamdi [4], Sami Ullah [5,6] and Ibrahim El-Tantawy El Sayed [3,*]

1 Department of Microbiology, National Organization for Drug Control and Research, Giza 12553, Egypt; sara_hussein_moh@yahoo.com
2 Clinical Pathology Department, National Liver Institute, Menoufia University, Shebin El-Kom 32511, Egypt; yasmine.moemen@gmail.com
3 Chemistry Department, Faculty of Science, Menoufia University, Shebin El-Kom 32511, Egypt; ghadyfathy96@gmail.com (G.F.); chemist_abdullah_2009@yahoo.com (A.A.S.A.)
4 Department of Physics, Faculty of Science, King Abdulaziz University, Jeddah 21589, Saudi Arabia; agamdi@kau.edu.sa
5 Research Center for Advanced Materials Science (RCAMS), King Khalid University, P.O. Box 9004, Abha 61413, Saudi Arabia; samiali@kku.edu.sa
6 Department of Chemistry, College of Science, King Khalid University, P.O. Box 9004, Abha 61413, Saudi Arabia
* Correspondence: salehneveen@yahoo.com (N.M.S.); ibrahimtantawy@yahoo.co.uk (I.E.-T.E.S.)

Citation: Saleh, N.M.; Moemen, Y.S.; Mohamed, S.H.; Fathy, G.; Ahmed, A.A.S.; Al-Ghamdi, A.A.; Ullah, S.; El Sayed, I.E.-T. Experimental and Molecular Docking Studies of Cyclic Diphenyl Phosphonates as DNA Gyrase Inhibitors for Fluoroquinolone-Resistant Pathogens. *Antibiotics* **2022**, *11*, 53. https://doi.org/10.3390/antibiotics11010053

Academic Editors: Helena Felgueiras and Jean-Marc Sabatier

Received: 15 October 2021
Accepted: 29 December 2021
Published: 1 January 2022

Abstract: DNA gyrase and topoisomerase IV are proven to be validated targets in the design of novel antibacterial drugs. In this study, we report the antibacterial evaluation and molecular docking studies of previously synthesized two series of cyclic diphenylphosphonates (**1a–e** and **2a–e**) as DNA gyrase inhibitors. The synthesized compounds were screened for their activity (antibacterial and DNA gyrase inhibition) against ciprofloxacin-resistant *E.coli* and *Klebsiella pneumoniae* clinical isolates having mutations (deletion and substitution) in QRDR region of DNA gyrase. The target compound (**2a**) that exhibited the most potent activity against ciprofloxacin Gram-negative clinical isolates was selected to screen its inhibitory activity against DNA gyrase displayed IC_{50} of 12.03 μM. In addition, a docking study was performed with inhibitor (**2a**), to illustrate its binding mode in the active site of DNA gyrase and the results were compatible with the observed inhibitory potency. Furthermore, the docking study revealed that the binding of inhibitor (**2a**) to DNA gyrase is mediated and modulated by divalent Mg^{2+} at good binding energy (–9.08 Kcal/mol). Moreover, structure-activity relationships (SARs) demonstrated that the combination of hydrazinyl moiety in conjunction with the cyclic diphenylphosphonate based scaffold resulted in an optimized molecule that inhibited the bacterial DNA gyrase by its detectable effect in vitro on gyrase-catalyzed DNA supercoiling activity.

Keywords: cyclic diphenylphosphonate; quinoline; antibacterial activity; DNA gyrase inhibitor; molecular docking; magnesium ion

1. Introduction

Infections are among the major causes of human morbidity and mortality. The pharmaceutical industry is unable to keep up with the growing need for effective novel antibacterial drugs [1]; The main reason for this situation is the rapid bacterial adaptation to antibiotics; which, results in resistance development after antibacterial drugs are introduced into clinical use. Antibiotic resistance (AR) has been deemed as one of the most threats to global public health by the World Health Organization [1]. In 2050, an estimated number of 10 million deaths per year will be attributed to AR, thus proper action needs to be applied to stop this negative development [2]. Around 50% of the antimicrobial drugs prescribed for human diseases, found to be unnecessary [3]. This use, misuse, overuse, or over-the-counter has driven the major source towards AR [4].

DNA gyrase and topoisomerase IV are essential bacterial enzymes that represent an important target for novel antibacterial drug development [5,6]. An important strategy in fighting antibiotic resistance is the discovery, development of novel antibiotics, and increasing the efficacy of the antibiotic that is already in a clinical study [7]. In this context, α-aminophosphonates gained great interest by medicinal chemists because of their diverse biological and industrial applications such as antibacterial [8–12], anticancer [13–15], enzyme inhibitors [16,17], and chelating material [18–21] which made them a promising drug candidate for further optimization. These compounds are phosphorus analogs of naturally occurring α-amino acids and therefore, are considered promising in the field of drug discovery and development [22]. Moreover, quinoline-containing heterocyclic compounds received much attention due to their wide pharmacological applications [23–25]. The hybridization of quinoline moiety with α-aminophsophonate is expected to have a noticeable synergistic effect on biological activity. The present work has been carried out as part of our ongoing program for developing novel antibacterial agents which are based on α-aminophsophonates. In our previous work, we have reported a new class of cyclic α-aminophophonates bearing quinoline and hydrazine moiety with potent antibacterial activity [26]. These results prompted us to further extend and evaluate their antibacterial activity to understand the mode of action of the active compounds, for example, the determination of DNA gyrase binding affinity as potential inhibitors. In addition, a molecular docking approach will be applied to select the most promising inhibitor(s) for further lead optimization. Moreover, the structure-activity relationships (SARs) will be investigated to identify the most potent inhibitor that can be used as a template to further design novel compounds targeting DNA gyrase and effective against resistant bacterial strains such as fluoroquinolone-resistant pathogens. Herein, we describe the discovery of bacterial DNA gyrase inhibitors via binding to, and stabilization of, DNA cleavage complexes.

2. Results and Discussion

2.1. *Chemistry*

A two series of cyclic diphenylphosphonates (**1a–e** and **2a–e**) were prepared by following the procedure previously reported by us starting from glutaraldehyde, amines, diphenylphosphite, and Lewis acid catalyst. The structures of the synthesized compounds were confirmed based on their spectral data and in good agreement with the proposed structures and with those reported in the literature [26]. The two synthesized series of compounds used for current biological screening are listed in the following Figure 1.

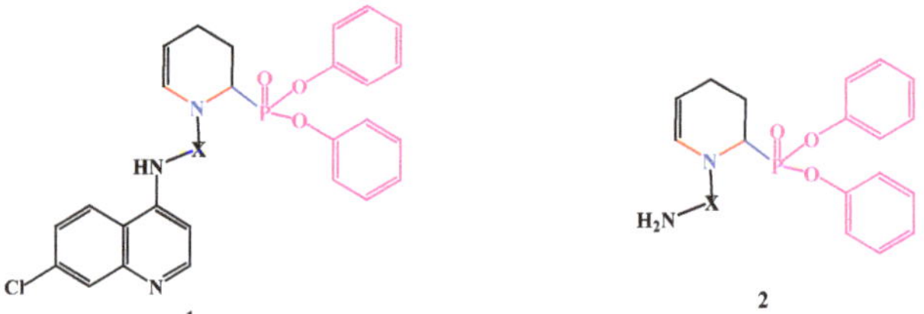

1 **2**

1		2	
1a: X =	0	2a: X =	0
b:	= -$(CH_2)_2$-	b:	= -$(CH_2)_2$-
c:	= -$(CH_2)_3$-	c:	= -$(CH_2)_3$-
d:	= 3 -C_6H_4-	d:	= 3 -C_6H_4-
e:	= 4 -C_6H_4-	e:	= 4 -C_6H_4-

Figure 1. Structures of cyclic diphenylphosphonates **1** and **2**.

2.2. *In Vitro Antibacterial Activity*

Recently, two series of synthetic chemical compounds (**1a–e** and **2a–e**) were tested against different highly virulent strains of clinical isolates *E.coli*, *K. pneumonia*, and *Staphylo-*

coccus aureus MRSA that previously showed resistance to ciprofloxacin [25,27–29], besides two reference strains (*Staphylococcus aureus* ATCC 25923, and *E. coli* ATCC 11229) and exhibited good antibacterial activity [26] as depicted in Figure 2 and Table S1 (cf. supplementary file).

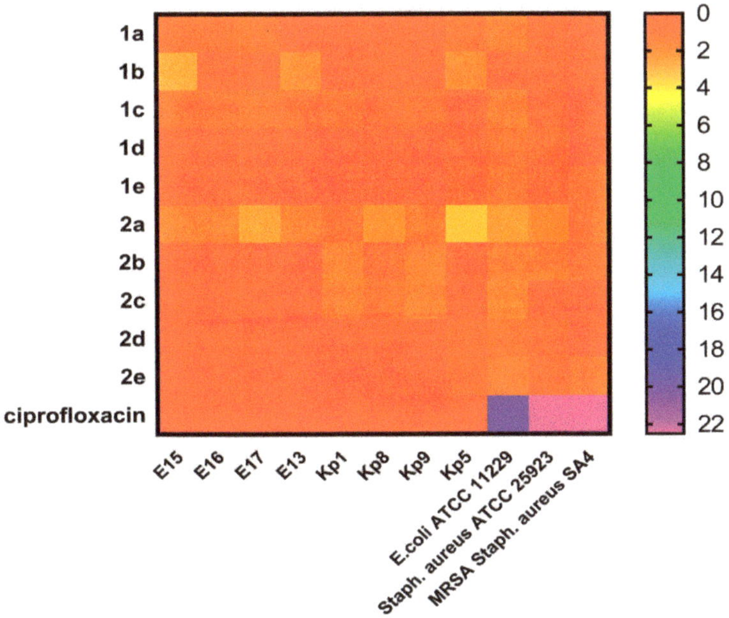

Figure 2. Heatmap Profile showed the sensitivity of tested MDR resistant Gram-positive and Gram-negative bacteria toward the tested two groups synthetic chemical compounds (**1a–e**, and **2a–e**) at a concentration (100 mg/mL) using agar well diffusion method. Scale from low inhibition zone diameter to high inhibition zone diameter. Red color represents low scale to violet color that represents a high scale.

The results of in vitro antibacterial activity from the heatmap (Figure 2, Table S1) and the structure-activity relationships study (SARs), revealed that the first series (**1a–e**) bearing quinoline moiety, compound **1c** with a 3-carbon spacer between the two nitrogen showed activity against almost all tested Gram-negative bacteria. Moreover, compound (**1a**) without spacer has potent activity against three pathogens of *E. coli* and one pathogen of *K. pneumonia*. On the other hand, compound (**1b**) with two carbon spacers has antibacterial activity against only two *E. coli* strains (E13 and E15), while compounds (**1d** and **1e**) with rigid phenyl ring spacer showed potent antibacterial activity against both Gram-positive and Gram-negative bacteria and compound (**1e**) showed activity against both sensitive and resistant strains. For the second synthesized series (**2a–e**), compound (**2a**) without quinoline ring and carbon spacer showed antibacterial activity against all tested Gram-positive and Gram-negative pathogens, followed by compounds (**2b** and **2c**) with flexible two and three carbon spacers, respectively, that have been shown activity against only three Gram-negative strains of *K. pneumonia*.

However, compounds (**2d** and **2e**) with rigid phenyl ring spacer showed the same activity as (**1d** and **1e**) from the first series. In addition, the results revealed that *K. pneumonia* (Kp5) was the sensitive isolate to almost all tested compounds. A comparison between cyclic diphenylphosphonate with quinoline motif and the corresponding ones without revealed that the former with quinoline was the most potent against MDR resistant Gram-positive and Gram-negative bacteria. From SARs study it was concluded that the difference in antibacterial activity between the two series of compounds was a result of the different substitutions on the cyclohexene ring nitrogen attached to the chiral carbon-bearing the diphenylphosphonate structural motif.

2.3. DNA Gyrase Mutation in Ciprofloxacin-Resistant Clinical Isolates E. coli (E17) and K. pneumonia (Kp8)

Exploring the resistance mechanism that bacteria used to resist the aaction of the antibiotic to show if the resistance was due to mutation in amino acids codon in quinolone resistance determining region that shas been associated with DNA gyrase where the structural topoisomerase changes reducing the affinity of this enzyme to fluoroquinolones are caused by mutations in the quinolone resistance-determining regions (QRDR) of *gyrA*/*gyrB*/*parC* and/or *parE* genes that will help to figure out the way to discover a new treatment approach.

We studied that mechanism in both clinical isolates *E. coli* (E17) and *K. pneumonia* (Kp8). To identify substitution and deletion mutations, manually *QRDR* sequences were compared with GenBank sequences. Nucleotide sequences coding amino acid 70–88 in the gyrA QRDR were analyzed. The National Institutes of Health (NCBI) Web site was used to perform BLASTP analysis. To map the relative locations of *gyrA*, NCBI BLASTN and BLASTX, accessed through (https://blast.ncbi.nlm.nih.gov/Blast.cgi, accessed on 5 May 2020), were used to search the *E. coli* and *K. pneumonia* genome for *gyrA* gene, and the alignment sequence for mutation was performed using Clustal W2 sequence alignment (Figures 3 and 4).

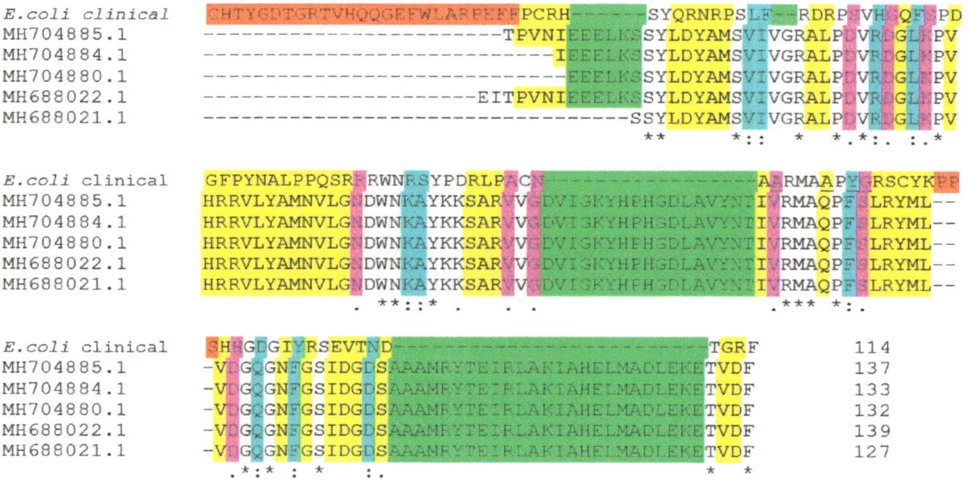

Figure 3. Amino Acid Multiple Sequence Alignment of *gyrA* (DNA gyrase subunit A) gene mutations in ciprofloxacin-resistant *Escherichia coli* clinical isolate (E17) compared with another *gyrA* gene in NCBI database. The alignment sequence was performed using Clustal W2 sequence alignment. Different colors indicates the difference in sequence aligment, red color indicates genes codon in our clinical isolte deleted in compared gene bank isolates, green colors indicates genes codon deleted in out tested isolates, "*" conserved sequences indicates amino acid have single, fully conserved residue (identical); "." violet color Indicates conservation between groups of strongly similar properties; ":" blue color indicates non-conservative mutations that amino acid have different properties.

```
Kl. pneumoniae  -MAQPFSLRYMLVDGQGNFG-SIDGDSAAAMRYTEIRLAKIAHELMADLEKETVDFVDNY 58
ACY02504.1      RMAGPFSLRYMLVDGGGNFG-SIDGDSAAAMRYTEIRLAKIAHELMADLEKETVDFVDNY 59
AUX13671.1      RMAGPFSLRYMLVDGGGNFGDSIDGDSAAAMRYTEIRLAKIAHELMADLEKETVDFVDNY 60
AUX13672.1      RMAGPFSLRYMLVDGGGNFG-SIDGDSAAAMRYTEIRLSKISHELMADLEKETVDFVDNY 59
VTM77560.1      RMAGPFSLRYMLVDGGGNFG-SIDGDSAAAMRYTEIRLAKIAHELMADLEKETVDFVDNY 59
AAG40200.1      RMAQPFSLRYMLVDGGGNFG-SIDGDSAAAMRYTEIRLAKIAHELMADLEKETVDFVDNY 59
                 ** *********** **** *****************:**:******************

Kl. pneumoniae  DGTERIPDVMPTKIPNLLVNGASGIAVGMA-------------      88
ACY02504.1      DGTERIPDVMPTKIPNLLV----------ATNIPPHNLTEVING     93
AUX13671.1      DGTERIPDVMPTKIPNLLVNGASGIAVGMATNIPPHNTLE----     100
AUX13672.1      DGTERIPDVMPTKIPNLLVNGASGIAVGMATNIPPHNLT-----     98
VTM77560.1      DGTERIPDVMPTKIPNLLVNGASGIAVGMAPTYRRIT-------     96
AAG40200.1      DGTERIPDVMPTKIPNLLVNGASGIAVGMATN------------     91
                *******************          *
```

Figure 4. Amino Acid Multiple Sequence Alignment of *gyrA* (DNA gyrase subunit A) gene mutations in ciprofloxacin-resistant *Klebsiella pneumoniae* clinical isolate (Kp8) compared with another *gyrA* gene in NCBI database, mutation by deletion from position 75 to 88 of QRDR. The alignment sequence was performed using Clustal W2 sequence alignment. Different colors indicates the difference in sequence aligment, red color indicates genes codon in our clinical isolte deleted in compared gene bank isolates, green colors indicates genes codon deleted in out tested isolates, "*" conserved sequences indicates amino acid have single, fully conserved residue (identical); ":" blue color indicates non-conservative mutations that amino acid have different properties.

By comparing *gyrA* gene of ciprofloxacin-resistant *E.coli* (E17) clinical isolate with other *gyrA* genes in NCBI database (Figure 3), the mutation was noted at codon positions 85 glutamine (Gln)→alanine (Ala), 87 phenylalanine (Phe)→tyrosine (Tyr), and 88 serine (Ser)→glycine (Gly) of QRDR, which resulted in a substitution of Glutamine, Phenylalanine, and serine with alanine, tyrosine, and glycine, respectively. Mutations in *gyrA* were defined as one of the most common mechanisms of fluoroquinolone-resistance in different bacterial species [6,30], and usually detected at either codon 83 or 87, and/or the *parC* gene [31]. Mutations of *gyrA* at codons 67, 81, 82, 83, 84, 87, and 106 are responsible for the development of quinolone resistance in *E. coli*, while in clinical isolates, the most common mutation is at codon 87 [32]. Accumulation of Ser83 Leu and Asp87Asn mutations in the *gyrA* gene of *E. coli* was common (48). In addition to some unique mutations in codons 60, 64, 111 of *gyrA*, silent mutations at codons 85, 86, and 91 in resistant strains were observed [33]. Different changes of amino acid residues (codon Asp-87) between isolates having the same genotype observed, which suggested that the amino acid mutations at codon 87 (and possibly the development of high-level fluoroquinolone-resistance) might have occurred after the transmission/sharing of a precursor strain carrying the Ser-83→Leu mutation [34].

In our study, mutation by deletion from position 75 to 88 of QRDR was detected in Kp8 clinical isolate (Figure 4). Acquisition of mutations in *gyrA*, as well as *parC* genes, suggested playing a significant role in causing high quinolones-resistance levels in certain claustral lineages of *K. pneumoniae* [6]. Isolates carrying such mutations were found to have high MICs (>16 µg/mL), which indicates that these alterations in *gyrA* are responsible for conferring high-level ciprofloxacin resistance [35]. Mutations at codons such as 83 and 87 in *gyrA* gene have been reported as the most common mutation points causing major alterations among clinical strains resulting in fluoroquinolone resistance [36].

Due to the useful characteristics of fluoroquinolone as potency, the spectrum of activity, oral bioavailability, and generally good safety profile, they were used extensively for multiple clinical indications throughout the world they still clinically valuable, but fluoroquinolone use has become limited in some clinical settings, as bacterial resistance has emerged over time, therefore, the screening of novel DNA gyrase inhibitor has been needed to solve this issue [37].

2.4. *DNA Supercoiling Assay of Compound (**2a**) against DNA Gyrase Enzyme Activity*

We rationalized the inhibitory effect of hydrazine linker exerts on the cell wall, as well as DNA gyrase inhibition. Reports stated that ciprofloxacin-resistance evolved in bacteria due to alterations in DNA gyrase/topoisomerase IV or due to a decrease in intracellular drug levels caused by changes in membrane permeability or overexpression of drug efflux pumps of the cell wall [6,38] and that what have been proved in our investigation, bacterial strains showed ciprofloxacin-resistance due to DNA alteration. To discover novel inhibitors that would act on microbial topoisomerases that are resistant to the known DNA gyrase inhibitors, we utilized synthetic chemical compound (**2a**) screening against gyrase of *E. coli* DNA as a model.

According to the screening results of the antibacterial activity, compound (**2a**) was selected to use as a gyrase enzyme inhibitor of *E. coli* DNA gyrase, the compound markedly inhibited both ciprofloxacin-resistant mutant and the wild-type strain with different behavior toward Gram-positive bacteria that was less susceptible in comparison with Gram-negative bacteria. Importantly, this inhibition was performed through this mechanism depending on genetic approaches to probe the nature of the mechanism action.

However, we postulated that compound **2a** may inhibit DNA gyrase which is considered the primary target in Gram-negative bacteria as well as topoisomerase V by inhibiting both wild-type and CIP-resistant *Staphylococcus aureus MRSA*. Our data was supported by Doddaga et al., 2013 who proved the inhibitory effect of α-aminophosphonate against DNA Gyrase [39].

In our study, we tested the effect of compound (**2a**) on supercoiling activity of DNA gyrase, using inhibition assay of *E. coli* Gyrase enzyme. Studying the dose-response inhibition as shown in (Figure 5), we calculated the 50% inhibition using inhibitor (**2a**) and it was 12.03 μM as compared with the standard antibiotic ciprofloxacin that showed IC_{50} 10.71 μM and with increasing the concentration, the inhibitory effect of the compound (**2a**) increases. The lower IC_{50} value indicates the relative affinity of inhibitor (**2a**) towards gyrase enzyme. Therefore, we postulated that compound (**2a**) was more specific towards DNA gyrase enzyme by inhibiting DNA binding to the enzyme and preventing the supercoiling reactions [40,41]. Further, the DNA gyrase cleavable complex is formed with the incubation of DNA and enzyme in the presence of compound (**2a**) that mediated stabilization of a cleavable complex through a cooperative drug binding process to a desaturated DNA pocket caused by the enzyme. This result is consistent with Otter and his co-works observation [40].

From the gel electrophoresis, we tested the effect of the inhibitor by showing the difference in the mobility between relaxed and supercoiled DNA. the result showed that the compound (**2a**) has potency in comparison with ciprofloxacin against the enzyme activity explored by inhibiting the DNA gyrase enzyme at different concentrations, where relaxed DNA substrate become completely negatively supercoiled at a lower concentration, and with increasing concentration to 50 μM inhibit supercoiling completely that is also noticed with the addition of ciprofloxacin at 25μM that showed by DNA supercoiling (Figure 6).

2.5. *Molecular Docking*

A molecular docking study was performed to offer a molecular basis for the potency and selectivity of the here reported compounds. We presume that understanding the interactions between cyclic-diphenylphosphonates and DNA gyrase is necessary for a good and selective antibacterial drug design and development. The inhibitor **2a** is considered the most fitting inhibitor to Active site 1 (AC1) pocket with good binding energy as discussed in the methodology part because of its small size when compared to the other analogs as shown in (Figures 7–9).

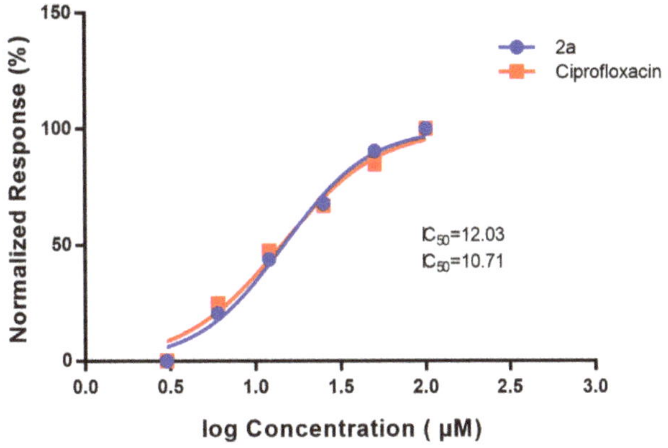

Figure 5. Dose-response inhibition curve for *E. coli* DNA gyrase-dependent supercoiling activity in the presence of cyclic diphenylphosphonate **2a**, ciprofloxacin with different concentrations of inhibitor (**2a**), and ciprofloxacin (standard) which showed 50% inhibition after 30 min as affecting DNA gyrase enzyme and the DNA was separated on a 1.0% (w/v) agarose gel. The fluorescence intensity of the supercoiled DNA band was normalized to the DMSO solvent control.

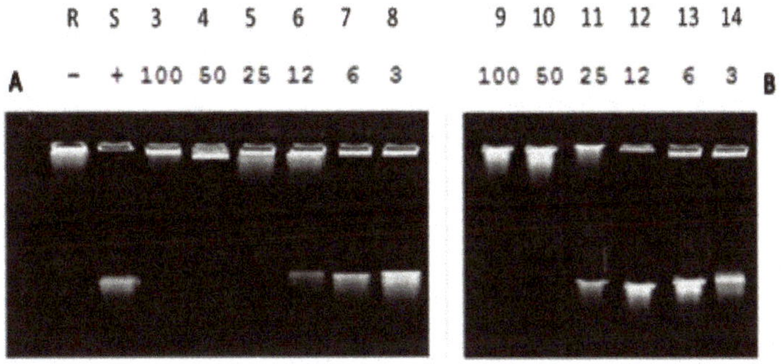

Figure 6. Supercoiling reactions at different concentrations of (**A**) ciprofloxacin (Standard) and (**B**) cyclic diphenylphosphonate **2a**. Lanes 3–14: different concentrations of compound **2a** and ciprofloxacin, respectively (3–14), Lane R: relaxed pNO1, Lane S: supercoiled pNO1 of *E. coli* DNA gyrase.

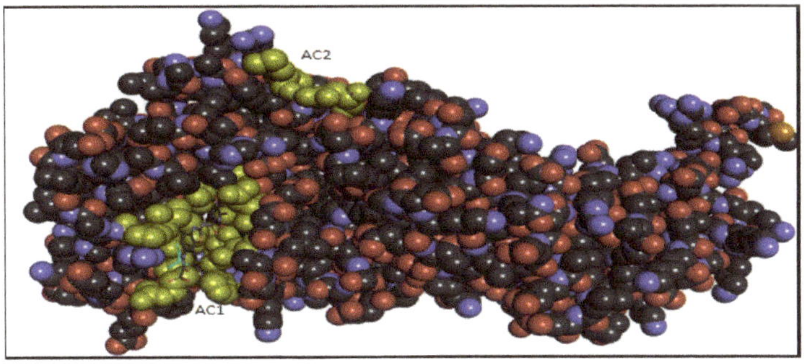

Figure 7. The Crystal structure of DNA gyrase (PDB ID 5L3J) showing two active sites AC1 and AC2.

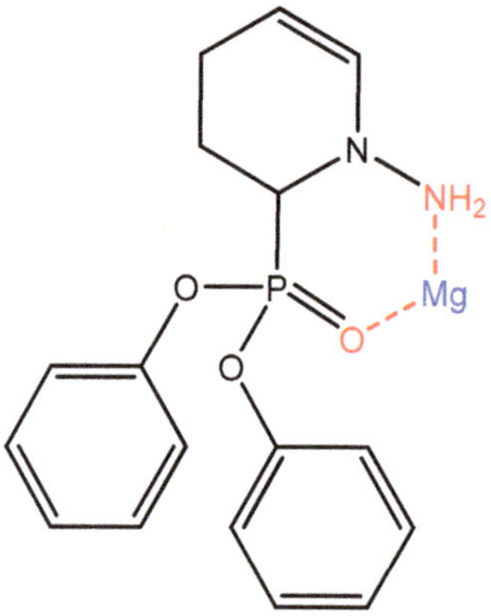

(2a)

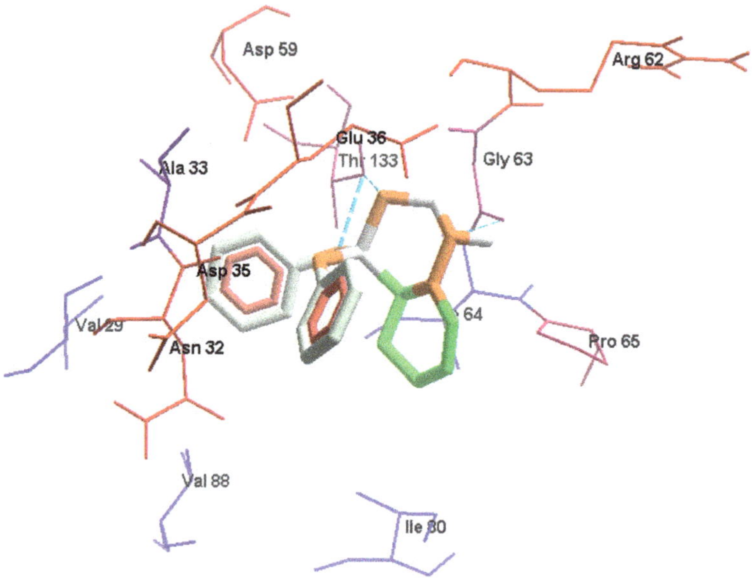

Figure 8. The first view demonstrates hydrogen bonds (blue dash), and hydrophobic interactions between **2a** and gyrase B residues. The hydrophobic parts of **2a** (2 light gray phenyl groups) were enclosed with red residues Asn32 and Asp35; Three hydrogen bonds (blue dash line) interaction one with NH group and Gly33 (NH-Gly63, 3 Å) besides 2 HBs with 2 oxygen atoms of phosphonate groups; Thr133(O-Thr133, 3.3 Å) and (O-Thr133, 2.8 Å). Figure 8 was mapped by Molegro Molecular Viewer, it uses the Kyte-Doolittle scale to rank amino acid hydrophobicity, where the color blue indicates the most hydrophilic, the color white is equal to 0.0, and orange-red color being the most hydrophobic. It also displays the amino acids of gyrase B as thin sticks while compound **2a** atoms are represented as bold sticks.

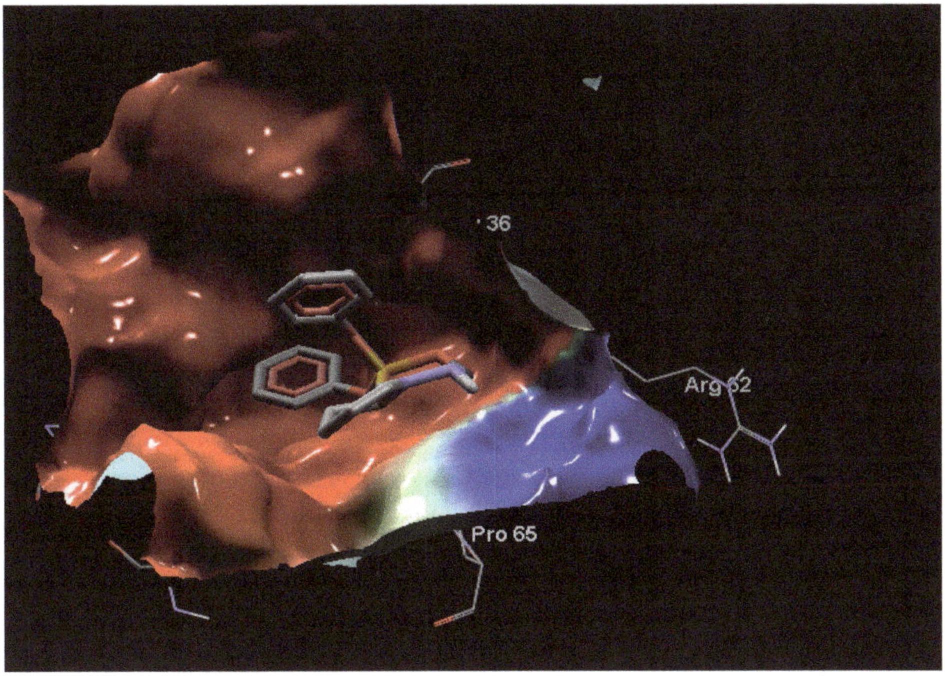

Figure 9. The second view represents the electrostatic interactions of **2a**-gyrase B complex. The second view displays the electrostatic charges, red surface refers to the negative charge while blue surface is the positive charge and the inhibitor **2a** is colored according to the atom type (carbon atom is dark gray, oxygen atoms are red while phosphorus is dark yellow and nitrogen for violet).

The docking results revealed that compound **2a** affects DNA supercoiling through N-terminal domain of gyrase B subunit targets ATP-binding sites that are supposed to compete with ATP for binding to gyrase B, Therefore, we suggest that the mode of action of compound **2a** was similar to the action/mechanism of antibacterial agents as aminocoumarins, novobiocin, and some bacterial toxins such as CcdB and microcin B17 (MccB17), and newly molecule benzothiazole exerting slow inhibition of DNA supercoiling which causing bacterial cell death [42–45]. Similar to coumarins that competitively inhibit ATP hydrolysis, whereas quinolones, such as ciprofloxacin were stabilizing the covalent gyrase-DNA cleavage complex. CcdB also stabilizes a cleavage complex but only in the presence of ATP [46]. The trapping of the gyrase-DNA cleavage complex by MccB17 is also reported to be ATP-dependent [45]. In addition, the rotatable bonds count has a synergistic effect on binding energy as listed in (Figure 10) and Table 1. A rotatable bond is any single non-ring bond, bound to a non-terminal heavy atom; it detects the conformational entropy change in protein-inhibitor interactions. Rotatable bonds are related to molecular flexibility, which is a good descriptor of oral bioavailability [47]. All the current compounds were bound to gyrase B in AC1 except **1e1** which is bound to Active site 2 (AC2) and different types of interactions were depicted as shown in the supplementary file (Figures S1–S11 cf. Supplementary File).

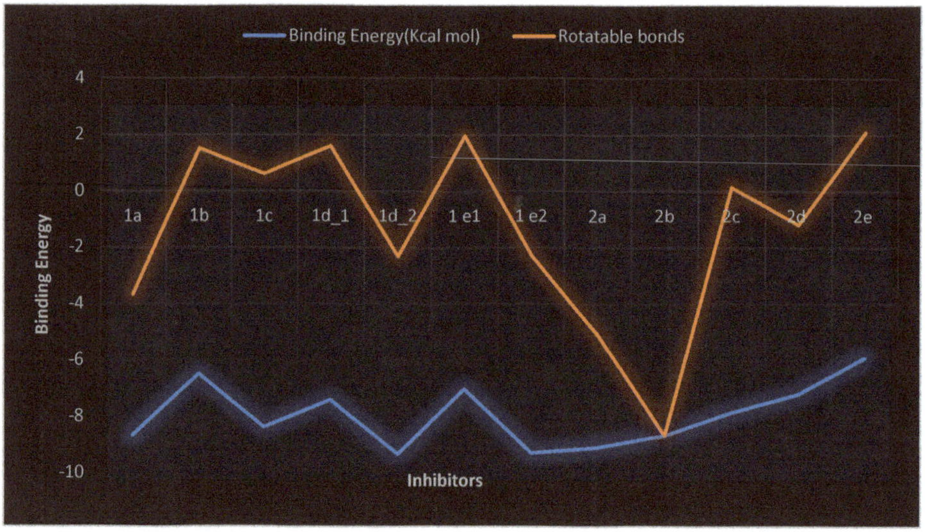

Figure 10. The rotatable bonds effect on the binding energy of gyrase B-inhibitor complex.

Table 1. Binding energy of the two series gyrase B inhibitors.

Compound	Binding Energy (Kcal mol)	Rotatable Bonds
1a	−8.65	5
1b	−6.49	8
1c	−8.38	9
1d1	−7.4	9
1d2	−9.32	7
1e1	−7.03	9
1e2	−9.28	7
2a	−9.08	4
2b	−8.67	0
2c	−7.85	8
2d	−7.2	6
2e	−5.9	8

From Table 1, compound (**2a**) is the most potent inhibitor while **2b**, **1a,** and **1c** are almost equal in their potency, **1d2** and **1e2** (red color) do not exist in the current experimental condition, they may have occurred at different experimental conditions, **2e** is least potent compound.

3. Materials and Methods

3.1. Microbiological Screening

3.1.1. Bacterial Strains

Nine clinical pathogenic Multi-Drug Resistance (MDR) isolates namely; *Klebsiella pneumonia, E. coli, and* Methicillin-resistant *Staphylococcus aureus* (*MRSA*) that have been previously identified and their antimicrobial susceptibility assay assessed [4,25,26] were used in our experminet. Bacterial isolates were stored in Brain Heart-Glycerol (Oxoid Ltd., Basingstoke, UK) at −80 °C until use. Bacterial isolates were refreshed by incubating overnight at 37 °C on nutrient broth media (Oxoid, Basingstoke, UK), and then sub-cultured on selective media (MacConkey and Mannitol agar, (Oxoid, Basingstoke, UK). Quality control assessment was carried out using standard reference bacterial strains; *Staphylococcus aureus* ATCC® 25923, and *E.coli* ATCC® 11229 that were obtained from Microbiology Lab's Unit of National Organization for Drug Control and Research (NODCAR).

3.1.2. Screening of Synthesized Compounds against Tested Isolates Using Agar Well Diffusion Method

Synthesized compounds were prepared for Antibacterial Activity by dissolving in Dimethyl Sulfoxide (DMSO) and then diluted in sterile distilled water to obtain a final concentration of 100 mg/mL. To check the effect of solvent on the growth of microorganisms, DMSO (100 μL) was used as negative control [48]. The antibacterial activity of different compounds was evaluated by agar well diffusion method. Briefly, 100 μL of 0.5 MacFarland bacterial suspensions (1.5×10^8 CFU/mL) was spread on Müller-Hinton agar (Oxoid, Basingstoke, UK). Wells were made on the agar plates using sterile cork borer, then 100 μL of each prepared compound was introduced into appropriately marked wells. The antibacterial activity was evaluated by measuring the diameter of the inhibition zone for each tested organism compared with the negative and positive control after an incubation period of 24 h at 37 °C. DMSO (100 μL) was used as a negative control, and an antibiotic disc of Ciprofloxacin (5 μg) was used as a positive control [48,49].

3.1.3. Quinolone Resistance Mechanism Detection (QRDR): Amplification and Sequencing of *gyrA* in QRDR DNA

QRDR regions of *gyrA* gene of both clinical isolate CIP-resistant *Klebsiella pneumoniae* (Kp8) and CIP-resistant *Escherichia coli* (E17) were amplified by PCR from the chromosomal DNA of quinolone-resistant isolates. A 344-bp region covering the QRDR of *gyrA* was amplified with primers 5′-AAATCTGCCCGTGTCGTTGGT-3′and 5′- GCCATACCTACTGCGATACC-3′ [50]. PCR was performed as recommended, and PCR products were visualized by 1% agarose gel electrophoresis using ethidium bromide [51]. PCR products were purified with high pure PCR product purification kits (QIAquick PCR Purification Kit, Qiagen, Hilden, Germany). Purified PCR products were sequenced using Applied Biosystems 3500 Genetic Analyzer (Hitachi, ThermoFisher, MA, USA) in Colors labs, Egypt. The primers used for sequencing were the same used for amplification. BigDye Terminator v3.1 Cycle Sequencing Kit and 5× Sequencing Buffer (ThermoFisher) were used.

3.1.4. Impact of Synthesized Compound (**2a**) against DNA Gyrase Activity Using DNA Supercoiling Assay

In vitro, the effect of synthesized compound (**2a**) as a quinolone inhibitor compared with ciprofloxacin (reference standard) at different concentrations was determined using *E. coli* Gyrase Microplate Assay Kit (Inspiralis, Norwich, UK) based on the DNA Supercoiling using DNA gyrase enzyme according to manufacturer's instructions [52]. The test was carried out in the confirmatory diagnostic unit, Vacsera, Egypt. The inhibition test was carried out using *E. coli* DNA gyrase to determine IC_{50} value. The compound (**2a**) and reference standard were dissolved in DMSO and serially diluted at different concentrations, the assay was carried out in three replicates. Briefly, the reaction was started by rehydrating the wells with 3 × 200 μL wash buffer then zimmobilize 100 μL of 500 nM TFO1 oligo in each well (5 μL of 10 μM TFO1 in 95 μL wash buffer), incubating for 5 min at room temperature. The excess of oligo Wash off with 3 × 200 μL with wash Buffer. 1.5 U of gyrase incubates with 0.75 μg of relaxed plasmid pNO1 in a reaction volume of 30 μL at 37 °C for 30 min in assay buffer. After incubation, we add 100 μL TF buffer to the well and incubate it for a further 30 min at room temperature to allow triplex formation. We remove the unbound plasmid from the well by washing it with 3 × 200 μL TF buffer. The reaction is stained with DNA-detection dye (diluted to 1× with T10 buffer) then we add 200 μL per well and incubate for 10–20 min, then mix and read in a fluorescence plate reader at Ex: 495 nm; Em: 537 nm).

A 10 μL sample was removed from the well for gel assay and was determined using a standard 1% agarose gel assay depending on quantitation of the gel using the intensity of the ethidium fluorescence of the supercoiled DNA band. The IC_{50} was defined as the concentration causing 50% inhibition of the supercoiling reaction. The average IC_{50} values (μM) of the replicate experiments were calculated for the target and reference standard using non-linear regression analysis in GraphPad Prism 7 (GraphPad softwear, San Diego, CA, USA).

3.2. *Molecular Docking*

The molecular docking technique involves receptor preparation, ligand preparations, detection of the active site, and re-establishing a complex of the 3 dimensions (3D) co-crystal structure of receptor and 3D modeled ligand structures.

3.2.1. Preparation of Macromolecules and Ligands

The protein structure was prepared for docking by The UCSF Chimera software [53]. The ligands were drawn and created using Avogadro software [54], Mg^{2+} was the metal-coordinating ligand due to the affinity of cyclic diphenylphosphonate nitrogen donor atoms toward metal ions. About two different chelation modes were produced with Mg^{2+} cation in some compounds. The complexation of ligand monomer with Mg^{2+} was 1:1 molar ratios and minimized by the Avogadro software. Metal chelation of Mg^{2+} with ligand monomer interacted through N3 atom in the imidazole group of the monomer.

3.2.2. Active Site Detection

The N-terminal fragment of the *E. coli* DNA gyrase B (residues Gly15 to Thr392) was discovered from the X-ray crystal structure 5L3J with resolution 2.83 Å [55], it was used to investigate the binding affinity of the current inhibitors to DNA gyrase B. The crystal structure 5L3J contains two active sites which are AC1 and AC2 where AC1 are: Val43, Asn46, Glu50, Gly77, Ile78, Pro79, Val120, Thr165, and Val167; while AC2 is Gly24 and Gln335, (Figure S12 cf. supplementary file).

Several interactions were shown in (Figure S12 cf. supplementary file), where amide Pi-stacked interaction was confirmed with residue Asn46; while van der Waals interaction exhibited through Glu50, His55, Asp73, Arg76, Gly77, Met 95, and Arg136. Pi-Sigma interaction was exhibited by Thr165 also, Pi-alkyl with Val43, Ala47, Val120, and Val167.

3.2.3. Molecular Docking Implementation Process

Targeting binding sites with automated docking [56,57] was used to dock ligands to identify the active entities and determine the binding sites in target proteins. Autodock 4.2 [58] was used for docking the current compounds understudy to 5L3J protein. Lamarckian Genetic Algorithm (LGA) was used to determine the globally optimized conformation. LGA for docking was implemented with defined parameters for determining the docking performance. Polar hydrogen atoms were added Kollman charge, atomic solvation parameters, and fragmental volumes were assigned to the protein using Autodock tools. The grid spacing was 0.375 Å for each spacing. Molegro Molecular Viewer packages [59] have been used to visualize 5L3J crystal structure and its binding mode. BIOVIA Discovery Studio 2020 [60] was used to illustrate enzyme-inhibitor interactions.

4. Conclusions

Two series of cyclic diphenylphsophonates (**1a–e** and **2a–e**) were synthesized and evaluated for their in vitro antibacterial activity against ciprofloxacin-resistant *E.coli* and *Klebsiella pneumoniae* clinical isolates. The results of in vitro antibacterial activity in combination with docking study revealed that installation of hydrazine moiety without quinoline and carbon spacer highly contributed to the activity as in compound (**2a**). Further SARs study, demonstrated that the difference in antibacterial activity was a result of the variation of substitutions on the ring nitrogen attached to the chiral carbon atom bearing diphenylphosphonate structural motif. In addition, the experimental and docking studies were compatible with the observed potency of compound (**2a**) as the most potent DNA gyrase inhibitor with an IC_{50} of 12.03 μM. Further variations in substitution patterns may be necessary to obtain more potent and selective DNA-gyrase inhibitors competent in facing the increasing antibacterial resistance.

Supplementary Materials: The following are available online at https://www.mdpi.com/article/10.3390/antibiotics11010053/s1, Figures S1–S11: display the hydrophobicity interaction of inhibitor for compounds 1 and 2 in AC1 site and their the electrostatic charges, Figure S12:The experimental ligand interaction and distance with the crystal structure 5L3J in AC1. Table S1: Antibacterial activity of cyclic diphenyl phosphonate against tested Gram-positive and Gram-Negative bacteria using agar well diffuion method towards tested two groups of synthetic chemical compounds at concentration 100 mg/mL A: 1 a–e, and B: 2 a–e.

Author Contributions: Conceptualization, N.M.S., and I.E.-T.E.S.; methodology, N.M.S., I.E.-T.E.S., and A.A.S.A.; software, Y.S.M.; validation, I.E.-T.E.S., A.A.A.-G., and S.U.; formal analysis, N.M.S., I.E.-T.E.S., S.H.M., and A.A.S.A.; investigation, N.M.S., I.E.-T.E.S., and A.A.S.A.; resources, I.E.-T.E.S.; data curation, N.M.S., S.H.M., and I.E.-T.E.S.; writing—original draft preparation, S.H.M., Y.S.M., A.A.S.A., and G.F.; writing—review and editing, N.M.S., and I.E.-T.E.S.; visualization, N.M.S., I.E.-T.E.S.; supervision, N.M.S., S.H.M., and I.E.-T.E.S.; project administration, A.A.A.-G., and S.U.; funding acquisition, A.A.A.-G., and S.U. All authors have read and agreed to the published version of the manuscript.

Funding: Authors acknowledge support and funding of King Khalid University Abha, Saudi Arabia and Research Center for Advanced Materials Science at King Khalid University Abha, Saudi Arabia, research grant no: RCAMS/KKU//008/21.

Data Availability Statement: The data used to support the findings of this study are available from the corresponding author upon request.

Acknowledgments: This work was funded by King Khalid University, Saudi Arabia, through Research Center for Advanced Materials Science (RCAMS) under grant no: RCAMS/KKU//008/21. The authors, therefore, gratefully acknowledge the technical and financial support.

Conflicts of Interest: The authors declare no conflict of interest.

References

1. World Health Organization (WHO). Fact Sheet. 2018. Available online: https://www.who.int/news-room/fact-sheets/detail/antibiotic-resistance (accessed on 20 August 2020).
2. De Kraker, M.E.A.; Stewardson, A.J.; Harbarth, S. Will 10 Million People Die a Year due to Antimicrobial Resistance by 2050? *PLoS Med.* **2016**, *13*, e1002184. [CrossRef] [PubMed]
3. Centers for Disease Control and Prevention (CDC). *Antibiotic Resistance Threats in the United States*; U.S. Department of Health and Human Services, Centers for Disease Control and Prevention (CDC): Atlanta, GA, USA, 2019. [CrossRef]
4. Mohamed, S.H.; Khalil, M.S.; Azmy, M. In Vitro Efficiency of Ampicillin, Thymol and Their Combinations against Virulence Strains of *Klebsiella pneumoniae*. *Int. J. Pharm. Sci.* **2019**, *11*, 315–321.
5. Norouzi, A.; Azizi, O.; Nave, H.H.; Shakibaie, S.; Shakibaie, M.R. Analysis of Amino Acid Substitution Mutations of gyrA and parC Genes in Clonal Lineage of *Klebsiella pneumoniae* Conferring High-level Quinolone Resistance. *Eur. J. Clin. Microbiol. Infect. Dis.* **2014**, *2*, 109–117.
6. Rushdy, A.A.; Mabrouk, M.I.; Abu-Sef, F.A.; Kheiralla, Z.H.; Abdel, S.M.; Saleh, N.M. Contribution of different mechanisms to the resistance to fluoroquinolones in clinical isolates of *Salmonella enterica*. *Braz. J. Infect. Dis.* **2013**, *17*, 431–437. [CrossRef]
7. Mohamed, S.H.; Mohamed, M.S.M.; Khalil, M.; Azmy, M.; Mabrouk, M. Combination of essential oil and ciprofloxacin to inhibit/eradicate biofilms in multidrug-resistant Klebsiella pneumoniae. *J. Appl. Microbiol.* **2018**, *125*, 84–95. [CrossRef] [PubMed]
8. Boshta, N.M.; Elgamal, E.A.; El-Sayed, I.E.T. Bioactive amide and α-aminophosphonate inhibitors for methicillin-resistant *Staphylococcus aureus* (MRSA). *Monatsh. Chem.* **2018**, *149*, 2349–2358. [CrossRef]
9. Elsherbiny, D.A.; Abdelgawad, A.M.; Elnaggar, M.; El-Sherbiny, R.A.; El-Rafie, M.H.; El Sayed, I.E.T. Synthesis, antimicrobial activity, and sustainable release of novel α-aminophosphonate derivatives loaded carrageenan cryogel. *Int. J. Biol. Macromol.* **2020**, *163*, 96–107. [CrossRef]
10. El Gokha, A.A.; Ahmed, A.A.S.; Abdelwahed, N.A.M.; El Sayed, I.E.T. Synthesis and antimicrobial activity of novel mono- and bis-α-aminophosphonate derivatives. *Int. J. Pharm. Sci. Rev. Res.* **2016**, *36*, 35–39.
11. Hamed, M.A.; El Gokha, A.A.; Ahmed, A.F.A.; Elsayed, M.S.A.E.; Tarabee, R.; El Megeed, A.S.; El Sayed, I.E.T. Synthesis and Antimicrobial Activity of Novel α-Aminophosphonates Bearing Pyrazoloquinoxaline Moiety. *Int. J. Pharm. Sci. Rev. Res.* **2015**, *34*, 205–213.

12. Ouf, N.H.; Hamed, M.A.; El Sayed, I.E.T.; Sakeran, M.I. Anti-cancer, Anti-inflammatory, Cytotoxic and Biochemical Activities of a Novel Phosphonotripeptide Synthesized from Formyl Pyrazolofuran using TUBU as Condensing Agent. *J. Adv. Chem.* **2014**, *6*, 1093–1102. [CrossRef]
13. Ahmed, A.A.S.; Awad, H.M.; El Sayed, I.E.T.; El Gokha, A.A. Synthesis and antiproliferative activity of new hybrids bearing neocryptolepine, acridine and α-aminophosphonate scaffolds. *J. Iran. Chem. Soc.* **2020**, *17*, 1211–1221. [CrossRef]
14. Azzam, M.A.; El-Boraey, H.A.L.; El Sayed, I.E.T. Transition metal complexes of α-aminophosphonates part II: Synthesis, spectroscopic characterization, and in vitro anticancer activity of copper (II) complexes of α-aminophosphonates. *Phosphorus Sulfur Silicon Relat. Elem.* **2020**, *195*, 339–347. [CrossRef]
15. El-Boraey, H.A.L.; El Gokha, A.A.; El Sayed, I.E.T.; Azzam, M.A. Transition metal complexes of α-aminophosphonates Part I: Synthesis, spectroscopic characterization, and in vitro anticancer activity of copper (II) complexes of α-aminophosphonates. *Med. Chem. Res.* **2015**, *24*, 2142–2153. [CrossRef]
16. Joossens, J.; van der Veken, P.; Surpateanu, G.; Lambeir, A.M.; El Sayed, I.E.T.; Ali, O.M.; Augustyns, K.; Haemers, A. Diphenyl phosphonate inhibitors for the urokinase-type plasminogen activator: Optimization of the P4 position. *J. Med. Chem.* **2006**, *49*, 5785–5793. [CrossRef]
17. Van der Veken, P.; El Sayed, I.E.T.; Joossens, J.; Stevens, C.V.; Augustyns, K.; Haemers, A. The Lewis acid catalyzed synthesis of N-protected diphenyl 1-aminoalkylphosphonates. *Synthesis* **2005**, 634–638. [CrossRef]
18. Galhoum, A.; Eisa, W.H.; El Sayed, I.E.T.; Tolba, A.A.; Shalaby, Z.M.; Mohamady, S.I.; Muhammad, S.S.; Hussien, S.S.; Akashi, T.; Guibal, E. A new route for manufacturing poly (aminophosphonic)-functionalized poly (glycidyl methacrylate)-magnetic nanocomposite-Application to uranium sorption from ore leachate. *Environ. Pollut.* **2020**, *264*, 114797–114812. [CrossRef]
19. Hamed, M.A.; Elkhabiry, S.; Kafafy, H.; El Gokha, A.A.; El Sayed, I.E.T. Synthesis and Characterization of Novel Azo Disperse Dyes Containing α-amino Phosphonate and Their Dyeing Performance on Polyester Fabric. *Egypt. J. Chem.* **2017**, *60*, 89–95. [CrossRef]
20. Imam, E.A.; El Sayed, I.E.T.; Mahfouz, M.A.A.; Tolba, T.; Akashi, A.; Galhoum, A.; Gubial, E. Synthesis of α-aminophosphonate functionalized chitosan sorbents: Effect of methyl vs phenyl group on uranium sorption. *Chem. Eng. J.* **2018**, *352*, 1022–1034. [CrossRef]
21. Mahmoud, M.E.; Adel, S.E.; El Sayed, I.E.T. Development of titanium oxide-bound-α-aminophosphonate nanocomposite for adsorptive removal of lead and copper from aqueous solution. *Water Resour. Ind.* **2020**, *23*, 100126–100138. [CrossRef]
22. Amira, A.; Aouf, Z.; Ktir, H.; Chemam, Y.; Ghodbane, R.; Zerrouki, R.; Aouf, N.-E. Recent Advances in the Synthesis of α-Aminophosphonates: A Review. *Chem. Select.* **2021**, *6*, 6137–6149. [CrossRef]
23. Kouznetsov, V.; Gómez, C.M.M.; Valencia Peña, J.L.; Vargas-Méndez, L.Y. Natural and synthetic quinoline molecules against tropical parasitic pathologies: An analysis of activity and structural evolution for developing new quinoline-based antiprotozoal agents. In *Discovery and Development of Therapeutics from Natural Products Against Neglected Tropical Diseases*; Elsevier: Amsterdam, The Netherlands, 2019; pp. 87–164.
24. Kukowska, M. Amino acid or peptide conjugates of acridine/acridone and quinoline/quinolone-containing drugs. A critical examination of their clinical effectiveness within a twenty-year timeframe in antitumor chemotherapy and treatment of infectious diseases. *Eur. J. Pharm. Sci.* **2017**, *15*, 587–615. [CrossRef] [PubMed]
25. Manjunath, G.; Mahesh, M.; Bheemaraju, G.; Ramana, P.V. Synthesis of New Pyrazole Derivatives Containing Quinoline Moiety via Chalcones: A Novel Class of Potential Antibacterial and Antifungal Agents. *Chem. Sci. Trans.* **2016**, *5*, 61–74.
26. El Sayed, I.E.T.; Fathy, G.; Ahmed, A.A.S. Synthesis and Antibacterial Activity of Novel Cyclic α-Aminophsophonates. *Biomed. J. Sci. Tech. Res.* **2019**, *23*, 17609–17614.
27. Mohamed, S.; Elshahed, M.; Saied, Y. Evaluation of Honey as an antibacterial agent against drug-resistant uropathogenic *E. coli* strains. *Research, J. Pharm. Tech.* **2020**, *13*, 3720–3724. [CrossRef]
28. Mohamed, S.H.; Elshahed, M.M.S.; Saied, Y.M.; Mohamed, M.S.M.; Osman, G.H. Detection of heavy metal tolerance among different MLSB resistance phenotypes of methicillin-resistant *S. aureus* (MRSA). *J. Pure. Appl. Microbiol.* **2020**, *5*, 1905–1916. [CrossRef]
29. Mohamed, S.H.; Khalil, M.S.; Mohamed, M.S.M.; Mabrouk, M.I. Prevalence of antibiotic resistance and biofilm formation in *Klebsiella pneumoniae* carrying fimbrial genes in Egypt. *Res. J. Pharm. Technol.* **2020**, *13*, 3051–3058. [CrossRef]
30. Li, Z.; Deguchi, T.; Yasuda, M.; Kawamura, T.; Kanematsu, E.; Nishino, Y.; Ishihara, S.; Kawada, Y. Alteration in the GyrA Subunit of DNA Gyrase and the ParC Subunit of DNA Topoisomerase IV in Quinolone-Resistant Clinical Isolates of *Staphylococcus epidermidis*. *Antimicrob. Agents Chemother.* **1998**, *42*, 3293–3295. [CrossRef] [PubMed]
31. Sekyere, J.O.; Amoako, D.G. Genomic and phenotypic characterisation of fluoroquinolone resistance mechanisms in Enterobacteriaceae in Durban South Africa. *PLoS ONE* **2017**, *12*, e0178888. [CrossRef]
32. Ruiz, J. Mechanisms of resistance to quinolones: Target alterations, decreased accumulation and DNA gyrase protection. *J. Antimicrob. Chemother.* **2003**, *51*, 1109–1117. [CrossRef]
33. Dasgupta, N.; Paul, D.; Chanda, D.D.; Chetri, S.; Chakravarty, A.; Bhattacharjee, A. Observation of a new pattern of mutations in gyrA and parC within *Escherichia coli* exhibiting fluroquinolone resistance. *Indian J. Med. Microbiol.* **2018**, *36*, 131–135. [CrossRef]
34. Conrad, S.; Oethinger, M.; Kaifel, K.; Klotz, G.; Marre, R.; Kern, W.V. gyrA Mutations in high-level fluoroquinolone-resistant clinical isolates of *Escherichia coli*. *J. Antimicrob. Chemother.* **1996**, *38*, 443–455. [CrossRef]

35. Fu, Y.; Guo, L.; Xu, Y.; Zhang, W.; Gu, J.; Xu, J.; Chen, X.; Zhao, Y.; Ma, J.; Liu, X.; et al. Alteration of GyrA Amino Acid Required for Ciprofloxacin Resistance in *Klebsiella pneumoniae* Isolates in China. *Antimicrob. Agents Chemother.* **2008**, *52*, 2980–2983. [CrossRef] [PubMed]
36. Hooper, D.; Jacoby, G. Mechanisms of drug resistance: Quinolone resistance. *Ann. N. Y. Acad. Sci.* **2017**, *1354*, 12–31. [CrossRef]
37. Chatterji, M. Effect of different classes of inhibitors on DNA gyrase from *Mycobacterium Smegmatis. J. Antimicrob. Chemother.* **2001**, *48*, 479–485. [CrossRef]
38. Vila, J.; Ruiz, J.; Goñi, P.; De Anta, T.J. Quinolone-resistance mutations in the topoisomerase IV parC gene of *Acinetobacter baumannii. J. Antimicrob. Chemother.* **1997**, *39*, 757–762. [CrossRef] [PubMed]
39. Doddaga, S.; Muttana, V.B.R.; Donka, R.; Meriga, B.; Chamarthi, N. Design, Synthesis and Antimicrobial Activity of α-Aminophosphonates of Quinoline and their Molecular Docking Studies Against DNA Gyrase A. *Lett. Drug Des. Discov.* **2013**, *10*, 967–976.
40. Otter, R.; Cozzarelli, N.R. Eschenichia coli DNA gyrase. *Method Enzymol.* **1983**, *100*, 171–180.
41. Heddle, J.G.; Blance, S.J.; Zamble, D.B.; Hollfelder, F.; Miller, D.A.; Wentzell, L.M.; Walsh, C.T.; Maxwell, A. The antibiotic microcin B17 is a DNA gyrase poison: Characterisation of the mode of inhibition. *J. Mol. Biol.* **2001**, *307*, 1223–1234. [CrossRef]
42. Oyamada, Y.; Yamagishi, J.I.; Kihara, T.; Yoshida, H.; Wachi, M.; Ito, H. Mechanism of inhibition of DNA gyrase by ES-1273, a novel DNA gyrase inhibitor. *Microbiol. Immunol.* **2007**, *51*, 977–984. [CrossRef]
43. Pierrat, O.A.; Maxwell, A. The Action of the Bacterial Toxin Microcin B17. *Biochimie* **2003**, *278*, 35016–35023. [CrossRef]
44. Zamble, D.B.; Miller, D.A.; Heddle, J.G.; Maxwell, A.; Walsh, C.T.; Hollfelder, F. In vitro characterization of DNA gyrase inhibition by microcin B17 analogs with altered bisheterocyclic sites. *Proc. Natl. Acad. Sci. USA* **2001**, *98*, 7712–7717. [CrossRef]
45. Bernard, P.; Kezdy, K.E.; van Melderen, L.; Steyaert, J.; Wyns, L.; Pato, M.L.; Higgins, N.P.; Couturier, M. The F Plasmid CcdB Protein Induces Efficient ATP-dependent DNA Cleavage by Gyrase. *J. Mol. Biol.* **1993**, *234*, 534–541. [CrossRef]
46. Kyte, J.; Doolittle, R.F. A simple method for displaying the hydropathic character of a protein. *J. Mol. Biol.* **1982**, *157*, 105–132. [CrossRef]
47. Zlatkov, A.B.; Peikov, P.T.; Momekov, G.C.; Pencheva, I.; Tsvetkova, B. Synthesis, stability and computational study of some ester derivatives of theophylline-7-acetic acid with antiproliferative activity. *Der Pharma Chem.* **2010**, *2*, 197–210.
48. Vinoda, B.; Bodke, Y.; Vinuth, M.; Aruna, S.M.; Venkatesh, T.; Sandeep, T. One Pot Synthesis, Antimicrobial and In Silico Molecular Docking Study of 1,3-Benzoxazole-5-Sulfonamide Derivatives. *Curr. Org. Chemie* **2016**, *5*, 1000163. [CrossRef]
49. Wayne, P.A. *Methods for Dilution Antimicrobial Susceptibility Tests for Bacteria That Grow Aerobically; Approved Standard—Tenth Edition*; CLSI document M07-A10; Clinical and Laboratory Standards Institute: Wayne, PA, USA, 2015.
50. Liao, C.; Hsueh, P.; Jacoby, G.A.; Hooper, D.C. Risk factors and clinical characteristics of patients with qnr -positive *Klebsiella pneumoniae* bacteraemia. *J. Antimicrob. Chemother.* **2013**, *68*, 2907–2914. [CrossRef]
51. Fàbrega, A.; du Merle, L.; Le Bouguénec, C.; de Anta, M.J.; Vila, J. Repression of Invasion Genes and Decreased Invasion in a High-Level Fluoroquinolone-Resistant *Salmonella Typhimurium* Mutant. *PLoS ONE* **2009**, *4*, e8029. [CrossRef] [PubMed]
52. Maxwell, A.; Burton, N.P.; Hagan, N.O. High-throughput assays for DNA gyrase and other topoisomerases. *Nucleic Acids Res. Spec. Publ.* **2006**, *34*, e104. [CrossRef] [PubMed]
53. Pettersen, E.F.; Goddard, T.D.; Huang, C.C.; Couch, G.S.; Greenblatt, D.M.; Meng, E.C.; Ferrin, T. E UCSF Chimera—A visualization system for exploratory research and analysis. *J. Comput. Chem.* **2004**, *25*, 1605–1612. [CrossRef] [PubMed]
54. Hanwell, M.D.; Curtis, D.E.; Lonie, D.C.; Vandermeerschd, T.; Zurek, E.; Hutchison, G.R. R. Avogadro: An advanced semantic chemical editor, visualization, and analysis platform. *J. Cheminform.* **2012**, *4*, 17. [CrossRef] [PubMed]
55. Gjorgjieva, M.; Tomasič, T.; Barancokova, M.; Katsamakas, S.; Ilas, J.; Tammela, P.; Masič, L.P.; Kikelj, D. Discovery of Benzothiazole Scaffold-Based DNA Gyrase B Inhibitors. *J. Med. Chem.* **2016**, *59*, 8941–8954. [CrossRef]
56. Alland, C.; Moreews, F.; Boens, D.; Carpentier, M.; Chiusa, S.; Lonquety, M.; Renault, N.; Wong, Y.; Cantalloube, H.; Chomilier, J.; et al. RPBS: A web resource for structural bioinformatics. *Nucleic Acids Res.* **2005**, *33*, W44–W49. [CrossRef]
57. Néron, B.; Ménager, H.; Maufrais, C.; Joly, N.; Maupetit, J.; Letort, S.; Carrere, S.; Tuffery, P.; Letondal, C. Mobyle: A new full web bioinformatics framework. *Bioinformatics* **2009**, *25*, 3005–3011. [CrossRef]
58. Forli, S.; Olson, A.J. A force field with discrete displaceable waters and desolvations entropy for hydrated ligand docking. *J. Med. Chem.* **2012**, *55*, 623–638. [CrossRef] [PubMed]
59. Moemen, Y.S.; El-Nahas, A.M.; Helmy, A.; Hassan, E.; Abdel-Azeim, S.; El-Bialy, S.A.A. Docking and 3D-QSAR Studies on Some HCV NS5b Inhibitors. *J. Drug Des. Med. Chem.* **2017**, *3*, 49–59.
60. Adeniji, S.E.; Arthur, D.E.; Abdullahi, M.; Haruna, A. Quantitative structure–activity relationship model, molecular docking simulation and computational design of some novel compounds against DNA gyrase receptor. *Chem. Afr.* **2020**, *3*, 391–408. [CrossRef]

antibiotics

Article

Co-Application of Allicin and Chitosan Increases Resistance of *Rosa roxburghii* against Powdery Mildew and Enhances Its Yield and Quality

Jiaohong Li [1,†], Rongyu Li [2,†], Cheng Zhang [2], Zhenxiang Guo [2], Xiaomao Wu [2,*] and Huaming An [3,*]

1 College of Forestry, Guizhou University, Guiyang 550025, China; xhli@gzu.edu.cn
2 Institute of Crop Protection, College of Agriculture, Guizhou University, Guiyang 550025, China; ryli@gzu.edu.cn (R.L.); 2111816013@stmail.ujs.edu.cn (C.Z.); zxguo3@gzu.edu.cn (Z.G.)
3 Research Center for Fruit Tree Engineering and Technology of Guizhou Province, College of Agriculture, Guizhou University, Guiyang 550025, China
* Correspondence: xmwu@gzu.edu.cn (X.W.); hman@gzu.edu.cn (H.A.)
† Jiaohong Li and Rongyu Li contributed equally to this work.

Abstract: Powdery mildew, caused by *Sphaerotheca* sp., annually causes severe losses in yield and quality in *Rosa roxburghii* production areas of southwest China. In this study, the role of the co-application of allicin and chitosan in the resistance of *R. roxburghii* against powdery mildew and its effects on growth, yield and quality of *R. roxburghii* were investigated. The laboratory toxicity test results show that allicin exhibited a superior antifungal activity against *Sphaerotheca* sp. with EC_{50} value of 148.65 mg kg^{-1}. In the field, the foliar application of allicin could effectively enhance chitosan against powdery mildew with control efficacy of 85.97% by spraying 5% allicin microemulsion (ME) 100–time liquid + chitosan 100–time liquid, which was significantly ($p < 0.01$) higher than 76.70% of allicin, 70.93% of chitosan and 60.23% of polyoxin. The co-application of allicin and chitosan effectively enhanced the photosynthetic rate and chlorophyll of *R. roxburghii* compared with allicin, chitosan or polyoxin alone. Moreover, allicin used together with chitosan was more effective than allicin or chitosan alone in enhancing *R. roxburghii* plant growth and fruit yield as well as improving *R. roxburghii* fruit quality. This work highlights that the co-application of allicin and chitosan can be used as a green, cost-effective and environmentally friendly alternative strategy to conventional antibiotics for controlling powdery mildew of *R. roxburghii*.

Keywords: allicin; chitosan; *Sphaerotheca* sp.; antibiotic; *Rosa roxburghii*

Citation: Li, J.; Li, R.; Zhang, C.; Guo, Z.; Wu, X.; An, H. Co-Application of Allicin and Chitosan Increases Resistance of *Rosa roxburghii* against Powdery Mildew and Enhances Its Yield and Quality. *Antibiotics* **2021**, *10*, 1449. https://doi.org/10.3390/antibiotics10121449

Academic Editor: Helena Felgueiras

Received: 2 November 2021
Accepted: 22 November 2021
Published: 25 November 2021

1. Introduction

Rosa roxburghii Tratt., an edible and medicinal fruit rich in vitamin C, flavonoids, superoxide dismutase (SOD) and various minerals, has high medicinal and nutritional values [1–5]. Recently, the *R. roxburghii* industry has developed rapidly in southwest China, especially in Guizhou Province, where the planting areas reached 170,000 hm^2 in 2020 [3,6]. Powdery mildew, caused by *Sphaerotheca* sp., is the most serious disease regarding *R. roxburghii* production [1]. In Guizhou Province of southwest China, powdery mildew seriously affects the growth, yield, and quality of *R. roxburghii*, and often causes 30~40% economic losses [7]. Although some chemical fungicides (triadimefon, myclobutanil, azoxystrobin and tebuconazole) [8] and conventional antibiotics (polyoxin and kasugamycin) [9] are frequently used to control powdery mildew, their residuals inevitably affect the environment, wildlife, and human beings [10]. Moreover, these chemicals and antibiotics easily generate resistance to pathogens with the increase in the use frequency [11,12]. Therefore, there is an urgent need to develop an alternative, cost-effective and environmentally friendly control strategy against powdery mildew of *R. roxburghii*.

It is generally believed that natural products are mild and basically harmless compared with chemical fungicides and conventional antibiotics. Although this view is not completely accurate, it has been suggested as one of the reasons for the growing preference of natural products by consumers, and their increasingly popular use in agriculture [13,14]. For instance, Yan et al. [8] reported that 6% ascorbic acid aqueous solutions could induce *R. roxburghii* against powdery mildew with the control effect of 61.45%. Chitosan, a natural resource substance for sustainable agriculture, can be used as a resistance inductor and biofungicide for controlling plant diseases and as a promoter for enhancing plant growth [15–20]. In our previous study, the foliar application of 1.0~1.5% chitosan could effectively control powdery mildew of *R. roxburghii* with an inducing control efficacy of 69.30~72.87%, and could notably induce the systemic disease resistance of *R. roxburghii*, as well as reliably enhancing its photosynthesis, growth, yield, and quality [7]. Although chitosan can be used as an effective, safe and economical inductor for controlling powdery mildew, its control effect is still relatively inferior. Thus, natural products enhancing chitosan against powdery mildew of *R. roxburghii* are worthy of further exploration and development.

Allicin, an oxygenated sulfur natural compound, was isolated and identified from garlic in 1944 by Cavallito and Bailey [21]. Since then, allicin has been widely used in agricultural plant protection and medical therapy due to its superior antimicrobial activity and ecofriendly advantage [13,14,22–25]. Allicin has a prominent reactivity, antioxidant activity and membrane permeability, and can undergo thiol–disulphide exchange reactions with free thiol groups of proteins in microorganisms [13,14,26–28]. In agriculture, allicin has been demonstrated to have satisfactory bioactivity against many plant-pathogenic fungi, such as *Plectospherella cucumerina, Botrytis cinerea, Phytophthora infestans, Xanthomonas axonopodis, Magnaporthe grisea* and *Alternaria brassicicola* [13,29]. However, to date, there are no documentations available about the application of allicin for controlling powdery mildew of *R. roxburghii* caused by *Sphaerotheca* sp. Moreover, whether allicin can be used as an adjuvant to enhance chitosan against powdery mildew of *R. roxburghii.* is worth further attention.

In this work, the bioactivity of allicin, chitosan and conventional antibiotics against *Sphaerotheca* sp. was firstly determined. Subsequently, the field control efficacy of the co-application of allicin and chitosan for powdery mildew of *R. roxburghii* was evaluated. Moreover, the effects of the co-application of allicin and chitosan on the powdery mildew resistance, growth, yield and quality of *R. roxburghii* were investigated. This study provides a green, cost-effective and environmentally friendly alternative strategy to conventional antibiotics for controlling powdery mildew of *R. roxburghii*.

2. Materials and Methods

2.1. Fungicides

5% allicin microemulsion (ME) was produced from Ciyuan Biotechnology Co. Ltd. (Xian, China). Chitosan (deacetylation ≥90.00%) was obtained from Huarun Bioengineering Co. Ltd. (Zhenzhou, China). Additionally, 3% polyoxin wettable powder (WP) and 6% kasugamycin WP were provided by Lvdun Biological Products Co. Ltd. (Xian, China).

2.2. Field Site

The field experiments were carried out in 2020 in an orchard of *R. roxburghii* with a 7-year-old 'Guinong 5' cultivar in Chaxiang village, Gujiao Town, Longli country, Guizhou Province, China (26°54′36″ N, 106°95′13″ E). The planting density of *R. roxburghii* trees was 106 plants per 666.7 m^2. The annual rainfall, mean temperature, annual sunshine duration, frostless season and mean altitude of field site were about 1100 mm, 13.9 °C, 1265 h, 280 days and 1384 m, respectively. The physical and chemical characteristics of planting soils are shown in Table 1.

Table 1. The physical and chemical characteristics of planting soils of *R. roxburghii*.

Parameters	Content	Parameters	Content
Organic matter	13.17 g·kg^{-1}	Exchangeable calcium	18.32 cmol·kg^{-1}
Total nitrogen	1.37 g kg^{-1}	Exchangeable magnesium	305.37 mg·kg^{-1}
Total phosphorus	1.72 g kg^{-1}	Available zinc	0.63 mg·kg^{-1}
Total potassium	1.11 g kg^{-1}	Available iron	6.42 mg·kg^{-1}
Available nitrogen	57.43 mg·kg^{-1}	Available manganese	15.33 mg·kg^{-1}
Available phosphorus	4.21 mg·kg^{-1}	Available boron	0.14 mg·kg^{-1}
Available potassium	26.75 mg·kg^{-1}	pH	6.89

2.3. *In Vitro Toxicity Tests*

The *Sphaerotheca* sp. pathogens of powdery mildew on *R. roxburghii* leaves were brushed into sterile water to produce a spore suspension with a concentration of about 100 spores per field of vision under a low power microscope. The healthy young leaves of *R. roxburghii* were washed, and their surface water was air-dried. No pathogen spores were found after microscopic examination. The healthy leaves were made into leaf discs with a diameter of 6 mm using a hole punch. The leaf discs were, respectively, immersed in the five gradient concentration solution of each tested fungicide for 10 s, and then placed in a Petri dish. Ten leaf discs were inoculated in each treatment with four replicates. Powdery mildew spores were inoculated on the front side of leaf discs by spray method, and the medium was sterile water. They were cultured in an artificial climate chamber at 20 °C for 7 days, with 10,000 lx of light intensity, 16 h/d of light duration and 70% relative humidity. The formula for calculating the inhibition rate of pathogens was as Equation (1):

$$\text{Inhibition rate (\%)} = 100 \times (1 - \text{Diseased leaf counts in treatment/Diseased leaf counts in control dish}) \quad (1)$$

EC_{50} (effective concentration of 50% inhibition rate) values were calculated statistically by a SPSS 18.0 software (SPSS Inc., Chicago, IL, USA).

2.4. *Field Control Experiment of Powdery Mildew of* R. roxburghii

The control experiment of powdery mildew of *R. roxburghii* was carried out using the foliar spray method. The experimental treatments included 5% allicin ME 100–time dilution liquid + chitosan 100–time dilution liquid, 5% allicin ME 100–time dilution liquid, chitosan 100–time dilution liquid, 3% polyoxin WP 100–time dilution liquid and clear water (control). A total of twenty plots were arranged randomly with four replicates and each plot had nine trees. Five trees on the diagonal of each plot were used for determination. Considering powdery mildew mainly damages the fresh young leaves and stems, as well as flower buds, flowers, and young fruits of *R. roxburghii*, about 1.50 L of fungicide dilution liquid was sprayed on each *R. roxburghii* plant (including leaves, stems, flowers and buds) on 31 March and 29 April 2020.

2.5. *Investigation of Control Effect of Powdery Mildew of* R. roxburghii*, and Determination of Its Resistance Parameters, Photosynthetic Rate and Chlorophyll*

The control effect of tested fungicides for powdery mildew of *R. roxburghii* was investigated on May 30 in 2020 according to Li et al. [7]. The incidence rate, disease index, and control effect of tested fungicides for powdery mildew of *R. roxburghii* were calculated according to Equations (2)–(4), respectively. The incidence degree: 0 = no incidence, 1 = 1~2 diseased lobules with thin hyphae, 2 = 3~4 diseased lobules with thick hyphae, 3 = 5~6 diseased lobules with dense hyphae, 4 = more than 7 diseased lobules with dense hyphae.

$$\text{Incidence rate (\%)} = 100 \times \text{Number of diseased leaves/Total number of leaves} \quad (2)$$

$$\text{Disease index} = 100 \times \sum (\text{Disease grade value} \times \text{Number of leaves within each grade})/(\text{Total number of leaves} \times \text{the highest grade}) \quad (3)$$

$$\text{Control effect (\%)} = 100 \times (1 - \text{Disease index of treatment}/\text{Disease index of control}) \quad (4)$$

The resistance parameters of *R. roxburghii* leaves, such as proline (Pro), soluble sugar, malonaldehyde (MDA), flavonoid, SOD activity and PPO activity, were determined on 30 May 2020 as described by Zhang et al. [30,31]. The photosynthetic rate (Pn) of leaves in *R. roxburghii* was monitored using a portable LI-6400XT photosynthesis measurement system (LI-COR Inc., Lincoln, NE, USA) at 8:00–10:00 a.m. on 30 May. Chlorophyll content of *R. roxburghii* leaves was determined by a UV-5800PC spectrophotometer at 645 nm (OD_{645}) and 663 nm (OD_{663}) with an acetone–ethanol (v/v, 2:1) extraction.

2.6. Determination of Yield and Quality of R. roxburghii

Fruits of *R. roxburghii* were randomly collected on 2 September in 2020, and then single fruit weight, yield per plant and quality of each plot were determined. The weighing method was used for determining single fruit weight and fruit yield per plant. Fruit quality of *R. roxburghii*, including vitamin C, soluble solid, soluble sugar, total acidity, soluble protein, flavonoid and SOD activity, were also determined as described by Zhang et al. [30,31].

2.7. Statistical Analyses

The mean ± standard deviation (SD) of four replicates were exhibited. SPSS 18.0 was used for analyses. Significant differences were determined by a one-way analysis of variance (ANOVA). Origin 10.0 was used for drawing the chart.

3. Results

3.1. Toxicity of Allicin and Chitosan against Sphaerotheca sp.

The toxicity of allicin, chitosan, polyoxin and kasugamycin against *Sphaerotheca* sp. is shown in Table 2. The 5% allicin ME treatment exhibited an outstanding toxicity against *Sphaerotheca* sp. of *R. roxburghii* with EC_{50} value of 148.65 mg kg^{-1}, which was higher by 2.80- 1.24- and 6.95-fold than chitosan, 3% polyoxin WP and 6% kasugamycin WP, respectively. Although chitosan had a relatively inferior toxicity against *Sphaerotheca* sp., its EC_{50} value was 2.48-fold higher than that of 6% kasugamycin WP. The results here indicate that allicin possessed a superior antimicrobial activity compared to conventional antibiotics including polyoxin and kasugamycin.

Table 2. The toxicity of allicin, chitosan, polyoxin and kasugamycin against *Sphaerotheca* sp.

Treatments	Regression Equation	Determination Coefficient (R^2)	EC_{50} (mg kg^{-1})
5% Allicin ME	$y = 2.3339 + 1.2274\,x$	0.9626	148.65
Chitosan	$y = 2.5343 + 0.9413\,x$	0.9748	416.21
3% Polyoxin WP	$y = 2.9799 + 0.8922\,x$	0.9937	183.68
6% Kasugamycin WP	$y = 2.4254 + 0.8542\,x$	0.9406	1032.88

y and *x* indicate the inhibition rate and fungicide concentration, respectively.

3.2. Field Control Effect of Allicin and Chitosan against Powdery Mildew of Rosa roxburghii

The field control effect of allicin + chitosan, allicin, chitosan and polyoxin against powdery mildew in *R. roxburghii* are shown in Table 3. Allicin + chitosan, allicin, chitosan and polyoxin significantly ($p < 0.01$) decreased the incidence rate and disease index of powdery mildew of *R. roxburghii*, and allicin + chitosan was the most effective. The control effect of allicin + chitosan against powdery mildew was 85.97%, which was significantly ($p < 0.01$) higher than 76.70% of allicin, 70.93% of chitosan and 60.23% of polyoxin. These results indicate that the co-application of allicin and chitosan effectively controlled powdery mildew of *R. roxburghii*, whose control effect was significantly better than that of allicin, chitosan, or polyoxin alone.

Table 3. The control effect of allicin and chitosan against powdery mildew of *R. roxburghii*.

Treatments	Incidence Rate (%)	Disease Index	Control Effect (%)
Allicin + Chitosan	11.00 ± 1.00 cC	2.14 ± 0.18 dD	85.97 ± 1.16 aA
Allicin	14.33 ± 1.53 cC	3.53 ± 0.22 cC	76.70 ± 1.10 bB
Chitosan	16.00 ± 3.61 cC	4.42 ± 0.10 cC	70.93 ± 2.12 cB
Polyoxin	26.67 ± 1.53 bB	6.04 ± 0.19 bB	60.23 ± 4.17 dC
Control	45.67 ± 4.51 aA	15.26 ± 1.12 aA	

Values indicate the mean ± SD of three replicates. Different small letters indicate significant differences at 5% level ($p < 0.05$), and different capital letters indicate significant differences at 1% level ($p < 0.01$).

3.3. *Effects of Allicin and Chitosan on Resistance Parameters of R. roxburghii Leaves*

Figure 1 depicts the effects of allicin + chitosan, allicin, chitosan and polyoxin on the Pro, soluble sugar, MDA, flavonoid, SOD activity and PPO activity of leaves in *R. roxburghii*. Compared to polyoxin or control, allicin + chitosan, allicin and chitosan significantly ($p < 0.01$) increased the contents of proline, soluble sugar, and flavonoid of *R. roxburghii* leaves, and significantly ($p < 0.01$) enhanced their SOD and PPO activities, as well as effectively reducing leaf MDA content. The enhancing effect of allicin + chitosan on Pro, flavonoid, SOD activity and PPO activity of *R. roxburghii* leaves were significantly ($p < 0.01$) higher than that of allicin or chitosan alone. Soluble sugar of *R. roxburghii* leaves treated by allicin + chitosan was significantly higher than that of allicin ($p < 0.05$) or chitosan ($p < 0.01$) alone. MDA of *R. roxburghii* leaves treated by allicin + chitosan was significantly ($p < 0.05$) lower than that of allicin, but had no significant difference to that of chitosan. These results indicate that the co-application of allicin and chitosan effectively improved enhancing or inhibiting effects of allicin or chitosan on the proline, soluble sugar, MDA, flavonoid, SOD activity and PPO activity of leaves in *R. roxburghii*.

3.4. *Effects of Allicin and Chitosan on Photosynthetic Rate and Chlorophyll Content of R. roxburghii Leaves*

The effects of allicin + chitosan, allicin, chitosan and polyoxin on photosynthetic rate and chlorophyll content in *R. roxburghii* leaves are shown in Figure 2. Compared to polyoxin or control, allicin + chitosan, allicin and chitosan significantly ($p < 0.01$) enhanced the photosynthetic rate of *R. roxburghii* leaves. *R. roxburghii* leaves treated by allicin + chitosan exhibited an excellent photosynthetic rate with 7.52 $\mu mol \cdot CO_2 \cdot m^{-2} \cdot s^{-1}$, which was significantly ($p < 0.01$) higher than 6.87 $\mu mol \cdot CO_2 \cdot m^{-2} \cdot s^{-1}$ of allicin, and 6.64 $\mu mol \cdot CO_2 \cdot m^{-2} \cdot s^{-1}$ of chitosan. Compared to control, allicin + chitosan, allicin and chitosan significantly ($p < 0.01$) increased the chlorophyll of *R. roxburghii* leaves, and there was no significant difference among the three treatments. Compared to polyoxin, allicin + chitosan could significantly ($p < 0.01$) increase the chlorophyll of *R. roxburghii* leaves, while allicin and chitosan could only significantly ($p < 0.05$) increase that of *R. roxburghii* leaves. The results presented here indicate that the co-application of allicin and chitosan effectively promoted leaf chlorophyll of *R. roxburghii*, thereby enhancing its photosynthesis.

3.5. *Effects of Allicin and Chitosan on Yield and Quality of R. roxburghii*

Figure 3 displays the effects of allicin + chitosan, allicin, chitosan and polyoxin on the single fruit weight and fruit yield per plant of *R. roxburghii*. Compared to polyoxin or control, allicin + chitosan, allicin and chitosan could significantly ($p < 0.01$) enhance the single fruit weight and fruit yield of *R. roxburghii*, and allicin + chitosan was the most efficient. The single fruit weight and fruit yield per plant of *R. roxburghii* treated by allicin + chitosan was 21.34 g and 7.62 kg, which significantly ($p < 0.01$) increased by 10.11% and 9.52%, 11.44% and 10.84%, 23.64% and 30.62%, and 44.68% and 66.11% compared to allicin, chitosan, polyoxin and control, respectively. The results of this work reveal that the co-application of allicin and chitosan effectively promoted fruit growth and yield formation of *R. roxburghii*.

The effects of allicin + chitosan, allicin, chitosan and polyoxin on quality of *R. roxburghii* fruits are displayed in Table 4. Allicin + chitosan, allicin, and chitosan could significantly ($p < 0.05$) increase vitamin C, soluble solid, soluble sugar, total acidity, soluble protein, flavonoid, and SOD activity of *R. roxburghii* fruits compared to polyoxin or control. Vitamin C, soluble solid, soluble sugar, total acidity and SOD activity of *R. roxburghii* fruits treated by allicin + chitosan was significantly ($p < 0.05$) higher than that of allicin or chitosan. In addition, there were no significant ($p < 0.05$) differences between treatments of allicin and chitosan. These findings show that allicin used together with chitosan could effectively improve *R. roxburghii* fruit quality, and allicin and chitosan should have a notably synergistic effect in improving quality of *R. roxburghii* fruits.

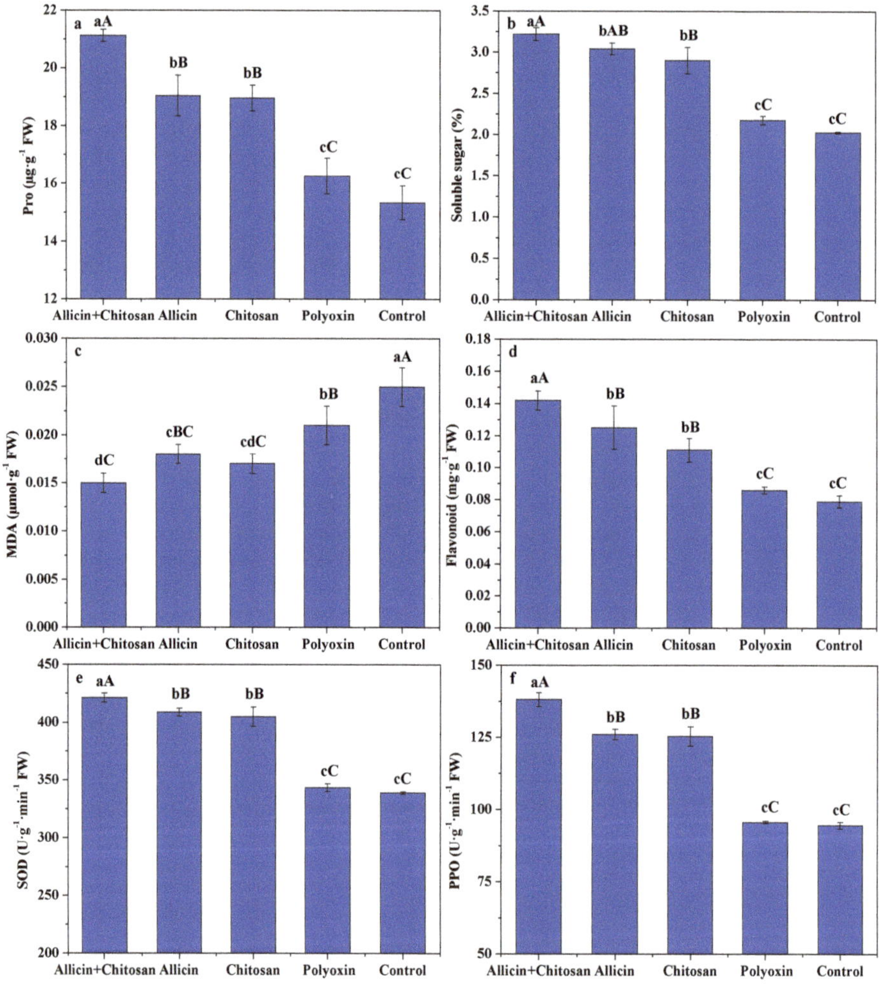

Figure 1. The effects of allicin and chitosan on the Pro (**a**), soluble sugar (**b**), malonaldehyde (**c**), flavonoid (**d**), SOD activity (**e**), and PPO activity (**f**) of leaves in *R. roxburghii*. Values and error bars indicate the mean and SD of three replicates, respectively. Different small letters indicate significant differences at 5% level ($p < 0.05$), and different capital letters indicate significant differences at 1% level ($p < 0.01$).

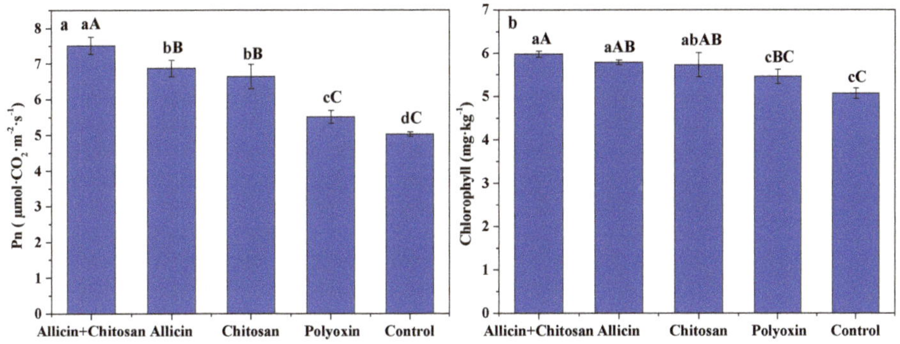

Figure 2. The effects of allicin and chitosan on the photosynthetic rate (**a**) and chlorophyll (**b**) of leaves in *R. roxburghii*. Values and error bars indicate the mean and SD of three replicates, respectively. Different small letters indicate significant differences at 5% level ($p < 0.05$), and different capital letters indicate significant differences at 1% level ($p < 0.01$).

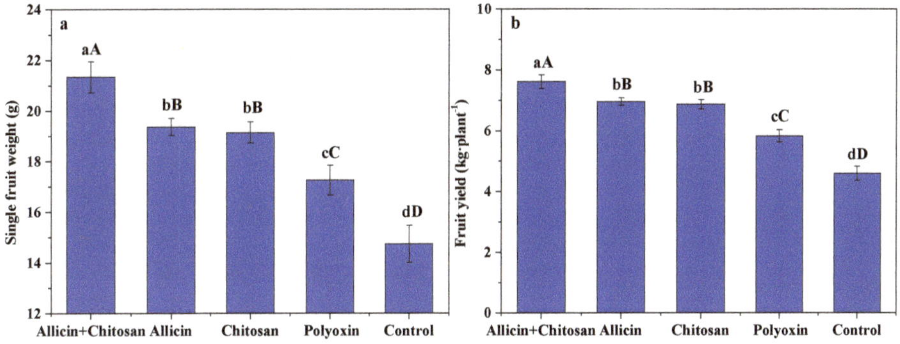

Figure 3. The effects of allicin and chitosan on single fruit weight (**a**) and fruit yield per plant (**b**) of *R. roxburghii*. Values and error bars indicate the mean and SD of three replicates, respectively. Different small letters indicate significant differences at 5% level ($p < 0.05$), and different capital letters indicate significant differences at 1% level ($p < 0.01$).

Table 4. The effects of allicin and chitosan on quality of *R. roxburghii* fruits.

Treatments	Vitamin C (mg·g^{-1})	Soluble Solid (%)	Soluble Sugar(%)	Total Acidity (%)	Soluble Protein(%)	Flavonoid ggx(mg·g^{-1})	SOD Activity ggx(U·g^{-1} FW)
Allicin + Chitosan	23.85 ± 0.16 ^{a}	12.65 ± 0.08 ^{a}	4.21 ± 0.10 ^{a}	3.94 ± 0.06 ^{a}	15.63 ± 0.47 ^{a}	0.127 ± 0.006 ^{a}	454.89 ± 2.05 ^{a}
Allicin	22.78 ± 0.66 ^{b}	12.18 ± 0.15 ^{b}	3.92 ± 0.04 ^{b}	3.62 ± 0.15 ^{b}	14.87 ± 0.72 ^{a}	0.119 ± 0.005 ^{a}	444.45 ± 4.89 ^{b}
Chitosan	22.56 ± 0.59 ^{b}	12.12 ± 0.11 ^{b}	3.87 ± 0.10 ^{b}	3.53 ± 0.14 ^{b}	14.59 ± 0.59 ^{a}	0.117 ± 0.004 ^{a}	441.12 ± 9.72 ^{b}
Polyoxin	19.64 ± 0.52 ^{c}	11.17 ± 0.13 ^{c}	3.26 ± 0.03 ^{c}	2.86 ± 0.09 ^{c}	13.42 ± 0.61 ^{b}	0.108 ± 0.008 ^{b}	407.62 ± 5.04 ^{c}
Control	17.88 ± 0.61 ^{d}	10.35 ± 0.22 ^{d}	3.14 ± 0.07 ^{c}	2.51 ± 0.14 ^{d}	12.65 ± 0.55 ^{b}	0.096 ± 0.003 ^{c}	376.95 ± 1.49 ^{d}

Values indicate the mean ± SD of three replicates. Different small letters indicate significant differences at 5% level ($p < 0.05$).

4. Discussion

Previous findings have demonstrated that allicin could effectively inhibit the growth of *Plectospherella cucumerina*, *Botrytis cinerea*, *Phytophthora infestans*, *Xanthomonas axonopodis*, *Magnaporthe grisea* and *Alternaria brassicicola*, etc. [13,29], and chitosan had antifungal activity against various fungal pathogens [15,16,32–35]. The results here show that 5% allicin ME displayed outstanding toxicity against *Sphaerotheca* sp., with an EC_{50} value of 148.65 mg kg^{-1}, which was 2.80-, 1.24- or 6.95-fold higher than chitosan, 3% polyoxin WP or 6% kasugamycin WP, respectively. This work extended the antimicrobial spectrum of allicin. Although chitosan exhibited a relatively inferior toxicity against *Sphaerotheca* sp., its EC_{50} value was still 2.48-fold higher than that of 6% kasugamycin WP. Moreover, the control effect of powdery mildew of *R. roxburghii* by allicin + chitosan was 85.97%, which was significantly ($p < 0.01$) higher than 76.70% of allicin, 70.93% of chitosan and 60.23% of polyoxin, respectively. Chitosan can trigger plant defense responses by inducing a variety of defense-related reactions [16,34–38]. Our previous results show that the inducing control effect of 1.0~1.5% chitosan against *Sphaerotheca* sp. was 69.30~72.87% [7]. In this study, the co-application of allicin and chitosan significantly ($p < 0.01$) enhanced the control effect of powdery mildew in *R. roxburghii* compared with allicin, chitosan or conventional antibiotic polyoxin alone. This suggests that allicin and chitosan had a notably synergetic effect in the control of powdery mildew of *R. roxburghii*. The effective control effect of allicin + chitosan was probably derived from the superior antimicrobial activity of allicin, as well as the excellent antimicrobial and induced resistance effect of chitosan.

The inducing of disease resistance is an effective agricultural practice for controlling plant diseases [39,40]. Pro and soluble sugar are important regulators of cell permeability, MDA is an important indicator of membrane lipid peroxidation and flavonoid is an important disease-resistant substance, as well as SOD and PPO being defense enzymes associated with plant disease resistance [38,40]. Many studies have also shown that chitosan could induce increases in sugar, Pro, flavonoid, polyphenolics and lignin in the plant and boost its defense enzyme activity, thereby enhancing its disease resistance [16,30–32,34–40]. Our previous results also indicate that the foliar application of 1.0~1.5% chitosan significantly ($p < 0.01$) increased Pro, soluble sugar and flavonoid contents, as well as SOD and POD activities of *R. roxburghii* leaves, and decreased their MDA [7]. The present results show that as compared with polyoxin or control, allicin + chitosan, allicin and chitosan could effectively increase Pro, soluble sugar, and flavonoid of *R. roxburghii* leaves, and enhance their SOD and PPO activities, as well as reduce their MDA, which is consistent with the above studies. Moreover, the enhancing or inhibiting effects of allicin + chitosan on Pro, soluble sugar, flavonoid and MDA contents, as well as SOD and PPO activities of *R. roxburghii* leaves were higher than those of allicin or chitosan alone. These results emphasize that the co-application of allicin and chitosan was more helpful in improving the disease resistance of *R. roxburghii*, and an obviously synergetic effect of allicin and chitosan was available.

Chlorophyll is an essential pigment for plant photosynthesis, and photosynthesis is the physiological basis of plant growth and development. Chitosan can promote plant growth and development by enhancing the photosynthetic rate by increasing chlorophyll content [16]. Our previous results show that foliar application of 0.5~1.5% chitosan effectively enhanced the photosynthetic rate, the content of chlorophyll a, chlorophyll b, and chlorophyll a + b of *R. roxburghii* leaves [7]. In this work, the co-application of allicin and chitosan more effectively promoted the chlorophyll and photosynthetic rate of *R. roxburghii* leaves compared with allicin, chitosan or polyoxin alone. This is closely related to the synergistic effect between allicin protecting plant leaf organs from pathogens and chitosan promoting plant growth. The growth and development of *R. roxburghii* determine its fruit yield and quality. Chitosan can also promote plant growth by activating the auxin and cytokinin signal transduction and gene expression, as well as increasing the nutrient intake [16,41]. Our previous results also indicate that the foliar application of 1.0~1.5% chitosan notably improved yield and quality of *R. roxburghii* fruits [7]. The present results indicate that the co-application of allicin and chitosan effectively enhance *R. roxburghii* fruit growth and yield formation. Moreover, vitamin C, soluble solid, soluble sugar, total acidity and SOD activity of *R. roxburghii* fruits treated by allicin + chitosan was significantly ($p < 0.05$) higher than that of treatments by allicin or chitosan alone. These notable effects were probably derived from their division of labor; allicin can protect *R. roxburghii* from pathogen infection and chitosan can induce the disease resistance of *R. roxburghii*, which guarantee the healthy growth of *R. roxburghii* plants.

At present, increasing attention has been focused on natural products as effective fungicides for controlling plant fungal disease, with high efficacy, nontoxicity and low food safety risks [24,42]. Therefore, natural products as an alternative to traditional antibiotics have been recognized by the public. Allicin, extracted from garlic, is used for daily consumption, and chitosan is a natural, nontoxic substance widely used in food, cosmetics and other fields. Moreover, the safe interval period (from April 29 to September 2, more than 120 days) of *R. roxburghii* was very long. Thus, the food safety risks caused by allicin or chitosan are almost nonexistent. This study highlights that the co-application of allicin and chitosan can be used as a green, cost-effective and environmentally friendly alternative approach to conventional antibiotics for controlling powdery mildew of *R. roxburghii* and enhancing its resistance, growth, yield and quality.

5. Conclusions

In conclusion, allicin displayed outstanding antifungal activity against *Sphaerotheca* sp. compared with conventional antibiotics including polyoxin and kasugamycin. The co-application of allicin and chitosan effectively controlled powdery mildew of *R. roxburghii*, and reliably enhanced Pro, soluble sugar and flavonoid contents, SOD and PPO activities in *R. roxburghii* leaves and reduced their MDA contents, as well as notably promoted the photosynthetic rate and chlorophyll contents of *R. roxburghii*. Moreover, the co-application of allicin and chitosan was more effective than allicin or chitosan alone in enhancing growth of *R. roxburghii* plants and improving quality *of R. roxburghii* fruits. This work highlights that the co-application of allicin and chitosan can be used as an ideal alternative to conventional antibiotics for controlling powdery mildew of *R. roxburghii*.

Author Contributions: X.W. constructed the project; X.W., H.A., J.L. and R.L. designed the experiments; J.L., R.L., C.Z. and Z.G. performed the experiments; J.L., R.L. and C.Z. analyzed the data; J.L., R.L., X.W. and H.A. wrote the paper. All authors have read and agreed to the published version of the manuscript.

Funding: This work was supported by the National Natural Science Foundation of China (no. 32160656), the Science-Technology Support Program of Guizhou Province (no. (2019)2407, (2020)1Y134, (2021) YB243), the "Hundred" Level Innovative Talent Foundation of Guizhou Province (no. 20164016), and the Cultivation Program of Guizhou University (no. (2019)09).

Institutional Review Board Statement: Not applicable.

Informed Consent Statement: Not applicable.

Data Availability Statement: The datasets used or analyzed during the current study available from the corresponding author upon reasonable request.

Conflicts of Interest: We declare that we do not have any commercial or associative interest that represents a conflict of interest in connection with the work submitted.

References

1. Wang, L.-T.; Lv, M.-J.; An, J.-Y.; Fan, X.-H.; Dong, M.-Z.; Zhang, S.-D.; Wang, J.-D.; Wang, Y.-Q.; Cai, Z.-H.; Fu, Y.-J. Botanical characteristics, phytochemistry and related biological activities of *Rosa roxburghii* Tratt fruit, and its potential use in functional foods: A review. *Food Funct.* **2021**, *12*, 1432–1451. [CrossRef] [PubMed]
2. Qi, L.L.; Zhou, R.L. The Healthcare Function and Development Trend of Toxburgh Rose. *Food Res. Dev.* **2016**, *37*, 212–214.
3. Wang, D.; Lu, M.; Ludlow, R.A.; Zeng, J.; Ma, W.; An, H. Comparative ultrastructure of trichomes on various organs of Rosa roxburghii. *Microsc. Res. Tech.* **2021**, *84*, 2095–2103. [CrossRef] [PubMed]
4. Liu, X.Z.; Zhao, H.B.; Li, Y.F.; Yu, Z.H.; Liu, X.H.; Huang, M.Z. Identification and Oenological Properties Analysis of a Strain of Hanseniaspora uvarum from *Rosa roxburghii*. *Food Ferment. Ind.* **2020**, *46*, 97–104.
5. Huang, X.; Yan, H.; Zhai, L.; Yang, Z.; Yi, Y. Characterization of the *Rosa roxburghii* Tratt transcriptome and analysis of MYB genes. *PLoS ONE* **2019**, *14*, e0203014. [CrossRef]
6. Fan, W.G.; Pan, X.J.; Chen, H.; Yang, H.R.; Gong, F.F.; Guan, J.Y.; Wang, M.L.; Mu, R. Effects of Oxalic Acid on the Nutrient of Calcareous Cultivated Soil and Leaf, Fruit Yield and Quality of *Rosa roxburghii* Tratt. *J. Fruit Sci.* **2021**, *38*, 1113–1122. [CrossRef]
7. Li, J.; Guo, Z.; Luo, Y.; Wu, X.; An, H. Chitosan Can Induce *Rosa roxburghii* Tratt. against *Sphaerotheca* sp. and Enhance Its Resistance, Photosynthesis, Yield, and Quality. *Horticulturae* **2021**, *7*, 289. [CrossRef]
8. Yan, K.; Wang, J.L.; Zhou, Y.; Fu, D.P.; Huang, R.M. Efficacy of Five Fungicides in *Rosa roxburghii* Tratt against *Sphaerotheca* sp. *Agrochemicals* **2018**, *57*, 609–610.

9. Xiang, J.; He, B. Toxicity Determination of Several Bio-fungicides to Powdery Mildew in Laboratory. *Sci. Technol. Modern Agric.* **2013**, *19*, 147.
10. Meena, R.S.; Kumar, S.; Datta, R.; Lal, R.; Vijayakumar, V.; Brtnicky, M.; Sharma, M.P.; Yadav, G.S.; Jhariya, M.K.; Jangir, C.K.; et al. Impact of Agrochemicals on Soil Microbiota and Management: A Review. *Land* **2020**, *9*, 34. [CrossRef]
11. Wang, Q.; Zhang, C.; Long, Y.; Wu, X.; Su, Y.; Lei, Y.; Ai, Q. Bioactivity and Control Efficacy of the Novel Antibiotic Tetramycin against Various Kiwifruit Diseases. *Antibiotics* **2021**, *10*, 289. [CrossRef]
12. Massi, F.; Torriani, S.F.F.; Borghi, L.; Toffolatti, S.L. Fungicide Resistance Evolution and Detection in Plant Pathogens: *Plasmopara viticola* as a Case Study. *Microorganisms* **2021**, *9*, 119. [CrossRef]
13. Slusarenko, A.J.; Patel, A.; Portz, D. Control of plant diseases by natural products: Allicin from garlic as a case study. *Eur. J. Plant Pathol.* **2008**, *121*, 313–322. [CrossRef]
14. Borlinghaus, J.; Albrecht, F.; Gruhlke, M.C.H.; Nwachukwu, I.; Slusarenko, A.J. Allicin: Chemistry and Biological Properties. *Molecules* **2014**, *19*, 12591–12618. [CrossRef]
15. Verlee, A.; Mincke, S.; Stevens, C.V. Recent developments in antibacterial and antifungal chitosan and its derivatives. *Carbohydr. Polym.* **2017**, *164*, 268–283. [CrossRef]
16. Chakraborty, M.; Hasanuzzaman, M.; Rahman, M.; Khan, A.R.; Bhowmik, P.; Mahmud, N.U.; Tanveer, M.; Islam, T. Mechanism of Plant Growth Promotion and Disease Suppression by Chitosan Biopolymer. *Agriculture* **2020**, *10*, 624. [CrossRef]
17. Torres-Rodriguez, J.A.; Reyes-Pérez, J.J.; Castellanos, T.; Angulo, C.; Quiñones-Aguilar, E.E.; Hernandez-Montiel, L.G. A biopolymer with antimicrobial properties and plant resistance inducer against phytopathogens: Chitosan. *Not. Bot. Horti Agrobot. Cluj-Napoca* **2021**, *49*, 12231. [CrossRef]
18. Rahman, M.; Mukta, J.A.; Sabir, A.A.; Gupta, D.R.; Mohi-Ud-Din, M.; Hasanuzzaman, M.; Miah, M.G.; Rahman, M.; Islam, M.T. Chitosan biopolymer promotes yield and stimulates accumulation of antioxidants in strawberry fruit. *PLoS ONE* **2018**, *13*, e0203769. [CrossRef]
19. Coutinho, T.C.; Ferreira, M.C.; Rosa, L.H.; de Oliveira, A.M.; Júnior, E.N.D.O. Penicillium citrinum and Penicillium mallochii: New phytopathogens of orange fruit and their control using chitosan. *Carbohydr. Polym.* **2020**, *234*, 115918. [CrossRef]
20. El Amerany, F.; Meddich, A.; Wahbi, S.; Porzel, A.; Taourirte, M.; Rhazi, M.; Hause, B. Foliar Application of Chitosan Increases Tomato Growth and Influences Mycorrhization and Expression of Endochitinase-Encoding Genes. *Int. J. Mol. Sci.* **2020**, *21*, 535. [CrossRef]
21. Cavallito, C.J.; Bailey, J.H. Allicin, the Antibacterial Principle of Allium sativum. I. Isolation, Physical Properties and Antibacterial Action. *J. Am. Chem. Soc.* **1944**, *66*, 1950–1951. [CrossRef]
22. Auger, J.; Arnault, I.; Diwo-Allain, S.; Ravier, N.; Molia, F.; Pettiti, M. Insecticidal and fungicidal potential of Allium substances as biofumigants. *Agroindustria* **2004**, *3*, 5–8.
23. Khodavandi, A.; Alizadeh, F.; Harmal, N.S.; Sidik, S.M.; Othman, F.; Jahromi, M.A.F.; Sekawi, Z.; Ng, K.-P.; Chong, P.P. Comparison between efficacy of allicin and fluconazole against Candida albicans in vitro and in a systemic candidiasis mouse model. *FEMS Microbiol. Lett.* **2011**, *315*, 87–93. [CrossRef] [PubMed]
24. Marchese, A.; Barbieri, R.; Sanches-Silva, A.; Daglia, M.; Nabavi, S.F.; Jafari, N.J.; Izadi, M.; Ajami, M.; Nabavi, S.M. Antifungal and antibacterial activities of allicin: A review. *Trends Food Sci. Technol.* **2016**, *52*, 49–56. [CrossRef]
25. Choo, S.; Chin, V.K.; Wong, E.H.; Madhavan, P.; Tay, S.T.; Yong, P.V.C.; Chong, P.P. Review: Antimicrobial properties of allicin used alone or in combination with other medications. *Folia Microbiol.* **2020**, *65*, 451–465. [CrossRef] [PubMed]
26. Omar, S.; Al-Wabel, N. Organosulfur compounds and possible mechanism of garlic in cancer. *Saudi Pharm. J.* **2010**, *18*, 51–58. [CrossRef] [PubMed]
27. Dwivedi, V.P.; Bhattacharya, D.; Singh, M.; Bhaskar, A.; Kumar, S.; Fatima, S.; Sobia, P.; Van Kaer, L.; Das, G. Allicin enhances antimicrobial activity of macrophages during Mycobacterium tuberculosis infection. *J. Ethnopharmacol.* **2019**, *243*, 111634. [CrossRef]
28. Buendía, A.S.A.; González, M.T.; Reyes, O.S.; Arroyo, F.E.G.; García, R.A.; Tapia, E.; Lozada, L.G.S.; Alonso, H.O. Immunomodulatory Effects of the Nutraceutical Garlic Derivative Allicin in the Progression of Diabetic Nephropathy. *Int. J. Mol. Sci.* **2018**, *19*, 3107. [CrossRef]
29. Curtis, H.; Noll, U.; Störmann, J.; Slusarenko, A.J. Broad-spectrum activity of the volatile phytoanticipin allicin in extracts of garlic (*Allium sativum* L.) against plant pathogenic bacteria, fungi and Oomycetes. *Physiol. Mol. Plant Pathol.* **2004**, *65*, 79–89. [CrossRef]
30. Zhang, C.; Long, Y.-H.; Wang, Q.-P.; Li, J.-H.; Wu, X.-M.; Li, M. The effect of preharvest 28.6% chitosan composite film sprays for controlling the soft rot on kiwifruit. *Hortic. Sci.* **2019**, *46*, 180–194. [CrossRef]
31. Zhang, C.; Long, Y.; Li, J.; Li, M.; Xing, D.; An, H.; Wu, X.; Wu, Y. A Chitosan Composite Film Sprayed before Pathogen Infection Effectively Controls Postharvest Soft Rot in Kiwifruit. *Agronomy* **2020**, *10*, 265. [CrossRef]
32. Xing, K.; Zhu, X.; Peng, X.; Qin, S. Chitosan antimicrobial and eliciting properties for pest control in agriculture: A review. *Agron. Sustain. Dev.* **2015**, *35*, 569–588. [CrossRef]
33. Berger, L.R.R.; Stamford, N.P.; Willadino, L.G.; Laranjeira, D.; de Lima, M.A.B.; Malheiros, S.M.M.; de Oliveira, W.J.; Stamford, T.C.M. Cowpea resistance induced against *Fusarium oxysporum* f. sp. tracheiphilum by crustaceous chitosan and by biomass and chitosan obtained from *Cunninghamella elegans*. *Biol. Control.* **2016**, *92*, 45–54. [CrossRef]
34. Obianom, C.; Romanazzi, G.; Sivakumar, D. Effects of chitosan treatment on avocado postharvest diseases and expression of phenylalanine ammonia-lyase, chitinase and lipoxygenase genes. *Postharvest Biol. Technol.* **2019**, *147*, 214–221. [CrossRef]

35. El-Mohamedya, R.S.R.; Abd El-Aziz, M.E.; Kamel, S. Antifungal Activity of Chitosan Nanoparticles against Some Plant Pathogenic Fungi In Vitro. *Agric. Eng. Int. CIGR J.* **2019**, *21*, 201–209.
36. Yan, J.; Cao, J.; Jiang, W.; Zhao, Y. Effects of preharvest oligochitosan sprays on postharvest fungal diseases, storage quality, and defense responses in jujube (*Zizyphus jujuba* Mill. cv. Dongzao) fruit. *Sci. Hortic.* **2012**, *142*, 196–204. [CrossRef]
37. Ma, Z.; Yang, L.; Yan, H.; Kennedy, J.F.; Meng, X. Chitosan and oligochitosan enhance the resistance of peach fruit to brown rot. *Carbohydr. Polym.* **2013**, *94*, 272–277. [CrossRef]
38. Wang, Q.; Zhang, C.; Wu, X.; Long, Y.; Su, Y. Chitosan Augments Tetramycin against Soft Rot in Kiwifruit and Enhances Its Improvement for Kiwifruit Growth, Quality and Aroma. *Biomolecules* **2021**, *11*, 1257. [CrossRef]
39. Vlot, A.C.; Sales, J.H.; Lenk, M.; Bauer, K.; Brambilla, A.; Sommer, A.; Chen, Y.; Wenig, M.; Nayem, S. Systemic propagation of immunity in plants. *New Phytol.* **2021**, *229*, 1234–1250. [CrossRef]
40. Lopez-Moya, F.; Suarez-Fernandez, M.; Lopez-Llorca, L.V. Molecular Mechanisms of Chitosan Interactions with Fungi and Plants. *Int. J. Mol. Sci.* **2019**, *20*, 332. [CrossRef]
41. Dzung, N.A.; Khanh, V.T.P.; Dzung, T.T. Research on impact of chitosan oligomers on biophysical characteristics, growth, development and drought resistance of coffee. *Carbohydr. Polym.* **2011**, *84*, 751–755. [CrossRef]
42. Newman, D.J.; Cragg, G.M. Natural Products as Sources of New Drugs over the 30 Years from 1981 to 2010. *J. Nat. Prod.* **2012**, *75*, 311–335. [CrossRef] [PubMed]

antibiotics

Review

Antibiotics- and Heavy Metals-Based Titanium Alloy Surface Modifications for Local Prosthetic Joint Infections

Jaime Esteban [1,2,*], María Vallet-Regí [3,4] and John J. Aguilera-Correa [2,3,*]

1 Clinical Microbiology Department, Jiménez Díaz Foundation Health Research Institute, Autonomous University of Madrid, Av. Reyes Católicos 2, 28040 Madrid, Spain
2 Networking Research Centre on Infectious Diseases (CIBER-ID), 28029 Madrid, Spain
3 Department of Chemistry in Pharmaceutical Sciences, Research Institute Hospital 12 de Octubre (i+12), School of Pharmacy, Complutense University of Madrid, Pza. Ramón y Cajal s/n, 28040 Madrid, Spain; vallet@ucm.es
4 Networking Research Centre on Bioengineering, Biomaterials and Nanomedicine (CIBER-BBN), 28029 Madrid, Spain
* Correspondence: jestebanmoreno@gmail.com (J.E.); john_j2a@hotmail.com (J.J.A.-C.); Tel.: +34-91-550-4900 (J.E.)

Abstract: Prosthetic joint infection (PJI) is the second most common cause of arthroplasty failure. Though infrequent, it is one of the most devastating complications since it is associated with great personal cost for the patient and a high economic burden for health systems. Due to the high number of patients that will eventually receive a prosthesis, PJI incidence is increasing exponentially. As these infections are provoked by microorganisms, mainly bacteria, and as such can develop a biofilm, which is in turn resistant to both antibiotics and the immune system, prevention is the ideal approach. However, conventional preventative strategies seem to have reached their limit. Novel prevention strategies fall within two broad categories: (1) antibiotic- and (2) heavy metal-based surface modifications of titanium alloy prostheses. This review examines research on the most relevant titanium alloy surface modifications that use antibiotics to locally prevent primary PJI.

Keywords: prosthetic joint infection; local prevention

Citation: Esteban, J.; Vallet-Regí, M.; Aguilera-Correa, J.J. Antibiotics- and Heavy Metals-Based Titanium Alloy Surface Modifications for Local Prosthetic Joint Infections. *Antibiotics* **2021**, *10*, 1270. https://doi.org/10.3390/antibiotics10101270

Academic Editors: Helena Felgueiras and Nicholas Dixon

Received: 21 September 2021
Accepted: 13 October 2021
Published: 19 October 2021

1. Introduction

The use of arthroplasty makes it possible to replace a natural joint with artificial material or a joint prosthesis. Although, arthroplasty is highly effective and has improved the quality of life of millions of patients [1], implant-related complications can appear during the lifetime of patients [2]. One of the most important complications is prosthetic joint infection (PJI), although others may occur. This is probably the most devastating complication due to the high morbidity, mortality, and costs associated with PJI. The mean cost per patient with knee PJI of is USD 52,555 (EUR 40,542), with a range of between USD 24,980 (EUR 19,270.80) for patients with early PJI, and USD 78,111 (EUR 60,257) for those with late PJI [3]. Incidence varies from country to country, between 0.5–2%. Thus, PJI incidence is ranged between 1 and 2% in the United States, and between 0.6% and 0.72% in Nordic countries [4,5]. It is important to know this incidence could be higher in patients undergoing a primary arthroplasty with a history of a PJI in another joint showing up to a three-fold higher risk of PJI [6]. Currently, the 5-year mortality rate associated with PJI is greater than that of breast cancer, melanoma, and Hodgkin's lymphoma [7].

The aim of this work is to review research on the most relevant titanium alloy surface modifications that use antibiotics to locally prevent primary PJI.

2. Etiopathology

Staphylococci, including *Staphylococcus aureus* (30–40%) and different species of coagulase-negative staphylococci (27–43%), among which *S. epidermidis* predominates, are the most common etiological agents associated with PJI [8–12]. Among Gram-negative bacteria (3–9%) [13], enterobacteria and non-fermenting Gram-negative bacilli stand out. However, there could be differences in these patterns according to the characteristics of the infection [9] or the affected joint [14,15]. Polymicrobial infections, or those caused by more than one microorganism, may occur in 10–35% of cases [2,13]. *Enterococcus* species, *Staphylococcus*, and various Gram-negative bacilli such as Enterobacteriaceae and *Pseudomonas aeruginosa* are often associated with these infections.

A problem of growing importance associated with bacterial infections is antibiotic resistance [16]. According to the Centers for Disease Control, approximately 2.8 million antibiotic-resistant bacterial infections take place in the United States and provoke more than 35,000 deaths every year [17]. The main bacteria related to this antibiotic resistance are (as declared by the WHO) *Acinetobacter baumannii*, *P. aeruginosa*, enterobacteria (e.g., *Klebsiella pneumoniae* and *Enterobacter cloacae*), *Enterococcus faecium*, *S. aureus*, *Helicobacter pylori*, *Campylobacter* spp., *Salmonella* spp., *Neisseria gonorrhoeae*, *Streptococcus pneumoniae*, *Haemophilus influenzae*, and *Shigella* spp. [16,18]. As can be seen, many of the listed bacteria are causative agents of PJI, e.g., *S. aureus*, *P. aeruginosa*, *K. pneumonia*, *E. cloacae*, and *E. faecium*, and for that, the antibiotic resistance is also an emerging threat for PJI and must be taken into account in the development of any preventive treatment against them.

One of the most important characteristics in all the aspects of PJI is the ability of microorganisms to form biofilms. A biofilm is a conglomerate of microbial cells of at least one species that is irreversibly attached or not on a surface or an interface, and embedded in a self-produced matrix of polymeric extracellular substances [19], where numerous complex sociomicrobiological interactions prevail [20–22]. It is estimated that at least 80% of chronic infections are directly related to the ability of the causative microorganism to develop a biofilm, likely including 100% of all implant-related infections [23,24]. Biofilm formation involves at least three different stages:

(1) Attachment. Microorganisms come into contact with the surface, a process that is at least partly stochastic, driven by physical and chemical forces [25–27]. Furthermore, host proteins rapidly coat the surface of medical devices, facilitating specific adhesion mediated by microbial surface components recognizing adhesive matrix molecules (MSCRAMMs), which are part of the surface of many bacteria, e.g., *Staphylococcus* spp. [28,29].

(2) Maturation is characterized by intercellular aggregation coupled to a variety of molecules such as proteins or, usually, exopolysaccharides of a polysaccharide nature, and structuring forces that rearrange the biofilm into three-dimensional structures of variable morphology depending on the species and with microchannels within them [28]. During this stage, one of the most important processes is the production of the exopolysaccharide matrix, whose composition is characteristic of each species, and even of each strain [28–31]. At this stage, the relatively simple structure that the pre-biofilm acquired in irreversible adhesion takes on a much more structurally complex three-dimensional organization [32]. The nutritional gradient inside the biofilm gives rise to a variety of cells with metabolic differences, including starved cells, dormant cells, viable non-cultivable cells, "persister" cells, and dead cells [27,33].

(3) Dispersal. This is the process by which mature biofilm cells disperse to adjacent areas passively or actively [23,27]. Through this stage, the infection spreads to adjacent niches in an environment or within the host once nutrients or space has been depleted [32], where it attaches again and restarts the cycle.

The implications of biofilms in treatment and outcomes are enormous, as they confer phenotypical resistance that required the use of new surgeries and prolonged treatments. It is therefore of utmost importance to avoid bacterial colonization of implants and thus avoid the appearance of infection. Moreover, the possibility of an interaction between biofilms, cells, and implanted biomaterials is also of great importance, as the reservoir in the tissue also needs to be removed to cure patients [34,35].

3. Conventional Prevention of Prosthetic Joint Infections

Conventional prevention of PJI includes all measures developed for preventing surgical site infections (SSIs) that have appeared in official guidelines and statements [36,37]. More specific measures for the prevention of PJI have also been published recently [38–41], and the importance of these measures was considered at the 2nd International Consensus Meeting at Philadelphia as a whole chapter in the General Assembly issues [42]. Factors increasing PJI risk can be grouped into three categories: preoperative, intraoperative, and postoperative [43]. Among the preoperative factors, some well-known ones are obesity, malnutrition, diabetes mellitus, smoking, skin decolonization before surgery, and nasal decolonization. Some important intraoperative factors are surgical-site hair removal, perioperative antibiotics whose use has been successful in reducing the risk of such infections by up to 80% [44,45], and perioperative antibiotic timing [13,46], surgical site skin decolonization, intraarticular irrigation by incorporating antiseptic substances, fibrinolytic agent use, wound closure, implant surface properties, and local antibiotic delivery, since, for instance, the use of a prosthesis cemented with antibiotic-loaded polymethyl-methacrylate cement has been proposed as a potentially useful method that diminishes the risk of PJI [47–50]. However, the use of antibiotic-loaded cements is not used in all patients so far, since its use has shown a high variability between cohorts, which is translated as a problem when comparing results [51] and requires the employment of specific heat-tolerant antibiotics. Among postoperative factors, some authors consider the typical temporal patterns of C-reactive protein, erythrocyte sedimentation rate test, interleukin 6, and D-Dimer in the early postoperative period [43].

However, even taking all those risk factors into account, there are still several patients who develop PJI after surgery. Several strategies have been devised to avoid this kind of infection.

4. Local Preventive Antibiotic-Based Strategies

During prosthetic implantation, the bone and surrounding tissue must be irrigated; in addition, after implantation, the periprosthetic tissue may be left damaged, avascular, or even, necrotic. These events inherent to surgery locally reduce the concentration of the antibiotic systemically administrated and make it necessary to use a local antibiotic approach with a period of action of hours or days.

On the other hand, the foreign body reaction after the implantation gives rise to an interstitial milieu or a *locus minus resistentiae*, which is an immunosuppressed fibro-inflammatory zone [52]. This zone is a relatively inaccessible environment for the immune response due to the absence of normal blood supply to the periprosthetic tissue [53], which impairs the ability of lymphocytes, antibodies, and certain antibiotics to properly reach the implant surface and thus prevent and fight infection via the systemic route. For this reason, any prosthesis would be susceptible to be infected not only during the perioperative period but also throughout its whole lifetime [54]. Therefore, a local antibiotic approach with an active period of months or years is required.

The ideal antibiotic-loaded titanium alloy surface modification would require two components: a titanium alloy component and an antibiotic component. The ideal titanium alloy surface modification must not compromise its good corrosion resistance, high strength, low weight, its Young's modulus of elasticity [55], or non-cytotoxicity. In addition, this titanium alloy surface should be a selective surface able to impair the bacterial adhesion and to favor bone tissue integration [56]. The ideal antibiotic to be loaded should be a broad-spectrum drug based on local prevalence of antibiotic resistance with no adverse local or systemic effects. Further, the ideal antibiotic-loaded titanium alloy should fulfil some market requirements such as an acceptable cost, wide availability, and be easy to manufacture and overcome regulatory issues [57].

The local prevention approach can be classified into two types according to the mechanism of action: passive and active modifications. Passive modifications are surface coatings that endow biomaterial with antibacterial (anti-adherent, bacteriostatic, and/or bactericide) properties without releasing any compound that is responsible for these properties.

The active modifications do endow biomaterials with antibacterial properties through a compound released from the material. These active modifications are divided into two groups: active surfaces and coatings. The most recent antibiotic-loaded surface modifications of titanium alloys are illustrated in Figure 1.

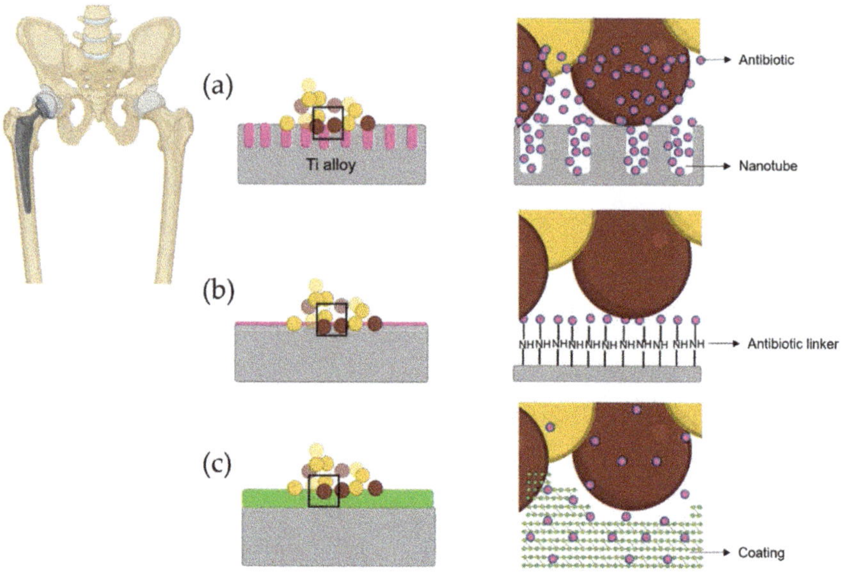

Figure 1. Different local antibiotic therapy strategies. (**a**) Antibiotic-loaded nanotubes. (**b**) Antibiotic covalently bound to titanium alloy. (**c**) Antibiotic-loaded coating. Yellow represents live bacteria. Red represents dead bacteria.

4.1. Active Titanium Surfaces Loaded with Antibiotics

The active titanium surfaces loaded with antibiotics can be divided into two categories: nanostructured surfaces and surfaces with covalently bound antibiotics.

The most representative nanostructured titanium surface approaches are summarized in Table 1. This strategy mainly consists of growing nanoscopic carriers made of the bulk alloy and loading them with at least one antibiotic. The most widely used nanostructure is the nanotube, a hollow cylinder without one of its circular faces. Nanotubes can be manufactured using different methods such as sol–gel synthesis, template-assisted synthesis, hydrothermal synthesis, and electrical anodization [58]. Among them, an exponential trend of the use of hydrothermal synthesis and electrical anodization can be observed over last two decades due to their multiple applications [59]. The hydrothermal synthesis modifies the crystallinity of the titanium precursor [60] and allows incorporating other chemical elements into the titanium nanotubes, which enhances their photoelectrochemical [1] properties [59] and confers interesting environmental applications involved, for instance, in the recalcitrant organic pollutant degradation [61]. However, between the two, the most versatile and used in the field of Biomaterials is electrical anodization due to its easy use and thrift.

This nanostructure allows its loading using different methods, mainly simplified lyophilization or soaking.

Bacterial and cellular adhesion are complex processes arising from the interaction between surface properties, biological factors, and environmental conditions. A recent systematic review concludes that there are three reasons why the relationship between surface topography and bacterial attachment can give rise to contradictory results: (i) roughness cannot be the sole descriptor of surface topography; (ii) topographical effects are influenced by the effects of other physicochemical factors, such as surface chemistry; and (iii) different anti-adherent mechanisms may take place at different topographical scales: nanoscale and microscale [62]. The last reason can be also applied to cell attachment. Some authors assert that titanium nanotubes increase the bacterial attachment but have excellent biocompatibility properties because of their enhanced protein interaction (including adsorption and conformation) what improves cellular adhesion and tissue growth [63]. Other authors, by contrast, assert that titanium nanostructures themselves can prevent [64] or reduce bacterial adhesion [65,66] or even biofilm development [67], and also promote cell adhesion and proliferation on the alloy [66,68]. Furthermore, nanotubes composition could be involved in part of these abilities. Thus, for instance, the incorporation of fluorine would be responsible for an anti-adherent ability [65], whilst the additional incorporation of phosphorus would be responsible for better osseointegration [69].

The nanotube diameter is pivotal for the release profile [70]; that is, the larger the diameter, the faster the release. Most of the nanotube-based approaches offer a constant antibiotic release for a few hours after surgery. As a result, this type of approach only guarantees local antibiotic with an active period of hours. The main antibiotic used for loading nanotubes are gentamicin [71–73] and vancomycin [74,75] in monotherapy since only few studies have used them in combination [76,77]. Gentamicin is a broad spectrum antibiotic effective against both Gram-positive and Gram-negative bacteria which has a great chemical stability since it remains stable at 4 °C for 30 days and at 23 °C for 7 days [78], and a great thermal stability due to this antibiotic retain its activity even after autoclaving [79]. For its part, vancomycin is a narrow spectrum antibiotic effective against Gram-positive bacteria, the main type of bacteria related to PJIs, and has a reduced chemical stability due to its the concomitant crystalline thermal degradation at physiologic condition [80], which can cause up to a 40% decrease in its activity in 3 weeks [81].

Table 1. Some of the most relevant studies based on titanium nanotubes loaded with antibiotics.

Year	Type of Surface Modification	Bacteria Evaluated	Bacterial State	Cytotoxicity (%)	Level Study	Cell Lines/Animal Used In Vivo	Reference
2014	Gentamicin-loaded nanotubes with different diameters	SA, SE	Biofilm	ND	In vitro	hBMMS cells	[71]
2016	Chitosan-coated gentamicin-loaded nanotubes	SA	Planktonic	20	In vitro	MG-63 osteoblasts	[72]
2017	Gentamicin-loaded nanotubes made with anodization	SA	Biofilm	ND	In vivo	-/rabbit	[73]
2018	Chitosan-hyaluronic acid-coated vancomycin-loaded nanotubes	SA	Planktonic/ Biofilm	0	In vitro/ in vivo	Primary osteoblasts/rat	[74]
	Vancomycin-loaded micro-patterning	MRSA	Biofilm	ND	In vivo	-/rabbit	[75]
	Gentamicin and/or vancomycin F-dopped nanotubes	SA, SE, EC	Planktonic	ND	In vitro	-/-	[66]
2019	Gentamicin plus vancomycin F- and P-dopped bottle-shaped nanotubes	SA	Biofilm	0	In vitro/ in vivo	MC3T3-E1 osteoblasts/rabbit	[76]

Abbreviation: SA: *S. aureus;* SE: *S. epidermidis*, EC: *E. coli;* MRSA: Methicillin-resistant *S. aureus;* ND: Not determined. hBMMS cells: Human marrow-derived mesenchymal stem cells.

Antibiotics covalently bound to titanium surfaces is another type of active titanium surfaces with antibiotics (Table 2). The main techniques for covalently bound of antibiotics onto titanium surfaces involve the covalent attachment of end-functionalized polymers incorporating an appropriate anchor, e.g., silane anchor, catechol anchor, and phosphor-based anchor [82]. To date, numerous antibiotics have been employed using this strategy such as daptomycin [83], ciprofloxacin [84], doxycycline [85], vancomycin [86], enoxacin [87], bacitracin [88], a new antibiotic such as SPI031 [89], and even antifungals such as caspofungin [86].

Table 2. Some of the most relevant studies based on antibiotic covalently bound to titanium surfaces.

Year	Antibiotic Covalently Bound	Bacteria Evaluated	Bacterial State	Cytotoxicity (%)	Level Study	Cell Lines/Animal Used In Vivo	Reference
2010	Daptomycin	SA	Biofilm	ND	In vitro	-/-	[90]
2014	Doxycycline	-	-	0– <40	In vitro/in vivo	MC3T3-E1 osteoblasts/rabbit	[85]
2015	Ciprofloxacin	PA	Biofilm	0	In vitro/in vivo	NIH3T3 fibroblasts/mouse	[84]
2016	Vancomycin/ caspofungin	SA, CA	Biofilm	0	In vitro/in vivo	hME cells/rat	[86]
	SPI031	SA, PA	Biofilm	0	In vitro/in vivo	hBMMS cells, hME cells/mouse	[89]
	Enoxacin	MRSA, SE, EC	Planktonic, Biofilm	0	In vitro/in vivo	hBMMS cells/rat	[87]
2017	Bacitracin	SA	Biofilm	ND	In vivo	-/rat	[88]

Abbreviations: SA: *S. aureus;* SE: *S. epidermidis,* EC: *E. coli;* PA: *P. aeruginosa;* MRSA: methicillin-resistant *S. aureus;* ND: Not determined. hBMMS cells: Human marrow-derived mesenchymal stem cells. hME cells: human microvascular endothelial cells.

4.2. Coating Loaded with Antibiotic for Titanium Alloys

Some of the most relevant coatings loaded with antibiotics described over the last 10 years are summarized in Table 3. In this period, strategies have focused on the design of coatings instead of nanostructures and the covalent binding of antibiotics. This reorientation of local antibiotic therapies may be justified by the huge versatility the coatings offer and their compatibility with not only titanium alloys, but also with almost any material from which a biomedical implant may be made.

Table 3. Some of the most relevant studies based on antibiotic loaded coating for titanium implants.

Year	Type of Coating	Evaluated Bacteria	Bacterial State	Cytotoxicity (%)	Level Study	Cell Lines/Animal Used In Vivo	Reference
2010	Vancomycin-loaded PMMA	SE	Biofilm	ND	In vitro	-/-	[91]
	Inorganic sol–gel with Polymyxin B covalently bound	EC	Planktonic	ND	In vitro	-/-	[92]
	Gentamicin-loaded polyelectrolyte multilayer	SA	Planktonic, Biofilm	0–80	In vitro/ in vivo	MC3T3-E1 osteoblasts/rabbit	[93]
2014	Rifampicin and fosfomycin-loaded Hydroxyapatite coating	MSSA, MRSA	Biofilm	ND	In vivo	-/rabbit	[94]
	Ciprofloxacin-loaded chitosan-nanoparticles coating	SA	Planktonic	<30	In vitro	MG63 osteoblast-like cells	[95]
	Chitosan–vancomycin composite coatings	SA	Planktonic	0	In vitro	MG63 osteoblast-like cells	[96]
	Vancomycin-loaded PLGA-coating	SA	Planktonic/ Biofilm	0	In vitro	MC3T3-E1 osteoblasts/rabbit	[97]
2015	Doxycycline-loaded polymer-lipid encapsulation matrix coating	MSSA, MRSA	Planktonic, Biofilm	ND	In vitro/ in vivo	-/mouse	[98]
2015	PLGA-gentamicin-hydroxyapatite-coating	SA, SE	Planktonic, Biofilm	ND	In vitro/ in vivo	-/rabbit	[99]
2016	Gentamicin-derivates coating	SA	Biofilm	ND	In vivo	-/rats	[100]
2016	Vancomycin-loaded phosphatidyl-choline	SA	Biofilm	ND	In vivo	-/rabbit	[101]
2016	Tetracycline loaded chitosan-gelatin nanosphere coating	SA	Biofilm	>90	In vitro/ in vivo	MC3T3-E1 osteoblasts/rabbit	[102]
2017	Doxycycline-loaded coaxial PCL-PVA nanofiber coating	SA	Biofilm	ND	In vivo	-/rat	[103]
	Tobramycin-loaded PDLLA coating	SA	Biofilm	ND	In vivo	-/rabbit	[1]

Table 3. *Cont.*

Year	Type of Coating	Evaluated Bacteria	Bacterial State	Cytotoxicity (%)	Level Study	Cell Lines/Animal Used In Vivo	Reference
2018	Vancomycin-loaded mesoporous bioglass-PLGA coating	SA	Planktonic, Biofilm	0	In vitro	hBMMS cells	[104]
	Vancomycin-loaded mesoporous silica nanoparticles-containing gelatin coating	SA	Biofilm	0	In vitro	hBMMS cells	[105]
2019	Gentamicin-loaded polyelectrolyte multilayer	SA, SE	Planktonic, Biofilm	<5	In vitro/ in vivo	MC3T3-E1 osteoblast/rats	[106]
	Tobramycin-loaded hydroxyapatite coating	SA	Planktonic, Biofilm	ND	In vitro/ in vivo	Endothelial cells, primary osteoblasts/rabbit	[107]
	Vancomycin plus tigecycline-loaded PEG-PPS coating	SA	Biofilm	ND	In vivo	-/mouse	[108]
	Gentamicin-loaded calcium phosphate-based coating	SA	Biofilm	ND	In vivo	-/rat	[109]
	Vancomycin-loaded polymethacrylate coating	SA	Planktonic/ Biofilm	ND	In vitro/ in vivo	-/mouse	[110]
2020	Cephalexin- and VEGF-loaded agarose-nanocrystalline apatite coating	SA	Planktonic	0	In vitro	MC3T3-E1 osteoblast	[111]
	Moxifloxacin-loaded organic-inorganic sol–gel	SA, SE, EC	Planktonic, Biofilm	0	In vitro/ in vivo	MC3T3-E1 osteoblasts/mouse	[112]
	Gentamicin loaded autologous blood glue	PA	Planktonic, Biofilm	0	In vitro	hBMMS cells	[113]
	Fluconazole/anidulafungin-loaded organic-inorganic sol–gel	CA, CP	Planktonic, Biofilm	0	In vitro	MC3T3-E1 osteoblasts	[114]
	Anidulafungin-loaded organic-inorganic sol–gel	CA	Biofilm	-	In vivo	-/mouse	[115]
	Vancomycin-loaded starch coating	SA	Planktonic	ND	In vitro	-/-	[116]

Abbreviations: PLGA: poly(lactic-co-glycolic acid); PCL-PVA: polycaprolactone/polyvinyl alcohol; PEG-PPS: poly(ethylene glycol-bl-propylene sulfide); PDLLA: poly (D, L-lactide); SA: *S. aureus;* SE: *S. epidermidis*, EC: *E. coli;* PA: *P. aeruginosa;* MRSA: methicillin-resistant *S. aureus;* MSSA: Methicillin-susceptible *S. aureus*; CA: *Candida albicans*; CP: *Candida parapsilosis*; ND: Not determined. hBMMS cells: human bone marrow mesenchymal stem cells.

Different approaches of deposition of antibiotic-loaded coatings such as sol–gel, covalent immobilization, spraying, electrophoretic, polyelectrolyte, and dip coating have been used on titanium surfaces [117]. Most of the coatings described are degradable over time and are composed of synthetic or natural polymers. The antibiotic release from these degradable coatings depends on their degradation or hydrolysis and the loaded antibiotic quantity depends on both the chemical composition of the coating and the chemical structure and chemical properties of the antibiotic used. The antibiotics that have been loaded onto these coatings are vancomycin [91,96,97,101,105,110,116], aminoglycosides (mainly gentamicin [93,99,100,106,109,113] and tobramycin), tetracyclines (especially doxycycline [98,103] and tetracycline) [102], cephalexin [111], moxifloxacin [112,118], and mixtures of antibiotics such as vancomycin plus tigecycline [108]. Further studies have demonstrated that antifungals, such as fluconazole and anidulafungin, loaded in a coating are effective to prevent *C. albicans* infection both in vitro [114] and in vivo [115].

The most commonly used synthetic polymers are poly (lactic-co-glycolic acid) (PLGA) (polycaprolactone/polyvinyl alcohol), poly (ethylene glycol-propylene sulphide), and poly-D,L-lactide. Most have been approved by the Food Drug Administration due to their biodegradability and biocompatibility in light of a vast number of recently reviewed studies [119,120]. New strategies based on the use of inorganic [92] and organo-inorganic sol–gels have recently emerged. Some of these organo-inorganic sol–gels have been shown to degrade into non-cytotoxic monomers [112], promote osteoblast proliferation [121], and can even prevent clotting [118]. The most representative natural polymers are based on the use of polysaccharides, e.g., chitosan and hyaluronic acid, and proteins, e.g., silk fibroin and collagen, whose use as drug delivery systems has been recently reviewed [122].

One of these coatings made of natural compounds, an antibiotic-loaded autologous blood glue [113], has attracted attention due to its enormous biocompatibility. This autologous blood glue is composed of a mixture of thrombin, platelet-rich plasma, and bone marrow aspirate and could therefore be loaded with gentamicin and become an antibacterial glue [113]. Several studies have evaluated the antibacterial efficacy of hybrid coatings made of biodegradable polymer and non-biodegradable material. Among them, it is important to consider gentamicin-loaded PLGA and hydroxyapatite, which improve the osteointegration of bone surrounding the implant [99]; vancomycin-loaded gelatin and mesoporous silica nanoparticles, which can carry antibiotic more efficiently [105]; and more complex coatings composed of agarose and nanocrystalline apatite for improved osseointegration, and with mesoporous silica nanoparticles loaded with cephalexin and vascular endothelial growth factor, able to promote vascularization surrounding the implant [123]. Hydroxyapatite coatings favor osteosynthesis [94,107] and prevent the development of fibrous tissue [124] surrounding the implant.

There are two marketed products based on the antibiotic-loaded degradable coating for titanium implants: gentamicin poly (D, L-lactide) (PLLA) coating, and a fast-resorbable hydrogel coating composed of covalently linked hyaluronan and PLLA. Gentamicin PLLA coating is based on a fully resorbable PLLA matrix loaded with gentamicin sulphate which releases 80% of its antibiotic load within the first 48 h [125]. Gentamicin PLLA coating is named PROtect Coating and is only marketed coating Expert Tibial Nail (DePuy Synthes, Bettlach, Switzerland). Though its use is limited to tibial intramedullary nail, it might be theoretically used on any titanium implant. In the first prospective study, Fuchs et al. [126] demonstrated that none of the 19 patients with closed or open tibial fractures who completed the 6-month follow-up showed implant-related infections. Similar results were obtained by Metsemakers et al. [98] in a single-center case series, where they demonstrated again its capacity of preventing implant-related infections in 16 patients with complex open tibia fracture and revision cases after an 18-month follow-up, but they also reported 25% of patients showed a nonunion, and 6.25% of them was a revision case. Finally, the most recent and largest study performed by Schmidmaier et al. [127] in a multicenter study analyzed the outcome of 99 patients with fresh open or closed tibial fractures or undergoing nonunion revision surgery. After an 18-month follow-up, deep SSI or osteomyelitis was only noted in 7.2% of patients after fresh fracture and in 7.7% of patients after revision surgery.

Fast-resorbable hydrogel coating is composed of covalently linked hyaluronan and PLLA and is marketed as Defensive Antibacterial Coating (DAC) (Novagenit Srl, Mezzolombardo, Italy). DAC is the first antimicrobial hydrogel specifically designed to avoid implant-related infections in orthopaedic surgery and trauma, dentistry, and maxillofacial surgery [128,129]. Its antimicrobial ability is due to the hyaluronic-based compounds that reduce microbial adhesion and biofilm formation of both bacteria and yeasts [130]. Moreover, the DAC has demonstrated itself to be capable of entrapping several antibacterial agents at concentrations ranging from 2–10%, released locally for up to 72 h [128]. The safety and efficacy of DAC have been demonstrated by using rabbit models that revealed the capacity of the vancomycin-loaded hydrogel to prevent implant-related infection [131,132]. In a further rabbit model, vancomycin-loaded DAC-coated implants showed no detrimental effects on the bone healing and implant osteointegration [133]. In the first large multicenter randomized prospective clinical trial reported by Romanò et al. [134], a total of 380 patients were included. The patients were randomly dived into two groups which received an implant with the DAC intraoperatively loaded with antibiotics (gentamicin, vancomycin, or vancomycin plus meropenem) or without the coating (control group). Overall, 96.5% of patients were available at a mean follow-up of 14.5 ± 5.5 months. Eleven SSIs were diagnosed in the control group (6%), whilst only one was observed in the treatment group (0.6%). Any patient from the treatment group showed no local or systemic side effects related to or detectable interference with implant osteointegration. In another multicenter prospective study performed by Malizos et al. [135], 256 patients undergoing osteosynthesis surgery for a closed fracture were randomly assigned to receive the DAC loaded with antibiotics (gentamicin, vancomycin, or vancomycin plus meropenem) or to a control group without coating. Six SSIs (4.6%) were observed in the control group compared with none (0%) in the treatment group after a mean follow-up of 18.1 ± 4.5 months. As in the previous study, any patient from the treatment group showed no local or systemic side effects related to or detectable interference with implant osseointegration.

Trentinaglia et al. [136] have recently described an algorithm to calculate the cost-effectiveness of different antibacterial coating strategies applied to joint prostheses, considering both direct and indirect hospital costs. According to their model, an antibacterial coating able to decrease post-surgical infection by 80%, at a cost per patient of EUR 600, would reduce hospital costs by EUR 200 per patient if routinely applied in a population that would theoretically show an expected PJI rate of 2% [137]. At a European level, considering that approximately 2.2 million joint arthroplasties are performed per year, they speculate that a year of delay in the routine use of this kind of coating would result in 35,200 PJI cases per year with associated annual costs of approximately EUR 440 million per year [137].

4.3. *The Antibiotic of Choice for Local Antibiotic-Based Therapy*

The use of almost any antibiotic in clinical practice is always followed by the development of resistant organisms, and the case of antibiotic-loaded titanium surfaces is not an exception. Antimicrobial resistance is the result of three major factors: (1) the increasing frequency of antimicrobial-resistant phenotypes among microbes resulting from selective pressure exerted by the widespread use of antimicrobials; (2) globalization, which favors the rapid spread of pathogens worldwide; and (3) improper use of antibiotics [138].

The antibiotic of choice for local antibiotic-based therapy should ideally be a broad-spectrum antibiotic that is the least allergenic possible and with no local adverse effects or cytotoxicity; furthermore, these antibiotics should not interfere with osseointegration or be essential for the treatment of PJI [56]. Most of the local antibiotics of choice are broad-spectrum antibiotics used in monotherapy, concretely gentamycin, tobramycin, and vancomycin. To date, there is no antibiotic that is evolution-proof [139,140], as any antibiotic monotherapy is associated with the emergence of antibiotic resistance to that particular antibiotic. This has been described previously, for instance, when a gentamicin-loaded spacer was used in a two-stage replacement which favored the emergence of gentamicin-resistant *S. aureus* [141] and *S. epidermidis* [142]. Therefore, the best prophylactic therapy should be based on the use of at least two antibiotics from different antibiotic families, as a handful of studies have done [76,94,108,143]. The microorganisms tested are staphylococci and, to a lesser extent, Gram-negative bacteria, such as *E. coli* and *P. aeruginosa*. Given the incidence of PJI (up to 40%) [144], Gram-negative bacteria should always be prevented by the local antibiotic approach.

5. Local Preventive Heavy Metals-Based Strategies

The increasing prevalence of antibiotic resistance among bacteria resulting in the selective pressure which the widespread use of antibiotics exerts on them, the globalization, and the inadequate use of antibiotics in many different settings [138] threaten to completely impede the development of an ideal preventive antibiotic therapy for any type of infection. Given this scenario, new non-antibiotic antimicrobials are gaining increasing importance in the field of PJI prevention strategies (Table 4).

Metals have been used by the Persians, Phoenicians, Greeks, Romans, and Egyptians for their antimicrobial properties for thousands of years [145,146]. Despite the fact that the exact mechanism involved in their broad-spread antibacterial mechanism remains unknown, metals show a higher number of unspecific targets within the bacteria, unlike the antibiotic, which is directly related to a reduced not null emergence of metal resistance. These targets are attacked by metallic cations and/or reactive oxygen species generated by both cations and by metallic oxide [147]. Thereby, the main antibacterial mechanisms of metals that show an antibacterial effect per se can be grouped into four categories: (outer and/or cytoplasmatic) membrane damage, protein blocking/inactivation, protein synthesis blocking, and DNA damage [145] (Figure 2). Different strategies have incorporated heavy metals into titanium surfaces. The main heavy metals used to provide titanium alloys with antimicrobial capacity are silver, copper, and gallium. The type of surface modification used to incorporate the metal on the titanium surfaces are mainly metallurgical addition, co-sputtering, ion implantation, and coatings.

Table 4. Some of the most relevant studies based on heavy metals incorporation for titanium implants.

Year	Type of Surface Modification	Incorporated Metal	Metal Incorporation	Bacteria Evaluated	Bacterial State	Cytotoxicity (%)	Level Study	Cell Lines/Animal Used In Vivo	Reference
2009	Metallurgical addition	Cu	Forge	SA, EC	Planktonic/ biofilm	Ctyocompatible	In vitro/ in vivo	V79 cell line/rabbits	[148]
2010	Co-sputtering	Cu-Mn-O, Ag-Mn-O	ternary and quaternary oxides	SA, SE	Planktonic	-	In vitro	-	[149]
	Single step silver plasma immersion ion implantation	Ag	Nanoparticles	SA, EC	Planktonic	Cytocompatible	In vitro	MG63 human osteoblast-like cells	[150]
2011	TiO_2-chitosan/heparin coating	Ag	Nanoparticles	SA	Biofilm	-	In vivo	-	[151]
	Hydroxyapatite coating	Ag	Nanoparticles	EC	Planktonic	-	In vitro	-	[152]
2013	Metallurgical addition	Cu	Powder metallurgy	SA, EC	Planktonic	-	In vitro	-	[153]
	Titanium nanotubular	Ag	Nanoparticle loading	SA, EC	Planktonic	-	In vitro	-	[154]
	Polydopamine-modified alloy surface	Ag	Silver inonic inmobilization	EC	Planktonic	-	In vitro	-	[155]
	Poly(ethylene glycol diacrylate)-co-acrylic acid coating	Ag	Nanoparticles	SA, EC, PA	Planktonic	Cytocompatible	In vitro	MG63 human osteoblast-like cells	[156]
2014	Metallurgical addition	Cu	Powder metallurgy	SA, EC	Planktonic	-	In vitro	-	[157]
	Metallurgical addition	Cu	Casting with post-treatment	SA, EC	Planktonic	Cytocompatible	In vitro	L929 cell line	[158]
	BMP-2/heparinchitosan-hydroxyapatite coating	Ag	Nanoparticles	SE, EC	Planktonic	Cytocompatible	In vitro	MC3T3-E1 cells, BMS cells	[159]
	Aminosilanized titanium alloy	Ag	Nanoparticles	SA	Planktonic	-	In vitro	-	[160]
2016	Metallurgical addition	Ag	Sintering	SA	Planktonic	-	In vitro	-	[161]
2017	Metallurgical addition	Ag	Sintering, casting, casting with appropiate post-treatment w/o surface tretament	SA	Planktonic	Cytocompatible	In vitro	MC3T3-E1 cells	[162]
2018	Metallurgical addition	Cu	Powder metallurgy	SA, EC	Planktonic	Cytocompatible	In vitro	HeLa cells	[163]
	Metallurgical addition	Ag	Spark plasma sintering and acid etching	SA	Planktonic	Cytocompatible	In vitro	MC3T3-E1 cells	[164]
	Metallurgical addition	Cu	Casting with post-treatment	SA	Planktonic	-	In vitro	-	[165]
2019	Metallurgical addition	Cu	Sintering	SA	Biofilm	-	In vivo	-	[166]
	Metallurgical addition	Ga	Powder metallurgy	MRSA	Planktonic/ biofilm	Cytocompatible	In vitro	ATCC CRL-11372 and ATCC HTB-96	[167]

Table 4. *Cont.*

Year	Type of Surface Modification	Incorporated Metal	Metal Incorporation	Bacteria Evaluated	Bacterial State	Cytotoxicity (%)	Level Study	Cell Lines/Animal Used In Vivo	Reference
2020	Metallurgical addition	Cu	Microwave sintering	SA, EC	Planktonic	-	In vitro	-	[168]
	Metallurgical addition	Cu	Powder metallurgy	EC	Planktonic	-	In vitro	-	[169]
	Metallurgical addition	Ag	Casting with appropiate post-treatment w/o surface tretament	SA	Planktonic	Cytocompatible	In vitro	MC3T3-E1 cells	[170]
2021	Metallurgical addition	Cu	As-cast	SA	Biofilm	-	In vitro/ in vivo	Mouse	[171]
	Metallurgical addition	Cu	As-cast	MRSA	Planktonic/ biofilm	Cytocompatible	In vitro/ in vivo	MC3T3-E1 cells/rat	[172]

Abbreviations: BMP-2: bone morphology protein-2; BMS: bone marrow stromal cells.

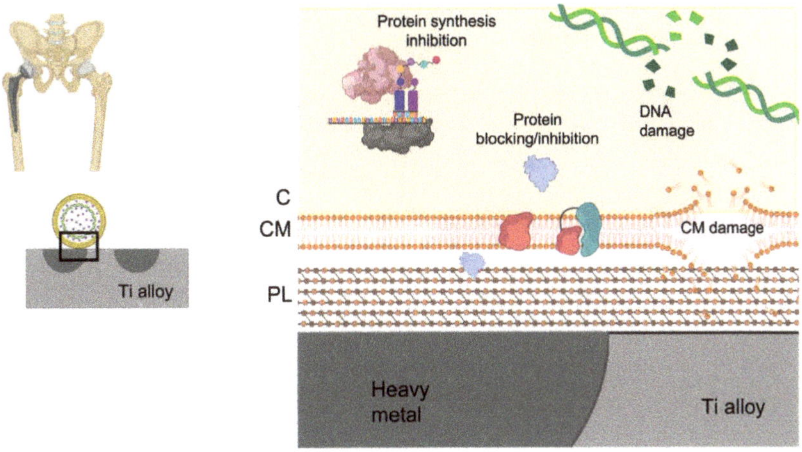

Figure 2. Main antibacterial mechanisms of heavy metals. PL: peptidoglycan layer. CM: cytoplasmatic membrane. C: cytoplasm.

Regarding the use of these metallic-based titanium alloy surface modifications in patients, it is noteworthy that there are no comparative or prospective studies and only retrospective cases of series have been published. Only silver has been proven in humans and has shown low infection risk in clinical studies. There are two technologies marketed nowadays for incorporated silver into titanium alloys: anodization and galvanic deposition. Titanium alloy prostheses with silver incorporated by anodizing is marketed under the name Agluna® (Accentus Medical, Oxfordshire, UK). Anodizing gives rise to the formation of 5 µm diameter circular tanks in the surface of the prosthesis, containing an amorphous titania species where the bulk of the ionic silver is stored. Silver galvanic deposition into titanium alloy prostheses is marketed under the name MUTARS® (tumor system components; Implantcast GmbH, Buxtehude, Germany). Its technology consists of a 15 $\pm$ 5 µm-thick silver coating deposited by galvanic deposition on a 200 nm layer of gold that acts as a carrier and bonding layer to the prosthesis. Recently, Deng et al. [173] have pointed out that some factors might underestimate the real anti-infective effect of silver-modified prostheses in clinical studies. First, most of indications published vouch for the use of this type of prosthesis in immunocompromised patients, those with musculoskeletal tumors [174–177] and/or with a previous PJI [175,176,178], and patients who are themselves more vulnerable to developing PJI [179]. Second, the antibiotherapy is usually administered to all patients, whether or not they carry silver-modified prostheses.

The use of heavy metals for PJI prevention may just be getting started, thus new promising metallic candidates with antimicrobial capacity are yet to be employed. This is the case for metals such as nickel [180,181], cerium [182], selenium [183,184], cesium [185], yttrium [186], palladium [187,188], or superparamagnetic Fe NPs [189].

6. Limitations Associated with Local PJI Prevention

Despite all the potential benefits offered by local prevention strategies for prosthetic joint infections, each has several limitations associated with its use. The advantages and disadvantages related to each preventive approach of PJI are summarized in Table 5.

Table 5. Some of the most important advantages and disadvantages related to each preventive approach of PJI.

Preventive Approach of PJI	Advantages	Disadvantages
Antibiotic-based strategies		
Nanostructured titanium surfaces	Possibility of increasing the osteointegration of the titanium surfaces	Reduced durability of antibiotic protection
		Unknown biomechanical stability
	Loaded antibiotic can act against both bacteria directly adhered on the titanium surface and bacteria near but not in contact with it	Unknown effects on the useful life of the implant, osteointegration, and coagulation profile
		Impossibility of intra-operative antibiotic load No clinical trials to support their use
Antibiotics covalently bound to titanium surfaces	Long durability of antibiotic protection, up to months or years	Loaded antibiotic can only act against bacteria directly adhered on the titanium surface
		Unknown durability of antibiotic protection
		Impossibility of intra-operative antibiotic load
		No clinical trials to support their use
Coatings loaded with antibiotic for titanium alloys	Possibility of increasing the osteointegration of the titanium surfaces	Incomplete surface protection
	Loaded antibiotic can act against both bacteria directly adhered on the titanium surface and bacteria near but not in contact with it	Unknown effects on the useful life of the implant, osteointegration, and coagulation profile
	Possibility of intra-operative antibiotic load	
	Clinical trials to support their use	Clinical trials that support their use has been carried out with few antibiotics
Heavy metals-based strategies	Broad spectrum antimicrobial effect (beyond antibacterial effect)	Local and systemic toxicity supported by clinical trials
	Loaded metals can act against both microorganisms directly adhered on the titanium surface and those near but not in contact with it	
	Long durability	
	Clinical trials to support their use	

Titanium nanotubular surfaces have at least five limitations. Firstly, the low drug concentration resulting from sustained release in a non-bacteria environment consumes antibiotic reserves and increases the possibility of developing drug-resistant bacteria in the vicinity of the implant [58]. Therefore, the ideal antibiotic release of a nanotube-based approach should terminate after the infection is eliminated until the next stimulus [58]. This perspective would require the use of self-responsive nanotubes able to release antibiotics before different infection scenarios. Secondly, any metallic implant in the human body degrades due to at least four fundamental phenomena: leaching, wear, corrosion, as well as the phenomenon resulting from the synergy between the latter two, tribocorrosion. Wear studies about the properties of nanostructured titanium surfaces are scarce, and it is known that wear proprieties of nanotubular titanium surfaces have to be hypothetically different as non-nanostructured surface and these nanostructures can be damaged during the prosthesis implantation; nanostructures pulled from the surface could act as debris, able to cause an aseptic loosening [190]. Nanotube fabrication increases the surface area and hence the corrodible area. Corrosion studies of Ti-6Al-4V implants in patients showed that the detection of elevated levels of titanium and normal levels of aluminum and vanadium (relative to a control group without loosening) in the serum or urine of wearers of a prosthesis made of this alloy was associated with the existence of aseptic loosening [191–194]. Thirdly, nothing is known about the repercussions that this corrosion may have on the useful life of the implant or its osseointegration. Fourthly, the current load methods require the employment of specific equipment (vacuum ovens, agitators, etc.) and long loading times, which make it impossible to load them in the operating theatre for the time being. Fifthly, this approach has no clinical trials to support its widespread use in humans and marketing.

Regarding antibiotics covalently bound to titanium surfaces, there are also important limitations associated with this approach. Unlike nanostructured surface, the antibiotics covalently bound to surfaces are not released into the milieu, and thus can only exert their action on bacteria in direct contact with the modified surface. There is no information about the exact durability of their protection or the hypothetical effect of the release of chemically modified antibiotic on the target bacteria and its role on the emergence of antibiotic resistance. The chemical reaction needed for obtaining these surfaces makes the intra-operative antibiotic load impossible. Finally, there are no clinical trials to back up their use in humans.

Antibiotic-loaded coatings also show limitations. The main limitation is the incomplete protection of the implant, since the intramedullary component of the prosthesis and some modular components (e.g., the acetabular component and the polyethylene insert) cannot be coated. Therefore, an area of susceptibility will exist, where a bacterial infection could proliferate. There is absence of knowledge about the long-term effect that the product resulting from its degradation could exert on the useful life of the implant, its osseointegration, or even, the patient coagulation profile. Although it is the only approach with clinical trials, few antibiotics loaded in such coatings have been used so far.

Heavy metals into titanium surfaces are also associated with some limitations. First, the price of these modified implants is high because they are indicated for a very low number of specific patients [173]. Second, the heavy metals are linked to both local and systemic toxicity. The main side effects of local toxicity are the immunosuppressive effect [195] and the poor or impaired osteointegration that has been reported by both in vitro [196] and in vivo [197] studies. The main systemic side effect related to a titanium alloy surface modified with heavy metals has been described for silver. Argyria, a disease caused by a high silver concentration in the human body, has been reported in up to 23% patients that underwent megaendoprostheses for infection or resection of malignant tumors [198]. In this cohort, no neurological, renal, or hepatic symptoms of silver poisoning were found, and neither a relationship between argyria and the size of the implant or levels of serum silver [198]. Therefore, more studies about the silver intoxication caused by silver-coated implants need to be performed.

Therefore, toxicity is the first concern pertaining to these modifications. With a silver coating, the elevated silver concentration in the blood or in organs has been proven by Gosheger et al. [34], while there were no detectable clinical side effects in this study. The silver ion concentration was lower than the reported harmful concentration, which could be an explanation. Argyria, a disease caused by physiologic silver cation overload, was reported in nearly 22% patients who have received silver-coated prostheses [67]. Therefore, the release of silver ions to the human body after implantation of silver-coated prostheses should be investigated [52]. Impaired osteointegration, which is a special concern for arthroplasty, was generally tested in in vitro co-culture models [68].

Other limitations include the selection of antimicrobial compound. For preventive use, narrow-spectrum antibiotics that cover most potential pathogens are recommended for chemoprophylaxis [36,37]. However, because some antibiotics, such as beta-lactams, can degrade with different factors, such as time or temperature, more stable antibiotics (for example, vancomycin, gentamicin, quinolones) are chosen in many studies. Another important problem not directly related to the biomaterial is the increasing burden of infections caused by antibiotic-resistant microorganisms [8]. The problem of antimicrobial resistance is currently considered one of the most important menaces facing modern medicine [199]. The recent appearance of multidrug-resistant microorganisms has become an extremely important problem with implications for all aspects of medical practice. In orthopaedic surgery, the increasing number of multidrug-resistant organisms, especially Gram-negative organisms, has been described in PJI [8]. This type of infections caused by these microorganisms implies a poor outcome in many cases [200–202]. Even silver or copper as heavy metals representants can give rise to heavy metal-resistant Gram-negative bacteria (mainly *E. coli* and *P. aeruginosa*) [203,204], one of the bacterial groups related with PJI that is increasing its incidence [205].

In this scenario, the selection of the antimicrobials necessary to prevent PJI infections should consider the existence of multidrug-resistant bacteria [206], which emphasizes the need to select a mixture of at least two antibiotics for preventing PJIs or even using more than one of the preventive approaches described here, e.g., an antibiotic-loaded and heavy metal-dopped surface modification, but also drives the search for new strategies based on the use of iodine-doped titanium alloys [207], antimicrobial peptides [208], and bacteriophages [209–211], among others.

7. Conclusions

Research into the development of locally antibiotic therapy approaches is broad and varied, though this review could mark the beginning of a promising journey towards the development of prostheses capable of complete PJI prevention. Despite the numerous preclinical studies that have been conducted, such as those using in vivo models, the move from bench to bedside continues to be hindered by at least two factors, including the low incidence of PJIs and the costs of clinical trials needed to demonstrate the efficacy of these approaches in human beings; indeed, these costs are so high that only large pharmaceutical companies can afford such an investment. These factors may be responsible for the fact that existing multicenter prospective clinical trials are poorly well-structured and often show contradictory or inconclusive results [212]. Thus, the only way patients can benefit from these promising approaches is by improving collaboration between governments, regulatory agencies, industry leaders, and health care payers [213].

Our review highlights that a trend from the antibiotic-loaded surface modifications of the bulk material to the biodegradable antibiotic-load coating can be observed since only two types of these coatings have come to be used in humans. Among heavy metals, silver-modified titanium surfaces are supported by numerous in vitro studies and clinical trials, though other metals such as copper or gallium might stand up as potential future candidates. Furthermore, there is no uniform way of evaluating the efficacy of such approaches. For that, we consider that at least cytotoxicity and cell proliferation should be evaluated in vitro, and that all be tested by using in vivo models. Due to the increasingly threatening emergence of antibiotic resistance, it would therefore be recommendable to use at least two antibiotics or heavy metals for functionalizing the titanium surfaces or antimicrobial substances whose antibacterial mechanisms do not lead to the development of resistant bacterial mutants. Finally, any of the PJI prevention approaches reviewed here are exempt of limitations, many of which should be elucidated by specifically designed studies.

Author Contributions: Conceptualization, J.E. and J.J.A.-C.; writing—original draft preparation, J.E. and J.J.A.-C.; writing—review and editing, J.E., M.V.-R., and J.J.A.-C.; project administration, J.E. and M.V.-R. All authors have read and agreed to the published version of the manuscript.

Funding: This research was partially funded by the European Research Council through an ERC-2015-AdG-694160 (VERDI) grant.

Institutional Review Board Statement: Not applicable.

Informed Consent Statement: Not applicable.

Data Availability Statement: The data presented in this study are available on request from the corresponding author. Some data are not publicly available since some articles are not open access.

Acknowledgments: We wish to acknowledge Oliver Shaw for his help in reviewing the manuscripts for language-related aspects. Figures 1 and 2 have been created with BioRender.com.

Conflicts of Interest: J.E. received travel grants from Pfizer and conference fees from Biomérieux and Heraeus. These funders had no role in the design of the study; in the collection, analyses, or interpretation of data; in the writing of the manuscript; or in the decision to publish the results.

References

1. Hawker, G.A.; Badley, E.M.; Borkhoff, C.M.; Croxford, R.; Davis, A.M.; Dunn, S.; Gignac, M.A.; Jaglal, S.B.; Kreder, H.J.; Sale, J.E.M. Which patients are most likely to benefit from total joint arthroplasty? *Arthritis Rheum.* **2013**, *65*, 1243–1252. [CrossRef] [PubMed]
2. Trampuz, A.; Zimmerli, W. Prosthetic joint infections: Update in diagnosis and treatment. *Swiss Med. Wkly.* **2005**, *135*, 243–251. [PubMed]
3. Garrido-Gómez, J.; Arrabal-Polo, M.A.; Girón-Prieto, M.S.; Cabello-Salas, J.; Torres-Barroso, J.; Parra-Ruiz, J. Descriptive analysis of the economic costs of periprosthetic joint infection of the knee for the public health system of Andalusia. *J. Arthroplasty* **2013**, *28*, 1057–1060. [CrossRef] [PubMed]
4. Dale, H.; Fenstad, A.M.; Hallan, G.; Havelin, L.I.; Furnes, O.; Overgaard, S.; Pedersen, A.B.; Kärrholm, J.; Garellick, G.; Pulkkinen, P.; et al. Increasing risk of prosthetic joint infection after total hip arthroplasty. *Acta Orthop.* **2012**, *83*, 449–458. [CrossRef] [PubMed]
5. Kurtz, S.M.; Lau, E.; Watson, H.; Schmier, J.K.; Parvizi, J. Economic burden of periprosthetic joint infection in the United States. *J. Arthroplasty* **2012**, *27*, 61–65. [CrossRef] [PubMed]
6. Chalmers, B.P.; Weston, J.T.; Osmon, D.R.; Hanssen, A.D.; Berry, D.J.; Abdel, M.P. Prior hip or knee prosthetic joint infection in another joint increases risk three-fold of prosthetic joint infection after primary total knee arthroplasty: A matched control study. *Bone Jt. J.* **2019**, *101*, 91–97. [CrossRef]
7. DeKeyser, G.J.; Anderson, M.B.; Meeks, H.D.; Pelt, C.E.; Peters, C.L.; Gililland, J.M. Socioeconomic status may not be a risk factor for periprosthetic joint infection. *J. Arthroplasty* **2020**, *35*, 1900–1905. [CrossRef]
8. Benito, N.; Franco, M.; Ribera, A.; Soriano, A.; Rodriguez-Pardo, D.; Sorlí, L.; Fresco, G.; Fernández-Sampedro, M.; del Toro, D.M.; Guío, L.; et al. Time trends in the aetiology of prosthetic joint infections: A multicentre cohort study. *Clin. Microbiol. Infect.* **2016**, *22*, 732.e1–732.e8. [CrossRef]
9. Benito, N.; Mur, I.; Ribera, A.; Soriano, A.; Rodríguez-Pardo, D.; Sorlí, L.; Cobo, J.; Fernández-Sampedro, M.; del Toro, M.D.; Guío, L.; et al. The different microbial etiology of prosthetic joint infections according to route of acquisition and time after prosthesis implantation, including the role of multidrug-resistant organisms. *J. Clin. Med.* **2019**, *8*, 673. [CrossRef]
10. Villa, J.M.; Pannu, T.S.; Theeb, I.; Buttaro, M.A.; Oñativia, J.I.; Carbo, L.; Rienzi, D.H.; Fregeiro, J.I.; Kornilov, N.N.; Bozhkova, S.A.; et al. International organism profile of periprosthetic total hip and knee infections. *J. Arthroplasty* **2021**, *36*, 274–278. [CrossRef]
11. Iqbal, F.; Shafiq, B.; Zamir, M.; Noor, S.; Memon, N.; Memon, N.; Dina, T.K. Micro-organisms and risk factors associated with prosthetic joint infection following primary total knee replacement-our experience in Pakistan. *Int. Orthop.* **2020**, *44*, 283–289. [CrossRef]
12. Yu, Y.; Kong, Y.; Ye, J.; Wang, A.; Si, W. Microbiological pattern of prosthetic hip and knee infections: A high-volume, single-centre experience in China. *J. Med. Microbiol.* **2021**, *70*. [CrossRef]
13. Tande, A.J.; Patel, R. Prosthetic joint infection. *Clin. Microbiol. Rev.* **2014**, *27*, 302–345. [CrossRef] [PubMed]
14. Tsai, Y.; Chang, C.-H.; Lin, Y.-C.; Lee, S.-H.; Hsieh, P.-H.; Chang, Y. Different microbiological profiles between hip and knee prosthetic joint infections. *J. Orthop. Surg. Hong Kong* **2019**, *27*. [CrossRef]
15. Paxton, E.S.; Green, A.; Krueger, V.S. Periprosthetic infections of the shoulder: Diagnosis and management. *J. Am. Acad. Orthop. Surg.* **2019**, *27*, e935–e944. [CrossRef]

16. Bloom, D.E.; Cadarette, D. Infectious disease threats in the twenty-first century: Strengthening the global response. *Front. Immunol.* **2019**, *10*, 549. [CrossRef] [PubMed]
17. Centers for Disease Control and Prevention (U.S.). *Antibiotic Resistance Threats in the United States, 2019*; Centers for Disease Control and Prevention (U.S.): Atlanta, GA, USA, 2019.
18. Tacconelli, E. Global priority list of antibiotic-resistant bacteria to guide research, discovery, and development of new antibiotics. *World Health Organ.* **2017**, *27*, 318–327.
19. Costerton, J.W.; Lewandowski, Z.; Caldwell, D.E.; Korber, D.R.; Lappin-Scott, H.M. Microbial biofilms. *Annu. Rev. Microbiol.* **1995**, *49*, 711–745. [CrossRef]
20. Diggle, S.P. Microbial communication and virulence: Lessons from evolutionary theory. *Microbiology* **2010**, *156*, 3503–3512. [CrossRef]
21. Nadell, C.D.; Xavier, J.B.; Foster, K.R. The sociobiology of biofilms. *FEMS Microbiol. Rev.* **2009**, *33*, 206–224. [CrossRef]
22. West, S.A.; Griffin, A.S.; Gardner, A.; Diggle, S.P. Social evolution theory for microorganisms. *Nat. Rev. Microbiol.* **2006**, *4*, 597–607. [CrossRef]
23. Monroe, D. Looking for chinks in the armor of bacterial biofilms. *PLoS Biol.* **2007**, *5*, e307. [CrossRef] [PubMed]
24. Høiby, N.; Ciofu, O.; Johansen, H.K.; Song, Z.; Moser, C.; Jensen, P.Ø.; Molin, S.; Givskov, M.; Tolker-Nielsen, T.; Bjarnsholt, T. The clinical impact of bacterial biofilms. *Int. J. Oral Sci.* **2011**, *3*, 55–65. [CrossRef] [PubMed]
25. Donlan, R.M. Biofilms: Microbial life on surfaces. *Emerg. Infect. Dis.* **2002**, *8*, 881–890. [CrossRef]
26. Kostakioti, M.; Hadjifrangiskou, M.; Hultgren, S.J. Bacterial biofilms: Development, dispersal, and therapeutic strategies in the dawn of the postantibiotic era. *Cold Spring Harb. Perspect. Med.* **2013**, *3*, a010306. [CrossRef] [PubMed]
27. Hall-Stoodley, L.; Costerton, J.W.; Stoodley, P. Bacterial biofilms: From the natural environment to infectious diseases. *Nat. Rev. Microbiol.* **2004**, *2*, 95–108. [CrossRef]
28. Otto, M. Staphylococcal Biofilms. *Microbiol. Spectr.* **2018**, *6*. [CrossRef] [PubMed]
29. Otto, M. Staphylococcus Epidermidis—The "accidental" pathogen. *Nat. Rev. Microbiol.* **2009**, *7*, 555–567. [CrossRef]
30. Laverty, G.; Gorman, S.P.; Gilmore, B.F. Biomolecular mechanisms of *Pseudomonas aeruginosa* and *Escherichia coli* biofilm formation. *Pathog. Basel Switz.* **2014**, *3*, 596–632. [CrossRef]
31. Büttner, H.; Mack, D.; Rohde, H. Structural basis of staphylococcus epidermidis biofilm formation: Mechanisms and molecular interactions. *Front. Cell. Infect. Microbiol.* **2015**, *5*, 14. [CrossRef]
32. McConoughey, S.J.; Howlin, R.; Granger, J.F.; Manring, M.M.; Calhoun, J.H.; Shirtliff, M.; Kathju, S.; Stoodley, P. Biofilms in periprosthetic orthopedic infections. *Future Microbiol.* **2014**, *9*, 987–1007. [CrossRef] [PubMed]
33. Flemming, H.-C.; Wingender, J.; Szewzyk, U.; Steinberg, P.; Rice, S.A.; Kjelleberg, S. Biofilms: An emergent form of bacterial life. *Nat. Rev. Microbiol.* **2016**, *14*, 563–575. [CrossRef] [PubMed]
34. Valour, F.; Trouillet-Assant, S.; Rasigade, J.-P.; Lustig, S.; Chanard, E.; Meugnier, H.; Tigaud, S.; Vandenesch, F.; Etienne, J.; Ferry, T.; et al. Staphylococcus epidermidis in orthopedic device infections: The role of bacterial internalization in human osteoblasts and biofilm formation. *PLoS ONE* **2013**, *8*, e67240. [CrossRef]
35. Ierano, C.; Stewardson, A.J.; Peel, T. *Prosthetic Joint Infections*; Peel, T., Ed.; Springer International Publishing: Berlin, Germany, 2018; ISBN 978-3-319-65249-8.
36. Berríos-Torres, S.I.; Umscheid, C.A.; Bratzler, D.W.; Leas, B.; Stone, E.C.; Kelz, R.R.; Reinke, C.E.; Morgan, S.; Solomkin, J.S.; Mazuski, J.E.; et al. Centers for disease control and prevention guideline for the prevention of surgical site infection, 2017. *JAMA Surg.* **2017**, *152*, 784–791. [CrossRef] [PubMed]
37. World Health Organization. *Global Guidelines for the Prevention of Surgical Site Infection*; WHO: Geneva, Switzerland, 2016; ISBN 978-92-4-154988-2.
38. Levy, D.M.; Wetters, N.G.; Levine, B.R. Prevention of periprosthetic joint infections of the hip and knee. *Am. J. Orthop. Belle Mead NJ* **2016**, *45*, E299–E307.
39. Alamanda, V.K.; Springer, B.D. The prevention of infection. *Bone Jt. J.* **2019**, *101*, 3–9. [CrossRef]
40. Berbari, E.; Segreti, J.; Parvizi, J.; Berríos-Torres, S.I. Future research opportunities in peri-prosthetic joint infection prevention. *Surg. Infect.* **2017**, *18*, 409–412. [CrossRef]
41. Goswami, K.; Stevenson, K.L.; Parvizi, J. Intraoperative and postoperative infection prevention. *J. Arthroplasty* **2020**, *35*, S2–S8. [CrossRef]
42. General Assembly. Available online: https://icmphilly.com/general-assembly/ (accessed on 26 April 2021).
43. Iannotti, F.; Prati, P.; Fidanza, A.; Iorio, R.; Ferretti, A.; Pèrez Prieto, D.; Kort, N.; Violante, B.; Pipino, G.; Schiavone Panni, A.; et al. Prevention of Periprosthetic joint infection (PJI): A clinical practice protocol in high-risk patients. *Trop. Med. Infect. Dis.* **2020**, *5*, 186. [CrossRef]
44. Jämsen, E.; Furnes, O.; Engesaeter, L.B.; Konttinen, Y.T.; Odgaard, A.; Stefánsdóttir, A.; Lidgren, L. Prevention of deep infection in joint replacement surgery. *Acta Orthop.* **2010**, *81*, 660–666. [CrossRef]
45. Siddiqi, A.; Forte, S.A.; Docter, S.; Bryant, D.; Sheth, N.P.; Chen, A.F. Perioperative antibiotic prophylaxis in total joint arthroplasty: A systematic review and meta-analysis. *J. Bone Jt. Surg. Am.* **2019**, *101*, 828–842. [CrossRef]
46. Del Pozo, J.L.; Patel, R. Clinical practice. Infection associated with prosthetic joints. *N. Engl. J. Med.* **2009**, *361*, 787–794. [CrossRef] [PubMed]
47. Fillingham, Y.; Greenwald, A.S.; Greiner, J.; Oshkukov, S.; Parsa, A.; Porteous, A.; Squire, M.W. Hip and knee section, prevention, local antimicrobials: Proceedings of international consensus on orthopedic infections. *J. Arthroplasty* **2019**, *34*, S289–S292. [CrossRef]
48. Baeza, J.; Cury, M.B.; Fleischman, A.; Ferrando, A.; Fuertes, M.; Goswami, K.; Lidgren, L.; Linke, P.; Manrique, J.; Makar, G.; et al. General assembly, prevention, local antimicrobials: Proceedings of international consensus on orthopedic infections. *J. Arthroplasty* **2019**, *34*, S75–S84. [CrossRef]

49. Schiavone Panni, A.; Corona, K.; Giulianelli, M.; Mazzitelli, G.; del Regno, C.; Vasso, M. Antibiotic-loaded bone cement reduces risk of infections in primary total knee arthroplasty? A systematic review. *Knee Surg. Sports Traumatol. Arthrosc. Off. J. ESSKA* **2016**, *24*, 3168–3174. [CrossRef]
50. Schmitt, D.R.; Killen, C.; Murphy, M.; Perry, M.; Romano, J.; Brown, N. The impact of antibiotic-loaded bone cement on antibiotic resistance in periprosthetic knee infections. *Clin. Orthop. Surg.* **2020**, *12*, 318–323. [CrossRef] [PubMed]
51. Wall, V.; Nguyen, T.-H.; Nguyen, N.; Tran, P.A. Controlling antibiotic release from polymethylmethacrylate bone cement. *Biomedicines* **2021**, *9*, 26. [CrossRef] [PubMed]
52. García-Gareta, E.; Davidson, C.; Levin, A.; Coathup, M.J.; Blunn, G.W. Biofilm formation in total hip arthroplasty: Prevention and treatment. *RSC Adv.* **2016**, *6*, 80244–80261. [CrossRef]
53. Rakow, A.; Perka, C.; Trampuz, A.; Renz, N. Origin and Characteristics of Haematogenous Periprosthetic Joint Infection. *Clinical Microbiology and Infection* **2019**, *25*, 845–850. [CrossRef]
54. Zimmerli, W.; Trampuz, A.; Ochsner, P.E. Prosthetic-joint infections. *N. Engl. J. Med.* **2004**, *351*, 1645–1654. [CrossRef] [PubMed]
55. Geetha, M.; Singh, A.K.; Asokamani, R.; Gogia, A.K. Ti based biomaterials, the ultimate choice for orthopaedic implants—A review. *Prog. Mater. Sci.* **2009**, *54*, 397–425. [CrossRef]
56. Campoccia, D.; Montanaro, L.; Speziale, P.; Arciola, C.R. Antibiotic-loaded biomaterials and the risks for the spread of antibiotic resistance following their prophylactic and therapeutic clinical use. *Biomaterials* **2010**, *31*, 6363–6377. [CrossRef]
57. Romanò, C.L.; Petrosillo, N.; Argento, G.; Sconfienza, L.M.; Treglia, G.; Alavi, A.; Glaudemans, A.W.J.M.; Gheysens, O.; Maes, A.; Lauri, C.; et al. The role of imaging techniques to define a peri-prosthetic hip and knee joint infection: Multidisciplinary consensus statements. *J. Clin. Med.* **2020**, *9*, 2548. [CrossRef] [PubMed]
58. Li, Y.; Yang, Y.; Li, R.; Tang, X.; Guo, D.; Qing, Y.; Qin, Y. Enhanced antibacterial properties of orthopedic implants by titanium nanotube surface modification: A review of current techniques. *Int. J. Nanomed.* **2019**, *14*, 7217–7236. [CrossRef] [PubMed]
59. Fu, Y.; Mo, A. A review on the electrochemically self-organized titania nanotube arrays: Synthesis, modifications, and biomedical applications. *Nanoscale Res. Lett.* **2018**, *13*, 187. [CrossRef]
60. López Zavala, M.Á.; Lozano Morales, S.A.; Ávila-Santos, M. Synthesis of stable TiO_2 nanotubes: Effect of hydrothermal treatment, acid washing and annealing temperature. *Heliyon* **2017**, *3*, e00456. [CrossRef]
61. Xie, Y. Photoelectrochemical application of nanotubular titania photoanode. *Electrochim. Acta* **2006**, *51*, 3399–3406. [CrossRef]
62. Cheng, Y.; Feng, G.; Moraru, C.I. Micro- and nanotopography sensitive bacterial attachment mechanisms: A review. *Front. Microbiol.* **2019**, *10*, 191. [CrossRef]
63. Puckett, S.D.; Taylor, E.; Raimondo, T.; Webster, T.J. The relationship between the nanostructure of titanium surfaces and bacterial attachment. *Biomaterials* **2010**, *31*, 706–713. [CrossRef] [PubMed]
64. Bartlet, K.; Movafaghi, S.; Dasi, L.P.; Kota, A.K.; Popat, K.C. Antibacterial activity on superhydrophobic titania nanotube arrays. *Colloids Surf. B Biointerfaces* **2018**, *166*, 179–186. [CrossRef]
65. Arenas, M.A.; Pérez-Jorge, C.; Conde, A.; Matykina, E.; Hernández-López, J.M.; Pérez-Tanoira, R.; de Damborenea, J.J.; Gómez-Barrena, E.; Esteba, J. Doped TiO_2 anodic layers of enhanced antibacterial properties. *Colloids Surf. B Biointerfaces* **2013**, *105*, 106–112. [CrossRef]
66. Aguilera-Correa, J.-J.; Mediero, A.; Conesa-Buendía, F.-M.; Conde, A.; Arenas, M.-Á.; de-Damborenea, J.-J.; Esteban, J. Microbiological and cellular evaluation of a fluorine-phosphorus-doped titanium alloy, a novel antibacterial and osteostimulatory biomaterial with potential applications in orthopedic surgery. *Appl. Environ. Microbiol.* **2018**, *85*, e02271-18. [CrossRef]
67. Perez-Jorge, C.; Arenas, M.-A.; Conde, A.; Hernández-Lopez, J.-M.; de Damborenea, J.-J.; Fisher, S.; Hunt, A.M.A.; Esteban, J.; James, G. Bacterial and fungal biofilm formation on anodized titanium alloys with fluorine. *J. Mater. Sci. Mater. Med.* **2017**, *28*, 8. [CrossRef]
68. Lozano, D.; Hernández-López, J.M.; Esbrit, P.; Arenas, M.A.; Gómez-Barrena, E.; de Damborenea, J.; Esteban, J.; Pérez-Jorge, C.; Pérez-Tanoira, R.; Conde, A. Influence of the nanostructure of F-doped TiO_2 films on osteoblast growth and function: Influence of the nanostructure of F-doped TiO_2 films. *J. Biomed. Mater. Res. A* **2015**, *103*, 1985–1990. [CrossRef]
69. Aguilera-Correa, J.-J.; Auñón, Á.; Boiza-Sánchez, M.; Mahillo-Fernández, I.; Mediero, A.; Eguibar-Blázquez, D.; Conde, A.; Arenas, M.-Á.; de-Damborenea, J.-J.; Cordero-Ampuero, J.; et al. Urine aluminum concentration as a possible implant biomarker of *Pseudomonas aeruginosa* Infection using a fluorine- and phosphorus-doped Ti-6Al-4V alloy with osseointegration capacity. *ACS Omega* **2019**, *4*, 11815–11823. [CrossRef]
70. Ercan, B.; Taylor, E.; Alpaslan, E.; Webster, T.J. Diameter of titanium nanotubes influences anti-bacterial efficacy. *Nanotechnology* **2011**, *22*, 295102. [CrossRef]
71. Lin, W.; Tan, H.; Duan, Z.; Yue, B.; Ma, R.; He, G.; Tang, T. Inhibited bacterial biofilm formation and improved osteogenic activity on gentamicin-loaded titania nanotubes with various diameters. *Int. J. Nanomed.* **2014**, *9*, 1215–1230. [CrossRef]
72. Feng, W.; Geng, Z.; Li, Z.; Cui, Z.; Zhu, S.; Liang, Y.; Liu, Y.; Wang, R.; Yang, X. Controlled release behaviour and antibacterial effects of antibiotic-loaded titania nanotubes. *Mater. Sci. Eng. C Mater. Biol. Appl.* **2016**, *62*, 105–112. [CrossRef]
73. Liu, D.; He, C.; Liu, Z.; Xu, W. Gentamicin coating of nanotubular anodized titanium implant reduces implant-related osteomyelitis and enhances bone biocompatibility in rabbits. *Int. J. Nanomed.* **2017**, *12*, 5461–5471. [CrossRef] [PubMed]
74. Yuan, Z.; Huang, S.; Lan, S.; Xiong, H.; Tao, B.; Ding, Y.; Liu, Y.; Liu, P.; Cai, K. Surface Engineering of titanium implants with enzyme-triggered antibacterial properties and enhanced osseointegration in vivo. *J. Mater. Chem. B* **2018**, *6*, 8090–8104. [CrossRef]
75. Zhang, H.; Wang, G.; Liu, P.; Tong, D.; Ding, C.; Zhang, Z.; Xie, Y.; Tang, H.; Ji, F. Vancomycin-loaded titanium coatings with an interconnected micro-patterned structure for prophylaxis of infections: An in vivo study. *RSC Adv.* **2018**, *8*, 9223–9231. [CrossRef]

76. Auñón, Á.; Esteban, J.; Doadrio, A.L.; Boiza-Sánchez, M.; Mediero, A.; Eguibar-Blázquez, D.; Cordero-Ampuero, J.; Conde, A.; Arenas, M.; de-Damborenea, J.; et al. *Staphylococcus aureus* prosthetic joint infection is prevented by a fluorine- and phosphorus-doped nanostructured Ti–6Al–4V alloy loaded with gentamicin and vancomycin. *J. Orthop. Res.* **2020**, *38*, 588–597. [CrossRef]
77. Aguilera-Correa, J.-J.; Doadrio, A.L.; Conde, A.; Arenas, M.-A.; de-Damborenea, J.-J.; Vallet-Regí, M.; Esteban, J. Antibiotic release from F-doped nanotubular oxide layer on TI6AL4V alloy to decrease bacterial viability. *J. Mater. Sci. Mater. Med.* **2018**, *29*, 118. [CrossRef]
78. Xu, Q.A.; Trissel, L.A.; Saenz, C.A.; Ingram, D.S. Stability of gentamicin sulfate and tobramycin sulfate in autodose infusion system bags. *Int. J. Pharm. Compd.* **2002**, *6*, 152–154.
79. Mullins, N.D.; Deadman, B.J.; Moynihan, H.A.; McCarthy, F.O.; Lawrence, S.E.; Thompson, J.; Maguire, A.R. The impact of storage conditions upon gentamicin coated antimicrobial implants. *J. Pharm. Anal.* **2016**, *6*, 374–381. [CrossRef]
80. Melichercik, P.; Klapkova, E.; Landor, I.; Judl, T.; Sibek, M.; Jahoda, D. The effect of vancomycin degradation products in the topical treatment of osteomyelitis. *Bratisl. Lek. Listy* **2014**, *115*, 796–799. [CrossRef]
81. Mousset, B.; Benoit, M.A.; Delloye, C.; Bouillet, R.; Gillard, J. Biodegradable implants for potential use in bone infection. An in vitro study of antibiotic-loaded calcium sulphate. *Int. Orthop.* **1995**, *19*, 157–161. [CrossRef] [PubMed]
82. Chouirfa, H.; Bouloussa, H.; Migonney, V.; Falentin-Daudré, C. Review of titanium surface modification techniques and coatings for antibacterial applications. *Acta Biomater.* **2019**, *83*, 37–54. [CrossRef]
83. Chen, C.-W.; Hsu, C.-Y.; Lai, S.-M.; Syu, W.-J.; Wang, T.-Y.; Lai, P.-S. Metal nanobullets for multidrug resistant bacteria and biofilms. *Adv. Drug Deliv. Rev.* **2014**, *78*, 88–104. [CrossRef]
84. Badar, M.; Rahim, M.I.; Kieke, M.; Ebel, T.; Rohde, M.; Hauser, H.; Behrens, P.; Mueller, P.P. Controlled drug release from antibiotic-loaded layered double hydroxide coatings on porous titanium implants in a mouse model: Antibiotic-loaded layered double hydroxide coatinGS. *J. Biomed. Mater. Res. A* **2015**, *103*, 2141–2149. [CrossRef]
85. Walter, M.S.; Frank, M.J.; Satué, M.; Monjo, M.; Rønold, H.J.; Lyngstadaas, S.P.; Haugen, H.J. Bioactive implant surface with electrochemically bound doxycycline promotes bone formation markers in vitro and in vivo. *Dent. Mater.* **2014**, *30*, 200–214. [CrossRef]
86. Kucharíková, S.; Gerits, E.; de Brucker, K.; Braem, A.; Ceh, K.; Majdič, G.; Španič, T.; Pogorevc, E.; Verstraeten, N.; Tournu, H.; et al. Covalent immobilization of antimicrobial agents on titanium prevents *Staphylococcus aureus* and *Candida albicans* colonization and biofilm formation. *J. Antimicrob. Chemother.* **2016**, *71*, 936–945. [CrossRef] [PubMed]
87. Nie, B.; Long, T.; Ao, H.; Zhou, J.; Tang, T.; Yue, B. Covalent immobilization of enoxacin onto titanium implant surfaces for inhibiting multiple bacterial species infection and In Vivo methicillin-resistant staphylococcus aureus infection prophylaxis. *Antimicrob. Agents Chemother.* **2017**, *61*, e01766-16. [CrossRef]
88. Nie, B.; Ao, H.; Long, T.; Zhou, J.; Tang, T.; Yue, B. Immobilizing bacitracin on titanium for prophylaxis of infections and for improving osteoinductivity: An in vivo study. *Colloids Surf. B Biointerfaces* **2017**, *150*, 183–191. [CrossRef]
89. Gerits, E.; Kucharíková, S.; van Dijck, P.; Erdtmann, M.; Krona, A.; Lövenklev, M.; Fröhlich, M.; Dovgan, B.; Impellizzeri, F.; Braem, A.; et al. Antibacterial activity of a new broad-spectrum antibiotic covalently bound to titanium surfaces. *J. Orthop. Res.* **2016**, *34*, 2191–2198. [CrossRef]
90. Chen, C.-P.; Wickstrom, E. Self-protecting bactericidal titanium alloy surface formed by covalent bonding of daptomycin bisphosphonates. *Bioconjug. Chem.* **2010**, *21*, 1978–1986. [CrossRef]
91. Lawson, M.C.; Hoth, K.C.; Deforest, C.A.; Bowman, C.N.; Anseth, K.S. Inhibition of Staphylococcus epidermidis biofilms using polymerizable vancomycin derivatives. *Clin. Orthop.* **2010**, *468*, 2081–2091. [CrossRef]
92. Mohorcič, M.; Jerman, I.; Zorko, M.; Butinar, L.; Orel, B.; Jerala, R.; Friedrich, J. Surface with antimicrobial activity obtained through silane coating with covalently bound polymyxin B. *J. Mater. Sci. Mater. Med.* **2010**, *21*, 2775–2782. [CrossRef]
93. Moskowitz, J.S.; Blaisse, M.R.; Samuel, R.E.; Hsu, H.-P.; Harris, M.B.; Martin, S.D.; Lee, J.C.; Spector, M.; Hammond, P.T. The effectiveness of the controlled release of gentamicin from polyelectrolyte multilayers in the treatment of *Staphylococcus aureus* infection in a rabbit bone model. *Biomaterials* **2010**, *31*, 6019–6030. [CrossRef] [PubMed]
94. Alt, V.; Kirchhof, K.; Seim, F.; Hrubesch, I.; Lips, K.S.; Mannel, H.; Domann, E.; Schnettler, R. Rifampicin–fosfomycin coating for cementless endoprostheses: Antimicrobial effects against methicillin-sensitive *Staphylococcus aureus* (MSSA) and methicillin-resistant *Staphylococcus aureus* (MRSA). *Acta Biomater.* **2014**, *10*, 4518–4524. [CrossRef] [PubMed]
95. Mattioli-Belmonte, M.; Cometa, S.; Ferretti, C.; Iatta, R.; Trapani, A.; Ceci, E.; Falconi, M.; de Giglio, E. Characterization and cytocompatibility of an antibiotic/chitosan/cyclodextrins nanocoating on titanium implants. *Carbohydr. Polym.* **2014**, *110*, 173–182. [CrossRef] [PubMed]
96. Ordikhani, F.; Tamjid, E.; Simchi, A. Characterization and antibacterial performance of electrodeposited chitosan–vancomycin composite coatings for prevention of implant-associated infections. *Mater. Sci. Eng. C* **2014**, *41*, 240–248. [CrossRef]
97. Zhang, L.; Yan, J.; Yin, Z.; Tang, C.; Guo, Y.; Li, D.; Wei, B.; Gu, Q.; Xu, Y.; Wang, L. Electrospun vancomycin-loaded coating on titanium implants for the prevention of implant-associated infections. *Int. J. Nanomed.* **2014**, *3027*. [CrossRef]
98. Metsemakers, W.-J.; Emanuel, N.; Cohen, O.; Reichart, M.; Potapova, I.; Schmid, T.; Segal, D.; Riool, M.; Kwakman, P.H.S.; de Boer, L.; et al. A doxycycline-loaded polymer-lipid encapsulation matrix coating for the prevention of implant-related osteomyelitis due to doxycycline-resistant methicillin-resistant *Staphylococcus Aureus*. *J. Control. Release* **2015**, *209*, 47–56. [CrossRef]
99. Neut, D.; Dijkstra, R.; Thompson, J.; Kavanagh, C.; van der Mei, H.; Busscher, H. A biodegradable gentamicin-hydroxyapatite-coating for infection prophylaxis in cementless hip prostheses. *Eur. Cell. Mater.* **2015**, *29*, 42–56. [CrossRef]

100. Diefenbeck, M.; Schrader, C.; Gras, F.; Mückley, T.; Schmidt, J.; Zankovych, S.; Bossert, J.; Jandt, K.D.; Völpel, A.; Sigusch, B.W.; et al. Gentamicin coating of plasma chemical oxidized titanium alloy prevents implant-related osteomyelitis in rats. *Biomaterials* **2016**, *101*, 156–164. [CrossRef]
101. Jennings, J.A.; Beenken, K.E.; Skinner, R.A.; Meeker, D.G.; Smeltzer, M.S.; Haggard, W.O.; Troxel, K.S. Antibiotic-loaded phosphatidylcholine inhibits staphylococcal bone infection. *World J. Orthop.* **2016**, *7*, 467. [CrossRef]
102. Ma, K.; Cai, X.; Zhou, Y.; Wang, Y.; Jiang, T. In vitro and in vivo evaluation of tetracycline loaded chitosan-gelatin nanosphere coatings for titanium surface functionalization. *Macromol. Biosci.* **2017**, *17*, 1600130. [CrossRef]
103. Song, W.; Seta, J.; Chen, L.; Bergum, C.; Zhou, Z.; Kanneganti, P.; Kast, R.E.; Auner, G.W.; Shen, M.; Markel, D.C.; et al. Doxycycline-loaded coaxial nanofiber coating of titanium implants enhances osseointegration and inhibits *Staphylococcus Aureus* infection. *Biomed. Mater.* **2017**, *12*, 045008. [CrossRef]
104. Cheng, T.; Qu, H.; Zhang, G.; Zhang, X. Osteogenic and antibacterial properties of vancomycin-laden mesoporous bioglass/PLGA composite scaffolds for bone regeneration in infected bone defects. *Artif. Cells Nanomed. Biotechnol.* **2017**, *46*, 1935–1947. [CrossRef]
105. Zhou, X.; Weng, W.; Chen, B.; Feng, W.; Wang, W.; Nie, W.; Chen, L.; Mo, X.; Su, J.; He, C. Mesoporous silica nanoparticles/gelatin porous composite scaffolds with localized and sustained release of vancomycin for treatment of infected bone defects. *J. Mater. Chem. B* **2018**, *6*, 740–752. [CrossRef]
106. Grohmann, S.; Menne, M.; Hesse, D.; Bischoff, S.; Schiffner, R.; Diefenbeck, M.; Liefeith, K. Biomimetic multilayer coatings deliver gentamicin and reduce implant-related osteomyelitis in rats. *Biomed. Eng. Biomed. Tech.* **2019**, *64*, 383–395. [CrossRef]
107. Janson, O.; Sörensen, J.H.; Strømme, M.; Engqvist, H.; Procter, P.; Welch, K. Evaluation of an alkali-treated and hydroxyapatite-coated orthopedic implant loaded with tobramycin. *J. Biomater. Appl.* **2019**, *34*, 699–720. [CrossRef] [PubMed]
108. Stavrakis, A.I.; Zhu, S.; Loftin, A.H.; Weixian, X.; Niska, J.; Hegde, V.; Segura, T.; Bernthal, N.M. Controlled release of vancomycin and tigecycline from an orthopaedic implant coating prevents *Staphylococcus Aureus* infection in an open fracture animal model. *BioMed Res. Int.* **2019**, *2019*, 1–9. [CrossRef]
109. Thompson, K.; Petkov, S.; Zeiter, S.; Sprecher, C.M.; Richards, R.G.; Moriarty, T.F.; Eijer, H. Intraoperative loading of calcium phosphate-coated implants with gentamicin prevents experimental *Staphylococcus Aureus* Infection in Vivo. *PLoS ONE* **2019**, *14*, e0210402. [CrossRef] [PubMed]
110. Zhang, B.; Braun, B.M.; Skelly, J.D.; Ayers, D.C.; Song, J. Significant suppression of *Staphylococcus aureus* colonization on intramedullary Ti6Al4V implants surface-grafted with vancomycin-bearing polymer brushes. *ACS Appl. Mater. Interfaces* **2019**, *11*, 28641–28647. [CrossRef]
111. Paris, J.L.; Vallet-Regí, M. Mesoporous silica nanoparticles for co-delivery of drugs and nucleic acids in oncology: A review. *Pharmaceutics* **2020**, *12*, 526. [CrossRef] [PubMed]
112. Aguilera-Correa, J.J.; Garcia-Casas, A.; Mediero, A.; Romera, D.; Mulero, F.; Cuevas-López, I.; Jiménez-Morales, A.; Esteban, J. A new antibiotic-loaded sol-gel can prevent bacterial prosthetic joint infection: From in vitro studies to an in vivo model. *Front. Microbiol.* **2019**, *10*, 2935. [CrossRef] [PubMed]
113. Ramalhete, R.; Brown, R.; Blunn, G.; Skinner, J.; Coathup, M.; Graney, I.; Sanghani-Kerai, A. A novel antimicrobial coating to prevent periprosthetic joint infection. *Bone Jt. Res.* **2020**, *9*, 848–856. [CrossRef]
114. Romera, D.; Toirac, B.; Aguilera-Correa, J.-J.; García-Casas, A.; Mediero, A.; Jiménez-Morales, A.; Esteban, J. A biodegradable antifungal-loaded sol–gel coating for the prevention and local treatment of yeast prosthetic-joint infections. *Materials* **2020**, *13*, 3144. [CrossRef]
115. Garlito-Díaz, H.; Esteban, J.; Mediero, A.; Carias-Cálix, R.A.; Toirac, B.; Mulero, F.; Faus-Rodrigo, V.; Jiménez-Morales, A.; Calvo, E.; Aguilera-Correa, J.J. A new antifungal-loaded sol-gel can prevent candida albicans prosthetic joint infection. *Antibiotics* **2021**, *10*, 711. [CrossRef]
116. Ujcic, A.; Krejcikova, S.; Nevoralova, M.; Zhigunov, A.; Dybal, J.; Krulis, Z.; Fulin, P.; Nyc, O.; Slouf, M. Thermoplastic starch composites with titanium dioxide and vancomycin antibiotic: Preparation, morphology, thermomechanical properties, and antimicrobial susceptibility testing. *Front. Mater.* **2020**, *7*, 9. [CrossRef]
117. Souza, J.G.S.; Bertolini, M.M.; Costa, R.C.; Nagay, B.E.; Dongari-Bagtzoglou, A.; Barão, V.A.R. Targeting implant-associated infections: Titanium surface loaded with antimicrobial. *iScience* **2021**, *24*, 102008. [CrossRef]
118. Aguilera-Correa, J.J.; Vidal-Laso, R.; Carias-Cálix, R.A.; Toirac, B.; García-Casas, A.; Velasco-Rodríguez, D.; Llamas-Sillero, P.; Jiménez-Morales, A.; Esteban, J. A new antibiotic-loaded sol-gel can prevent bacterial intravenous catheter-related infections. *Materials* **2020**, *13*, 2946. [CrossRef]
119. da Silva, A.C.; Córdoba de Torresi, S.I. Advances in conducting, biodegradable and biocompatible copolymers for biomedical applications. *Front. Mater.* **2019**, *6*, 98. [CrossRef]
120. Ramot, Y.; Haim-Zada, M.; Domb, A.J.; Nyska, A. Biocompatibility and safety of PLA and its copolymers. *Adv. Drug Deliv. Rev.* **2016**, *107*, 153–162. [CrossRef]
121. Garcia-Casas, A.; Aguilera-Correa, J.J.; Mediero, A.; Esteban, J.; Jimenez-Morales, A. Functionalization of sol-gel coatings with organophosphorus compounds for prosthetic devices. *Colloids Surf. B Biointerfaces* **2019**, *181*, 973–980. [CrossRef]
122. Tong, X.; Pan, W.; Su, T.; Zhang, M.; Dong, W.; Qi, X. Recent advances in natural polymer-based drug delivery systems. *React. Funct. Polym.* **2020**, *148*, 104501. [CrossRef]
123. Paris, J.L.; Lafuente-Gómez, N.; Cabañas, M.V.; Román, J.; Peña, J.; Vallet-Regí, M. Fabrication of a nanoparticle-containing 3D porous bone scaffold with proangiogenic and antibacterial properties. *Acta Biomater.* **2019**, *86*, 441–449. [CrossRef]

124. Aebli, N.; Krebs, J.; Schwenke, D.; Stich, H.; Schawalder, P.; Theis, J.C. Degradation of hydroxyapatite coating on a well-functioning femoral component. *J. Bone Jt. Surg. Br.* **2003**, *85*, 499–503. [CrossRef]
125. Schmidmaier, G.; Wildemann, B.; Stemberger, A.; Haas, N.P.; Raschke, M. Biodegradable poly(D,L-lactide) coating of implants for continuous release of growth factors. *J. Biomed. Mater. Res.* **2001**, *58*, 449–455. [CrossRef]
126. Fuchs, T.; Stange, R.; Schmidmaier, G.; Raschke, M.J. The use of gentamicin-coated nails in the tibia: Preliminary results of a prospective study. *Arch. Orthop. Trauma Surg.* **2011**, *131*, 1419–1425. [CrossRef]
127. Schmidmaier, G.; Kerstan, M.; Schwabe, P.; Südkamp, N.; Raschke, M. Clinical experiences in the use of a gentamicin-coated titanium nail in tibia fractures. *Injury* **2017**, *48*, 2235–2241. [CrossRef]
128. Drago, L.; Boot, W.; Dimas, K.; Malizos, K.; Hänsch, G.M.; Stuyck, J.; Gawlitta, D.; Romanò, C.L. Does implant coating with antibacterial-loaded hydrogel reduce bacterial colonization and biofilm formation in vitro? *Clin. Orthop.* **2014**, *472*, 3311–3323. [CrossRef] [PubMed]
129. Romanò, C.L.; de Vecchi, E.; Bortolin, M.; Morelli, I.; Drago, L. Hyaluronic acid and its composites as a local antimicrobial/antiadhesive barrier. *J. Bone Jt. Infect.* **2017**, *2*, 63–72. [CrossRef] [PubMed]
130. Ardizzoni, A.; Neglia, R.G.; Baschieri, M.C.; Cermelli, C.; Caratozzolo, M.; Righi, E.; Palmieri, B.; Blasi, E. Influence of hyaluronic acid on bacterial and fungal species, including clinically relevant opportunistic pathogens. *J. Mater. Sci. Mater. Med.* **2011**, *22*, 2329–2338. [CrossRef] [PubMed]
131. Giavaresi, G.; Meani, E.; Sartori, M.; Ferrari, A.; Bellini, D.; Sacchetta, A.C.; Meraner, J.; Sambri, A.; Vocale, C.; Sambri, V.; et al. Efficacy of antibacterial-loaded coating in an in vivo model of acutely highly contaminated implant. *Int. Orthop.* **2014**, *38*, 1505–1512. [CrossRef] [PubMed]
132. Boot, W.; Vogely, H.C.; Jiao, C.; Nikkels, P.G.; Pouran, B.; van Rijen, M.H.; Ekkelenkamp, M.B.; Hänsch, G.M.; Dhert, W.J.; Gawlitta, D. Prophylaxis of implant-related infections by local release of vancomycin from a hydrogel in rabbits. *Eur. Cell. Mater.* **2020**, *39*, 108–120. [CrossRef]
133. Boot, W.; Gawlitta, D.; Nikkels, P.G.J.; Pouran, B.; van Rijen, M.H.P.; Dhert, W.J.A.; Vogely, H.C. Hyaluronic acid-based hydrogel coating does not affect bone apposition at the implant surface in a rabbit model. *Clin. Orthop.* **2017**, *475*, 1911–1919. [CrossRef]
134. Romanò, C.L.; Malizos, K.; Capuano, N.; Mezzoprete, R.; D'Arienzo, M.; van der Straeten, C.; Scarponi, S.; Drago, L. Does an antibiotic-loaded hydrogel coating reduce early post-surgical infection after joint arthroplasty? *J. Bone Jt. Infect.* **2016**, *1*, 34–41. [CrossRef]
135. Malizos, K.; Blauth, M.; Danita, A.; Capuano, N.; Mezzoprete, R.; Logoluso, N.; Drago, L.; Romanò, C.L. Fast-resorbable antibiotic-loaded hydrogel coating to reduce post-surgical infection after internal osteosynthesis: A multicenter randomized controlled trial. *J. Orthop. Traumatol. Off. J. Ital. Soc. Orthop. Traumatol.* **2017**, *18*, 159–169. [CrossRef]
136. Trentinaglia, M.T.; van der Straeten, C.; Morelli, I.; Logoluso, N.; Drago, L.; Romanò, C.L. Economic evaluation of antibacterial coatings on healthcare costs in first year following total joint arthroplasty. *J. Arthroplasty* **2018**, *33*, 1656–1662. [CrossRef] [PubMed]
137. Romanò, C.L.; Tsuchiya, H.; Morelli, I.; Battaglia, A.G.; Drago, L. Antibacterial coating of implants: Are we missing something? *Bone Jt. Res.* **2019**, *8*, 199–206. [CrossRef] [PubMed]
138. Michael, C.A.; Dominey-Howes, D.; Labbate, M. The antimicrobial resistance crisis: Causes, consequences, and management. *Front. Public Health* **2014**, *2*, 145. [CrossRef] [PubMed]
139. Raymond, B. Five rules for resistance management in the antibiotic apocalypse, a road map for integrated microbial management. *Evol. Appl.* **2019**, *12*, 1079–1091. [CrossRef]
140. Bell, G.; MacLean, C. The search for 'evolution-proof' antibiotics. *Trends Microbiol.* **2018**, *26*, 471–483. [CrossRef] [PubMed]
141. Ma, D.; Shanks, R.M.Q.; Davis, C.M.; Craft, D.W.; Wood, T.K.; Hamlin, B.R.; Urish, K.L. Viable bacteria persist on antibiotic spacers following two-stage revision for periprosthetic joint infection. *J. Orthop. Res. Off. Publ. Orthop. Res. Soc.* **2018**, *36*, 452–458. [CrossRef] [PubMed]
142. Schmolders, J.; Hischebeth, G.T.; Friedrich, M.J.; Randau, T.M.; Wimmer, M.D.; Kohlhof, H.; Molitor, E.; Gravius, S. Evidence of MRSE on a gentamicin and vancomycin impregnated polymethyl-methacrylate (PMMA) bone cement spacer after two-stage exchange arthroplasty due to periprosthetic joint infection of the knee. *BMC Infect. Dis.* **2014**, *14*, 144. [CrossRef]
143. Aguilera-Correa, J.-J.; Conde, A.; Arenas, M.-A.; de-Damborenea, J.-J.; Marin, M.; Doadrio, A.L.; Esteban, J. Bactericidal activity of the Ti-13Nb-13Zr alloy against different species of bacteria related with implant infection. *Biomed. Mater.* **2017**, *12*, 045022. [CrossRef]
144. da Silva, R.B.; Salles, M.J. Outcomes and risk factors in prosthetic joint infections by multidrug-resistant gram-negative bacteria: A retrospective cohort study. *Antibiotics* **2021**, *10*, 340. [CrossRef]
145. Lemire, J.A.; Harrison, J.J.; Turner, R.J. Antimicrobial activity of metals: Mechanisms, molecular targets and applications. *Nat. Rev. Microbiol.* **2013**, *11*, 371–384. [CrossRef] [PubMed]
146. Alexander, J.W. History of the medical use of silver. *Surg. Infect.* **2009**, *10*, 289–292. [CrossRef] [PubMed]
147. Djurišić, A.B.; Leung, Y.H.; Ng, A.M.C.; Xu, X.Y.; Lee, P.K.H.; Degger, N.; Wu, R.S.S. Toxicity of metal oxide nanoparticles: Mechanisms, characterization, and avoiding experimental artefacts. *Small* **2015**, *11*, 26–44. [CrossRef] [PubMed]
148. Shirai, T.; Tsuchiya, H.; Shimizu, T.; Ohtani, K.; Zen, Y.; Tomita, K. Prevention of Pin tract infection with titanium-copper alloys. *J. Biomed. Mater. Res. B Appl. Biomater.* **2009**, *91B*, 373–380. [CrossRef]
149. Pérez-Tanoira, R.; Pérez-Jorge, C.; Endrino, J.L.; Gómez-Barrena, E.; Horwat, D.; Pierson, J.F.; Esteban, J. Antibacterial properties of biomedical surfaces containing micrometric silver islands. *J. Phys. Conf. Ser.* **2010**, *252*, 012015. [CrossRef]
150. Cao, H.; Liu, X.; Meng, F.; Chu, P.K. Biological actions of silver nanoparticles embedded in titanium controlled by micro-galvanic effects. *Biomaterials* **2011**, *32*, 693–705. [CrossRef]

151. Secinti, K.D.; Özalp, H.; Attar, A.; Sargon, M.F. Nanoparticle silver ion coatings inhibit biofilm formation on titanium implants. *J. Clin. Neurosci.* **2011**, *18*, 391–395. [CrossRef]
152. Ionita, D.; Grecu, M.; Ungureanu, C.; Demetrescu, I. Antimicrobial activity of the surface coatings on TiAlZr implant biomaterial. *J. Biosci. Bioeng.* **2011**, *112*, 630–634. [CrossRef] [PubMed]
153. Zhang, E.; Li, F.; Wang, H.; Liu, J.; Wang, C.; Li, M.; Yang, K. A new antibacterial titanium–copper sintered alloy: Preparation and antibacterial property. *Mater. Sci. Eng. C* **2013**, *33*, 4280–4287. [CrossRef]
154. Zhao, C.; Feng, B.; Li, Y.; Tan, J.; Lu, X.; Weng, J. Preparation and antibacterial activity of titanium nanotubes loaded with Ag nanoparticles in the dark and under the UV light. *Appl. Surf. Sci.* **2013**, *280*, 8–14. [CrossRef]
155. Saidin, S.; Chevallier, P.; Abdul Kadir, M.R.; Hermawan, H.; Mantovani, D. Polydopamine as an intermediate layer for silver and hydroxyapatite immobilisation on metallic biomaterials surface. *Mater. Sci. Eng. C* **2013**, *33*, 4715–4724. [CrossRef] [PubMed]
156. De Giglio, E.; Cafagna, D.; Cometa, S.; Allegretta, A.; Pedico, A.; Giannossa, L.C.; Sabbatini, L.; Mattioli-Belmonte, M.; Iatta, R. An innovative, easily fabricated, silver nanoparticle-based titanium implant coating: Development and analytical characterization. *Anal. Bioanal. Chem.* **2013**, *405*, 805–816. [CrossRef] [PubMed]
157. Liu, J.; Li, F.; Liu, C.; Wang, H.; Ren, B.; Yang, K.; Zhang, E. Effect of Cu Content on the antibacterial activity of titanium–copper sintered alloys. *Mater. Sci. Eng. C* **2014**, *35*, 392–400. [CrossRef] [PubMed]
158. Ren, L.; Ma, Z.; Li, M.; Zhang, Y.; Liu, W.; Liao, Z.; Yang, K. Antibacterial properties of Ti–6Al–4V–XCu alloys. *J. Mater. Sci. Technol.* **2014**, *30*, 699–705. [CrossRef]
159. Xie, C.-M.; Lu, X.; Wang, K.-F.; Meng, F.-Z.; Jiang, O.; Zhang, H.-P.; Zhi, W.; Fang, L.-M. Silver nanoparticles and growth factors incorporated hydroxyapatite coatings on metallic implant surfaces for enhancement of osteoinductivity and antibacterial properties. *ACS Appl. Mater. Interfaces* **2014**, *6*, 8580–8589. [CrossRef]
160. Rodríguez-Cano, A.; Pacha-Olivenza, M.-Á.; Babiano, R.; Cintas, P.; González-Martín, M.-L. Non-covalent derivatization of aminosilanized titanium alloy implants. *Surf. Coat. Technol.* **2014**, *245*, 66–73. [CrossRef]
161. Chen, M.; Zhang, E.; Zhang, L. Microstructure, mechanical properties, bio-corrosion properties and antibacterial properties of Ti–Ag sintered alloys. *Mater. Sci. Eng. C* **2016**, *62*, 350–360. [CrossRef]
162. Chen, M.; Yang, L.; Zhang, L.; Han, Y.; Lu, Z.; Qin, G.; Zhang, E. Effect of nano/micro-ag compound particles on the bio-corrosion, antibacterial properties and cell biocompatibility of Ti-Ag alloys. *Mater. Sci. Eng. C* **2017**, *75*, 906–917. [CrossRef]
163. Yamanoglu, R.; Efendi, E.; Kolayli, F.; Uzuner, H.; Daoud, I. Production and mechanical properties of Ti–5Al–2.5Fe– *x* Cu alloys for biomedical applications. *Biomed. Mater.* **2018**, *13*, 025013. [CrossRef] [PubMed]
164. Lei, Z.; Zhang, H.; Zhang, E.; You, J.; Ma, X.; Bai, X. Antibacterial activities and biocompatibilities of Ti-Ag alloys prepared by spark plasma sintering and acid etching. *Mater. Sci. Eng. C* **2018**, *92*, 121–131. [CrossRef] [PubMed]
165. Peng, C.; Zhang, S.; Sun, Z.; Ren, L.; Yang, K. Effect of annealing temperature on mechanical and antibacterial properties of Cu-bearing titanium alloy and its preliminary study of antibacterial mechanism. *Mater. Sci. Eng. C* **2018**, *93*, 495–504. [CrossRef]
166. Wang, X.; Dong, H.; Liu, J.; Qin, G.; Chen, D.; Zhang, E. In vivo antibacterial property of Ti-Cu sintered alloy implant. *Mater. Sci. Eng. C* **2019**, *100*, 38–47. [CrossRef]
167. Cochis, A.; Azzimonti, B.; Chiesa, R.; Rimondini, L.; Gasik, M. Metallurgical gallium additions to titanium alloys demonstrate a strong time-increasing antibacterial activity without any cellular toxicity. *ACS Biomater. Sci. Eng.* **2019**, *5*, 2815–2820. [CrossRef]
168. Tao, S.C.; Xu, J.L.; Yuan, L.; Luo, J.M.; Zheng, Y.F. Microstructure, mechanical properties and antibacterial properties of the microwave sintered porous Ti–3Cu alloys. *J. Alloys Compd.* **2020**, *812*, 152142. [CrossRef]
169. Bolzoni, L.; Alqattan, M.; Peters, L.; Alshammari, Y.; Yang, F. Ternary Ti alloys functionalised with antibacterial activity. *Sci. Rep.* **2020**, *10*, 22201. [CrossRef]
170. Shi, A.; Zhu, C.; Fu, S.; Wang, R.; Qin, G.; Chen, D.; Zhang, E. What controls the antibacterial activity of Ti-Ag alloy, Ag ion or Ti2Ag particles? *Mater. Sci. Eng. C* **2020**, *109*, 110548. [CrossRef]
171. Yang, J.; Qin, H.; Chai, Y.; Zhang, P.; Chen, Y.; Yang, K.; Qin, M.; Zhang, Y.; Xia, H.; Ren, L.; et al. Molecular mechanisms of osteogenesis and antibacterial activity of Cu-bearing Ti alloy in a bone defect model with infection in vivo. *J. Orthop. Transl.* **2021**, *27*, 77–89. [CrossRef]
172. Zhuang, Y.; Ren, L.; Zhang, S.; Wei, X.; Yang, K.; Dai, K. Antibacterial effect of a copper-containing titanium alloy against implant-associated infection induced by methicillin-resistant *Staphylococcus aureus*. *Acta Biomater.* **2021**, *119*, 472–484. [CrossRef] [PubMed]
173. Deng, W.; Shao, H.; Li, H.; Zhou, Y. Is surface modification effective to prevent periprosthetic joint infection? A systematic review of preclinical and clinical studies. *Orthop. Traumatol. Surg. Res.* **2019**, *105*, 967–974. [CrossRef] [PubMed]
174. Hardes, J.; von Eiff, C.; Streitbuerger, A.; Balke, M.; Budny, T.; Henrichs, M.P.; Hauschild, G.; Ahrens, H. Reduction of periprosthetic infection with silver-coated megaprostheses in patients with bone sarcoma: Silver-coated prostheses in sarcoma patients. *J. Surg. Oncol.* **2010**, *101*, 389–395. [CrossRef]
175. Hussmann, B.; Johann, I.; Kauther, M.D.; Landgraeber, S.; Jäger, M.; Lendemans, S. Measurement of the silver ion concentration in wound fluids after implantation of silver-coated megaprostheses: Correlation with the clinical outcome. *BioMed. Res. Int.* **2013**, *2013*, 1–11. [CrossRef]
176. Wafa, H.; Grimer, R.J.; Reddy, K.; Jeys, L.; Abudu, A.; Carter, S.R.; Tillman, R.M. Retrospective Evaluation of the Incidence of Early Periprosthetic Infection with Silver-Treated Endoprostheses in High-Risk Patients: Case-Control Study. *Bone Jt. J.* **2015**, *97*, 252–257. [CrossRef]

177. Schmolders, J.; Koob, S.; Schepers, P.; Pennekamp, P.H.; Gravius, S.; Wirtz, D.C.; Placzek, R.; Strauss, A.C. Lower limb reconstruction in tumor patients using modular silver-coated megaprostheses with regard to perimegaprosthetic joint infection: A case series, including 100 patients and review of the literature. *Arch. Orthop. Trauma Surg.* **2017**, *137*, 149–153. [CrossRef] [PubMed]
178. Zajonz, D.; Birke, U.; Ghanem, M.; Prietzel, T.; Josten, C.; Roth, A.; Fakler, J.K.M. Silver-coated modular megaendoprostheses in salvage revision arthroplasty after periimplant infection with extensive bone loss—A pilot study of 34 patients. *BMC Musculoskelet. Disord.* **2017**, *18*, 383. [CrossRef] [PubMed]
179. Tan, T.L.; Maltenfort, M.G.; Chen, A.F.; Shahi, A.; Higuera, C.A.; Siqueira, M.; Parvizi, J. Development and evaluation of a preoperative risk calculator for periprosthetic joint infection following total joint arthroplasty. *J. Bone Jt. Surg.* **2018**, *100*, 777–785. [CrossRef] [PubMed]
180. Jeyaraj Pandian, C.; Palanivel, R.; Dhanasekaran, S. Screening antimicrobial activity of nickel nanoparticles synthesized using *Ocimum sanctum* leaf extract. *J. Nanoparticles* **2016**, *2016*, 1–13. [CrossRef]
181. Ahghari, M.R.; Soltaninejad, V.; Maleki, A. Synthesis of nickel nanoparticles by a green and convenient method as a magnetic mirror with antibacterial activities. *Sci. Rep.* **2020**, *10*, 12627. [CrossRef]
182. Bellio, P.; Luzi, C.; Mancini, A.; Cracchiolo, S.; Passacantando, M.; Di Pietro, L.; Perilli, M.; Amicosante, G.; Santucci, S.; Celenza, G. Cerium oxide nanoparticles as potential antibiotic adjuvant. Effects of CeO_2 nanoparticles on bacterial outer membrane permeability. *Biochim. Biophys. Acta BBA—Biomembr.* **2018**, *1860*, 2428–2435. [CrossRef]
183. Vahdati, M.; Tohidi Moghadam, T. Synthesis and characterization of selenium nanoparticles-lysozyme nanohybrid system with synergistic antibacterial properties. *Sci. Rep.* **2020**, *10*, 510. [CrossRef]
184. Geoffrion, L.D.; Hesabizadeh, T.; Medina-Cruz, D.; Kusper, M.; Taylor, P.; Vernet-Crua, A.; Chen, J.; Ajo, A.; Webster, T.J.; Guisbiers, G. Naked selenium nanoparticles for antibacterial and anticancer treatments. *ACS Omega* **2020**, *5*, 2660–2669. [CrossRef]
185. Kang, S.-M.; Jang, S.-C.; Heo, N.S.; Oh, S.Y.; Cho, H.-J.; Rethinasabapathy, M.; Vilian, A.T.E.; Han, Y.-K.; Roh, C.; Huh, Y.S. Cesium-induced inhibition of bacterial growth of pseudomonas aeruginosa PAO1 and their possible potential applications for bioremediation of wastewater. *J. Hazard. Mater.* **2017**, *338*, 323–333. [CrossRef]
186. Banin, E.; Friedman, A.; Gedanken, A. Lellouche antibacterial and antibiofilm properties of yttrium fluoride nanoparticles. *Int. J. Nanomed.* **2012**, *7*, 5611. [CrossRef]
187. Adams, C.P.; Walker, K.A.; Obare, S.O.; Docherty, K.M. Size-dependent antimicrobial effects of novel palladium nanoparticles. *PLoS ONE* **2014**, *9*, e85981. [CrossRef]
188. Mohana, S.; Sumathi, S. Multi-functional biological effects of palladium nanoparticles synthesized using agaricus bisporus. *J. Clust. Sci.* **2020**, *31*, 391–400. [CrossRef]
189. Xu, C.; Akakuru, O.U.; Zheng, J.; Wu, A. Applications of iron oxide-based magnetic nanoparticles in the diagnosis and treatment of bacterial infections. *Front. Bioeng. Biotechnol.* **2019**, *7*, 141. [CrossRef]
190. Ren, K.; Dusad, A.; Zhang, Y.; Wang, D. Therapeutic intervention for wear debris-induced aseptic implant loosening. *Acta Pharm. Sin. B* **2013**, *3*, 76–85. [CrossRef]
191. Jacobs, J.J.; Gilbert, J.L.; Urban, R.M. Corrosion of metal orthopaedic implants. *J. Bone Jt. Surg. Am.* **1998**, *80*, 268–282. [CrossRef]
192. Jacobs, J.J.; Skipor, A.K.; Black, J.; Urban, R.M.; Galante, J.O. Release and excretion of metal in patients who have a total hip-replacement component made of titanium-base alloy. *J. Bone Jt. Surg. Am.* **1991**, *73*, 1475–1486. [CrossRef]
193. Jacobs, J.J.; Silverton, C.; Hallab, N.J.; Skipor, A.K.; Patterson, L.; Black, J.; Galante, J.O. Metal release and excretion from cementless titanium alloy total knee replacements. *Clin. Orthop.* **1999**, *358*, 173–180. [CrossRef]
194. Jacobs, J.J.; Skipor, A.K.; Patterson, L.M.; Hallab, N.J.; Paprosky, W.G.; Black, J.; Galante, J.O. Metal release in patients who have had a primary total hip arthroplasty. A prospective, controlled, longitudinal study. *J. Bone Jt. Surg.* **1998**, *80*, 1447–1458. [CrossRef] [PubMed]
195. AshaRani, P.V.; Low Kah Mun, G.; Hande, M.P.; Valiyaveettil, S. Cytotoxicity and genotoxicity of silver nanoparticles in human cells. *ACS Nano* **2009**, *3*, 279–290. [CrossRef] [PubMed]
196. Pauksch, L.; Hartmann, S.; Rohnke, M.; Szalay, G.; Alt, V.; Schnettler, R.; Lips, K.S. Biocompatibility of silver nanoparticles and silver ions in primary human mesenchymal stem cells and osteoblasts. *Acta Biomater.* **2014**, *10*, 439–449. [CrossRef] [PubMed]
197. De Jong, W.H.; van der Ven, L.T.M.; Sleijffers, A.; Park, M.V.D.Z.; Jansen, E.H.J.M.; van Loveren, H.; Vandebriel, R.J. Systemic and immunotoxicity of silver nanoparticles in an intravenous 28 days repeated dose toxicity study in rats. *Biomaterials* **2013**, *34*, 8333–8343. [CrossRef]
198. Glehr, M.; Leithner, A.; Friesenbichler, J.; Goessler, W.; Avian, A.; Andreou, D.; Maurer-Ertl, W.; Windhager, R.; Tunn, P.-U. Argyria following the use of silver-coated megaprostheses: No association between the development of local argyria and elevated silver levels. *Bone Jt. J.* **2013**, *95*, 988–992. [CrossRef]
199. O'Neill, J. Antimicrobial Resistance: Tackling a Crisis for the Health and Wealth of Nations/the Review on Antimicrobial Resistance Chaired by Jim O'Neill. Available online: https://wellcomecollection.org/works/rdpck35v (accessed on 20 May 2021).
200. Lora-Tamayo, J.; Murillo, O.; Iribarren, J.A.; Soriano, A.; Sánchez-Somolinos, M.; Baraia-Etxaburu, J.M.; Rico, A.; Palomino, J.; Rodríguez-Pardo, D.; Horcajada, J.P.; et al. A large multicenter study of methicillin-susceptible and methicillin-resistant *Staphylococcus aureus* prosthetic joint infections managed with implant retention. *Clin. Infect. Dis. Off. Publ. Infect. Dis. Soc. Am.* **2013**, *56*, 182–194. [CrossRef]
201. Pfang, B.G.; García-Cañete, J.; García-Lasheras, J.; Blanco, A.; Auñón, Á.; Parron-Cambero, R.; Macías-Valcayo, A.; Esteban, J. Orthopedic implant-associated infection by multidrug resistant enterobacteriaceae. *J. Clin. Med.* **2019**, *8*, 220. [CrossRef]

202. Papadopoulos, A.; Ribera, A.; Mavrogenis, A.F.; Rodriguez-Pardo, D.; Bonnet, E.; Salles, M.J.; del Toro, D.M.; Nguyen, S.; Blanco-García, A.; Skaliczki, G.; et al. Multidrug-resistant and extensively drug-resistant gram-negative prosthetic joint infections: Role of surgery and impact of colistin administration. *Int. J. Antimicrob. Agents* **2019**, *53*, 294–301. [CrossRef]
203. Randall, C.P.; Gupta, A.; Jackson, N.; Busse, D.; O'Neill, A.J. Silver resistance in gram-negative bacteria: A dissection of endogenous and exogenous mechanisms. *J. Antimicrob. Chemother.* **2015**, *70*, 1037–1046. [CrossRef]
204. Bondarczuk, K.; Piotrowska-Seget, Z. Molecular basis of active copper resistance mechanisms in gram-negative bacteria. *Cell Biol. Toxicol.* **2013**, *29*, 397–405. [CrossRef]
205. Runner, R.P.; Mener, A.; Roberson, J.R.; Bradbury, T.L.; Guild, G.N.; Boden, S.D.; Erens, G.A. Prosthetic joint infection trends at a dedicated orthopaedics specialty hospital. *Adv. Orthop.* **2019**, *2019*, 1–9. [CrossRef] [PubMed]
206. Perez-Jorge, C.; Gomez-Barrena, E.; Horcajada, J.-P.; Puig-Verdie, L.; Esteban, J. Drug treatments for prosthetic joint infections in the era of multidrug resistance. *Expert Opin. Pharmacother.* **2016**, *17*, 1233–1246. [CrossRef] [PubMed]
207. Tsuchiya, H.; Shirai, T.; Nishida, H.; Murakami, H.; Kabata, T.; Yamamoto, N.; Watanabe, K.; Nakase, J. Innovative antimicrobial coating of titanium implants with iodine. *J. Orthop. Sci.* **2012**, *17*, 595–604. [CrossRef] [PubMed]
208. Browne, K.; Chakraborty, S.; Chen, R.; Willcox, M.D.; Black, D.S.; Walsh, W.R.; Kumar, N. A new era of antibiotics: The clinical potential of antimicrobial peptides. *Int. J. Mol. Sci.* **2020**, *21*, E7047. [CrossRef] [PubMed]
209. Morris, J.L.; Letson, H.L.; Elliott, L.; Grant, A.L.; Wilkinson, M.; Hazratwala, K.; McEwen, P. Evaluation of bacteriophage as an adjunct therapy for treatment of peri-prosthetic joint infection caused by *Staphylococcus aureus*. *PLoS ONE* **2019**, *14*, e0226574. [CrossRef]
210. Van Belleghem, J.D.; Manasherob, R.; Międzybrodzki, R.; Rogóż, P.; Górski, A.; Suh, G.A.; Bollyky, P.L.; Amanatullah, D.F. The rationale for using bacteriophage to treat and prevent periprosthetic joint infections. *Front. Microbiol.* **2020**, *11*, 591021. [CrossRef]
211. Doub, J.B.; Ng, V.Y.; Wilson, E.; Corsini, L.; Chan, B.K. Successful treatment of a recalcitrant *Staphylococcus epidermidis* prosthetic knee infection with intraoperative bacteriophage therapy. *Pharm. Basel Switz.* **2021**, *14*, 231. [CrossRef]
212. Campoccia, D.; Montanaro, L.; Arciola, C.R. A review of the biomaterials technologies for infection-resistant surfaces. *Biomaterials* **2013**, *34*, 8533–8554. [CrossRef]
213. Romanò, C.L.; Scarponi, S.; Gallazzi, E.; Romanò, D.; Drago, L. Antibacterial coating of implants in orthopaedics and trauma: A classification proposal in an evolving panorama. *J. Orthop. Surg.* **2015**, *10*, 157. [CrossRef]

antibiotics

Article

Prevalence, Patterns, Association with Biofilm Formation, Effects on Milk Quality and Risk Factors for Antibiotic Resistance of Staphylococci from Bulk-Tank Milk of Goat Herds

Daphne T. Lianou [1], Efthymia Petinaki [2], Peter J. Cripps [1], Dimitris A. Gougoulis [1], Charalambia K. Michael [1], Katerina Tsilipounidaki [2], Anargyros Skoulakis [2], Angeliki I. Katsafadou [3], Natalia G. C. Vasileiou [4], Themis Giannoulis [4], Eleni I. Katsarou [1], Chrysoula Voidarou [5], Vasia S. Mavrogianni [1], Mariangela Caroprese [6] and George C. Fthenakis [1,*]

[1] Veterinary Faculty, University of Thessaly, 43100 Karditsa, Greece; dlianou@vet.uth.gr (D.T.L.); peterjohncripps@gmail.com (P.J.C.); dgoug@vet.uth.gr (D.A.G.); cmichail@vet.uth.gr (C.K.M.); elekatsarou@vet.uth.gr (E.I.K.); vmavrog@vet.uth.gr (V.S.M.)
[2] University Hospital of Larissa, 41110 Larissa, Greece; petinaki@med.uth.gr (E.P.); tsilipoukat@gmail.com (K.T.); skulakis@gmail.com (A.S.)
[3] Faculty of Public and One Health, University of Thessaly, 43100 Karditsa, Greece; agkatsaf@vet.uth.gr
[4] Faculty of Animal Science, University of Thessaly, 41110 Larissa, Greece; vasileiounat@gmail.com (N.G.C.V.); themisgia@gmail.com (T.G.)
[5] Department of Agriculture, University of Ioannina, 47132 Arta, Greece; xvoidarou@uoi.gr
[6] Department of Agriculture, Food, Natural Resources and Engineering (DAFNE), University of Foggia, 71122 Foggia, Italy; mariangela.caroprese@unifg.it
* Correspondence: gcf@vet.uth.gr

Citation: Lianou, D.T.; Petinaki, E.; Cripps, P.J.; Gougoulis, D.A.; Michael, C.K.; Tsilipounidaki, K.; Skoulakis, A.; Katsafadou, A.I.; Vasileiou, N.G.C.; Giannoulis, T.; et al. Prevalence, Patterns, Association with Biofilm Formation, Effects on Milk Quality and Risk Factors for Antibiotic Resistance of Staphylococci from Bulk-Tank Milk of Goat Herds. *Antibiotics* **2021**, *10*, 1225. https://doi.org/10.3390/antibiotics10101225

Academic Editor: Helena Felgueiras

Received: 17 September 2021
Accepted: 6 October 2021
Published: 8 October 2021

Abstract: The objectives of this work were to study the prevalence and the patterns of antibiotic resistance of staphylococcal isolates from bulk-tank milk of goat herds across Greece, to assess possible associations of the presence of antibiotic resistance with the quality of milk in these herds and to evaluate herd-related factors potentially associated with the presence of antibiotic resistance among these staphylococcal isolates. A cross-sectional study was performed on 119 goat herds in Greece. Bulk-tank milk samples were collected for bacteriological examination; staphylococcal isolates were evaluated for resistance to 20 antibiotics. Oxacillin-resistant, resistant to at least one antibiotic, and multi-resistant staphylococcal isolates were recovered from 5.0%, 30.3%, and 16.0% of herds, respectively. Of 80 isolates, 7.5% were resistant to oxacillin, 50.0% were resistant to at least one antibiotic and 27.5% were multi-resistant. Resistance was seen more frequently among coagulase-negative staphylococci (59.3%) than among *Staphylococcus aureus* (23.8%). Resistance was more frequent against penicillin and ampicillin (41.3% of isolates) and fosfomycin (27.5%). No association was found with biofilm formation by staphylococci. For recovery of oxacillin-resistant isolates, the presence of working staff in the herds emerged as a significant factor; respective factors for the isolation of staphylococci resistant to at least one antibiotic were part-time farming and high (>10) number of systemic disinfections in the farm annually. The same three factors concurrently were also identified to be significant for the recovery of multi-resistant isolates.

Keywords: bulk-tank milk; mastitis; methicillin; milk; goat; somatic cell counts; staphylococcus; tetracycline; total bacterial counts

1. Introduction

In Greece, goat farming for milk production is a significant sector of the agricultural industry. Goat milk production in the country amounted to 143,270,500 L in 2019 [1], which accounts for 10% of European and 3% of world goat milk production [2]. The product is consumed as a drink or used in cheese manufacturing. Among the various cheese types produced, an important part is exported (e.g., 'feta' cheese), which indicates the international significance of the goat farming industry in the country.

The quality of raw milk is important because it contributes to the quality of cheese and is significant for public health. Among the various factors that account for the quality of raw goat milk, antibiotic-resistant bacteria are of prime importance.

Staphylococci are frequently recovered from bulk-tank milk of goat herds [3–5]. Most previous studies that examined staphylococcal isolates from bulk-tank milk of goat farms, evaluated mostly methicillin-resistance, with variable results. For example, in Pakistan, Altaf et al. [6] reported that 19% of 122 *S. aureus* recovered from the milk of goats showed resistance to methicillin, whilst Caruso et al. [7] reported that they recovered only one such isolate from bulk-tank milk of 66 goat farms in Italy. In research that evaluated more antibiotics, the proportion of resistant isolates was found to be up to 100% in Brazil [8] and Jordan [9]. Thus far, all studies related to the resistance of staphylococci from goat milk have focused on the patterns of resistance of the staphylococcal isolates; herd management factors that are potentially associated with the development of resistance have not been thoroughly studied.

The objectives of this work were (a) to study the prevalence and the patterns of antibiotic resistance of staphylococcal isolates from bulk-tank milk of goat herds across Greece, (b) to assess possible associations of the presence of antibiotic resistance with the quality of milk in these herds, and (c) to evaluate herd-related factors potentially associated with the presence of antibiotic resistance among these staphylococcal isolates.

2. Results

2.1. Staphylococcal Recovery and Presence of Antibiotic Resistance

In total, staphylococci were recovered from bulk-tank milk samples from 75 herds (63.0%, 95% CI: 54.1–71.2%). Of these, *Staphylococcus aureus* was isolated from samples from 21 (17.6%) herds and coagulase-negative staphylococci were isolated from samples from 54 (45.4%) herds. A total of 80 staphylococcal isolates were recovered (21 *S. aureus* and 59 coagulase-negative staphylococci) (Table 1).

Table 1. Frequency of staphylococcal species recovered from bulk-tank milk of 119 goat herds in Greece.

Staphylococcal Species	Frequency of Staphylococcal Isolates			
	All Isolates [1]	Resistant Isolates [2,3]	Multi-Resistant Isolates [3]	Biofilm-Forming Isolates [3]
Staphylococcus aureus	21 (0.263)	5 (0.238)	0 (0.000)	17 (0.810)
Staphylococcus equorum	11 (0.138)	9 (0.818)	8 (0.727)	8 (0.727)
Staphylococcus simulans	9 (0.113)	1 (0.111)	0 (0.000)	6 (0.667)
Staphylococcus capitis	6 (0.075)	5 (0.833)	2 (0.333)	5 (0.833)
Staphylococcus lentus	5 (0.063)	2 (0.400)	2 (0.400)	1 (0.200)
Staphylcoccus haemolyticus	4 (0.050)	1 (0.250)	0 (0.000)	2 (0.500)
Staphylococcus vitulinus	4 (0.050)	4 (1.000)	4 (1.000)	3 ().750)
Staphylococcus kloosii	3 (0.038)	2 (0.667)	2 (0.667)	2 (0.667)
Staphylococcus pettenkoferi	3 (0.038)	3 (1.000)	0 (0.000)	3 (1.000)
Staphylococcus cohnii subsp. *urealyticum*	2 (0.025)	1 (0.500)	1 (0.500)	1 (0.500)
Staphylococcus lugdunensis	2 (0.025)	2 (1.000)	0 (0.000)	1 (0.500)
Staphylococcus warneri	2 (0.025)	2 (1.000)	1 (0.500)	2 (1.000)
Staphylococcus xylosus	2 (0.025)	1 (0.500)	1 (0.500)	2 (1.000)
Staphylococcus auricularis	1 (0.012)	0 (0.000)	0 (0.000)	1 (1.000)
Staphylococcus chromogenes	1 (0.012)	0 (0.000)	0 (0.000)	1 (1.000)
Staphylococcus cohnii subsp. *cohnii*	1 (0.012)	1 (1.000)	1 (1.000)	0 (0.000)
Staphylococcus epidermidis	1 (0.012)	1 (1.000)	0 (0.000)	1 (1.000)
Staphylococcus hominis	1 (0.012)	0 (0.000)	0 (0.000)	1 (1.000)
Staphylococcus intermedius	1 (0.012)	0 (0.000)	0 (0.000)	1 (1.000)
Total	80	40 (0.500)	22 (0.275)	58 (0.725)

[1] in brackets: proportion of isolates of the species among all isolates; [2] resistant to any (at least one) antibiotic; [3] in brackets: proportion of resistant, multi-resistant, or biofilm-forming isolates among the isolates of the respective species.

Resistant (to at least one (any) antibiotic) or multi-resistant staphylococci were obtained from 36 (30.3%, 95% CI: 22.7–39.0%) or 19 (16.0%, 95% CI: 10.5–23.6%) herds, respectively. There was no difference in the proportion of farms in which resistant staphylococcal isolates were recovered according to their geographic part of the country, where they were located ($p = 0.39$) (Table 2).

Table 2. Recovery of resistant staphylococcal isolates from bulk-tank milk of 119 goat herds in Greece, according to the part of the country from which the herds originated.

Location of Herds (Part of the Country)	Herds (*n*)	Herds in Which Resistant Staphylococcal Isolates Were Recovered (*n*) [1]
Central part	36	13 (0.361)
Islands	16	2 (0.125)
Northern part	36	11 (0.306)
Southern part	31	10 (0.323)

[1] in brackets: proportion of herds in which resistant staphylococcal isolates were recovered among all herds.

Of the 80 staphylococcal isolates, 40 (50.0%, 95% CI: 39.3–60.7%) (5 *S. aureus* and 35 coagulase-negative isolates, $p = 0.005$ for comparison between *S. aureus* and coagulase-negative staphylococci; $p = 0.026$ for comparison between the various coagulase-negative species) were resistant to antibiotics. Further, 22 isolates (27.5%, 95% CI: 18.9–38.1%) (all coagulase-negative isolates, $p = 0.001$ for comparison between *S. aureus* and coagulase-negative staphylococci; $p = 0.030$ for comparison between the various coagulase-negative species) were multi-resistant. Details are presented in Table 1.

At isolate level, resistance was found more frequently against penicillin and ampicillin (33 isolates, 41.3% of all isolates), fosfomycin (22 isolates, 27.5% of all isolates), clindamycin (19 isolates, 23.8% of all isolates), erythromycin (16 isolates, 20.0% of all isolates), tetracycline (12 isolates, 15.0% of all isolates) and oxacillin (6 isolates, 7.5% of all isolates) (Table S1).

At herd level, staphylococci resistant to penicillin and ampicillin were isolated from 30 (25.2%, 95% CI: 18.3–33.7%) herds, to fosfomycin from 20 (16.8%, 95% CI: 11.2–24.5%), to clindamycin from 17 (14.3%, 95% CI: 9.1–21.7%), to erythromycin from 14 (11.8%, 95% CI: 7.1–18.8%), to tetracycline from 9 (7.6%, 95% CI: 4.0–13.8%), and to oxacillin from 6 (5.0%, 95% CI: 2.3–10.6%) herds.

Among the staphylococcal species, *S. aureus* was found to be resistant more frequently to penicillin (3/21 isolates), *S. equorum* was found to be resistant more frequently to ampicillin, erythromycin, penicillin, fosfomycin, and clindamycin (8/11, 8/11, 8/11, 7/11, and 6/11 isolates, respectively), and *S. capitis* to ampicillin, fosfomycin and penicillin (5/6 isolates for each antibiotic) (Table S1).

2.2. Biofilm Formation

Of the 80 isolates, 58 (72.5%, 95% CI: 61.9–81.1%) were found to be biofilm forming (Table 1). No association was seen between biofilm formation and resistance to antibiotics. Of the 40 resistant isolates, 28 (70.0%, 95% CI: 54.6–81.9%) (4 *S. aureus* and 24 coagulase-negative isolates) were biofilm forming ($p = 0.62$). Of the 22 multi-resistant isolates, 14 (63.6%, 95% CI: 43.0–80.3%) (all coagulase-negative isolates) were biofilm forming ($p = 0.27$). Further, no association was found with specific resistance to the antibiotics evaluated ($p > 0.14$ for all comparisons) (Table S2), as well as no association was found for specific staphylococcal species ($p > 0.12$ for all comparisons).

2.3. Associations with Milk Quality

Increased total bacterial counts (i.e., $>1500 \times 10^3$ cfu mL^{-1}, which is the threshold set in the European Union for milk to undergo thermal processing [10]) were seen more commonly among herds from bulk-tank milk of which resistant staphylococcal isolates were recovered: 12/36 (33.3%) herds versus 17/83 (20.5%) herds without isolation of resistant staphylococci ($p = 0.010$). No other association of milk quality with the isolation of resistant staphylococci was found (Table S3).

2.4. Variables Associated with Isolation of Resistant or Multi-Resistant Staphylococcal Isolates from Bulk-Tank Milk

2.4.1. Isolation of Oxacillin-Resistant Staphylococcal Isolates

During the univariable analysis, a significant association with isolation of oxacillin-resistant staphylococcal isolates from bulk-tank milk was evident for 2 of the 25 variables evaluated (Table S4). These were the following: education of the farmer and presence of working staff in the herd.

Among the variables included in the multivariable analysis (Tables S4 and S5), only the following emerged as a significant factor: presence of working staff in the herd (Figure 1) ($p = 0.005$) (Table 3).

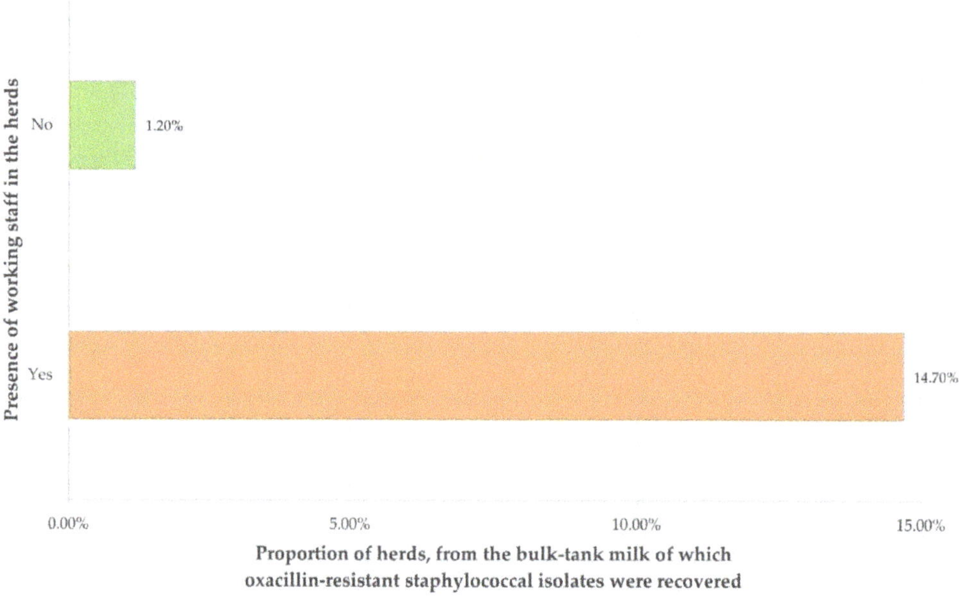

Figure 1. The proportion of herds from which oxacillin-resistant staphylococcal isolates were recovered, in terms of the presence of working staff in these herds.

Table 3. Results of multivariable analysis for isolation of oxacillin-resistant staphylococcal isolates from bulk-tank milk of 119 goat herds in Greece.

Variable ($n = 1$)	Odds Ratio [1] (95% Confidence Intervals)	p
Presence of working staff in the herd		0.005
Yes ($n = 34$)	14.483 (1.624–129.171)	0.017
No ($n = 85$)	reference	-

[1] odds ratio calculated against the lowest prevalence associations of variables.

2.4.2. Isolation of Staphylococcal Isolates Resistant to at Least One Antibiotic

During the univariable analysis, a significant association with isolation of resistant staphylococcal isolates from bulk-tank milk was evident for 6 of the 25 variables evaluated (Table S6). These were the following: management system applied in the herd, annual frequency of systemic disinfections in the farm, routine administration of antimicrobials in newborns, administration of 'dry-ewe' treatment at the end of the lactation period, farmer by profession, and presence of working staff in the herd.

Among the variables included in the multivariable analysis (Tables S5 and S6), the following two emerged as significant factors: (a) farmer by profession ($p = 0.001$) and (b) annual frequency of systemic disinfections in the farm ($p = 0.018$) (Figure 2) (Table 4).

Figure 2. Frequency (shown by the circle diameter) of herds from which resistant staphylococcal isolates were (orange circles, $n = 36$) or were not (blue circles, $n = 83$) recovered from bulk-tank milk, in relation to the number of systemic disinfections performed annually in the herd (vertical axis; 0–1 occasions, $n = 33$, 2–10 occasions, $n = 76$, >10 occasions, $n = 10$) and the professional capacity of the farmer (solid pattern of circles: full-time farmers, $n = 105$; motif pattern of circles: part-time farmers, $n = 14$).

Table 4. Results of multivariable analysis for isolation of resistant staphylococcal isolates from bulk-tank milk of 119 goat herds in Greece.

Variable ($n = 2$)	Odds Ratios [1] (95% Confidence Intervals)	p
Farmer by profession		0.001
Full-time ($n = 105$)	reference	-
Part-time ($n = 14$)	5.200 (1.602–16.882)	0.006
Annual frequency of systemic disinfectionsin the farm		0.018
0–1 occasion ($n = 33$)	reference	-
2–10 occasions ($n = 76$)	1.327 (0.499–3.529)	0.57
>10 occasions ($n = 10$)	33.429 (3.601–310.331)	0.002

[1] odds ratio calculated against the lowest prevalence associations of variables.

2.4.3. Isolation of Multi-Resistant Staphylococcal Isolates

During the univariable analysis, a significant association with isolation of multi-resistant staphylococcal isolates from bulk-tank milk was evident for 3 of the 12 variables evaluated (Table S7). These were the following: annual frequency of systemic disinfections in the farm, farmer by profession, and presence of working staff in the herd.

Additionally, the same three emerged as significant among the variables included in the multivariable analysis (Tables S5 and S7): (a) annual frequency of systemic disinfections in the farm ($p = 0.002$), (b) presence of working staff in the herd ($p = 0.016$), and (c) farmer by profession ($p = 0.022$) (Table 5).

Table 5. Results of multivariable analysis for isolation of multi-resistant staphylococcal isolates from bulk-tank milk of 119 goat herds in Greece.

Variable ($n = 3$)	Odds Ratio [1] (95% Confidence Intervals)	p
Annual frequency of systemic disinfectionsin the farm		0.002
0–1 occasion ($n = 33$)	reference	-
2–10 occasions ($n = 76$)	1.343 (0.339–5.317)	0.67
>10 occasions ($n = 10$)	23.333 (3.859–141.077)	0.0006
Presence of working staff in the herd		0.016
Yes ($n = 34$)	3.519 (1.281–9.668)	0.015
No ($n = 85$)	reference	-
Farmer by profession		0.022
Yes ($n = 105$)	reference	-
No ($n = 14$)	3.611 (1.056–12.349)	0.041

[1] odds ratio calculated against the lowest prevalence associations of variables.

3. Discussion

The European Food Safety Authority has published a scientific opinion [11] that pointed out the public health significance of antibiotic resistance of bacteria isolated from raw milk. Hence, it is relevant to study the patterns of resistance in goat farms. Moreover, the evaluation and identification of predictors related to management could allow the implementation of procedures that help to limit the presence of antibiotic resistance in the farms.

This study included goat farms from all parts of Greece. Thus, conditions prevailing throughout the country were taken into account, and factors of regional importance weighed less. In order to minimise possible bias, the study also used consistent methodologies and ensured that specific tasks were always performed by the same investigators.

3.1. Presence of Antibiotic Resistance in Staphylococcal Isolates

In previous studies of caprine mastitis, *S. caprae*, *S. chromogenes*, *S. epidermidis*, *S. simulans*, *S. warneri*, and *S. xylosus* predominated as causal agents of the infection [12,13]. This indicates that many of the recovered isolates in the current study possibly originated from sources outside the animals. Apart from the milk of the goats (i.e., as agents of mastitis), the staphylococci could have originated from the skin udder and teat or from the equipment for milk handling and storage (e.g., teat cups, pipelines, milk tank) [14]. Further, in herds in which hand milking is applied, the staphylococci might have also originated from the hands of the milkers [15].

The extent of antibiotic resistance was, in general, similar to that presented in other relevant reports from the para-Mediterranean region where dairy goats are kept and milk is produced for human consumption. The results of this study showed low-level resistance among *S. aureus* isolates but a significantly greater problem among the coagulase-negative isolates. *S. aureus* is a significant causal agent of clinical mastitis in goats; it can be diagnosed easily and then followed by the initiation of appropriate treatment. In contrast, coagulase-negative isolates cause subclinical mastitis, an infection of lesser severity, which is difficult to diagnose and thus is treated infrequently. These organisms are also present in the environment or are part of a carrier state [16] in the animals; therefore, there are more opportunities for exposure to factors that lead to the development of resistance. These results are in line with those of a recent study that we performed on the antibiotic resistance patterns of ovine mastitis pathogens, where *S. aureus* isolates showed significantly less frequent resistance than the coagulase-negative isolates [17]. It is also possible that some of the coagulase-negative isolates originated from people (e.g., farm personnel), as some species (e.g., *S. hominis* or *S. haemolyticus*) are confirmed human pathogens. Moreover, the detection of resistance to fosfomycin, which is not licenced for veterinary use, further supports the suggestion that some of the recovered isolates likely were of human origin.

Limited associations were found between the recovery of resistant staphylococcal isolates from the milk and its quality. The increased total bacterial counts may also reflect a difficulty in treating cases of mastitis, due to the presence of resistant isolates [18] or also, possibly, the development of resistance by relevant bacteria in the farm. As total bacterial counts over the threshold of 1500×10^3 cfu mL^{-1} could result in penalties in the milk price paid to farmers, the presence of resistant isolates would have tangible adverse consequences to farmers.

3.2. Predictors for Antibiotic-Resistant Staphylococcal Isolates

Three factors were found to be associated with the presence of resistance in the staphylococcal isolates recovered during the study. This suggests that there are many aspects of farm systems that can influence the development of antibiotic resistance.

Professional farmers have obviously appreciated the importance of preventing the development of antibiotic resistance in their herds. This had been repeatedly underlined in many relevant campaigns in Greece, staged by various public and private organisations within their areas of responsibility [19]. One such campaign was initiated by the Hellenic Veterinary Association [20] and involved the production of leaflets for farmers and the distribution to professionals to inform them about the significance of resistant bacterial isolates for the animals (e.g., increased animal morbidity and adverse financial effects) and the potential transmission to humans. Additionally, veterinarians would discuss with farmers and highlight the importance of preventing antibiotic resistance. We can thus postulate that part-time farmers were not fully aware of the importance of the problem and were following practices and procedures that promoted the development of resistance.

The increased number of disinfections performed in the herds was also identified as a significant predictor for the recovery of resistant isolates. The long-standing use of disinfectants has been found to lead to the development of resistance to these by staphylococcal isolates, especially given that many isolates bear genes specific for the development of resistance to these biocides (e.g., *qac*, which encodes for resistance to quaternary ammonium compounds [21]). The use of disinfectants in goat farms is related to cleaning and to the maintenance of biosecurity, aiming to protect animals and people against harmful biological agents. In piggeries also, the development of methicillin-resistance of staphylococcal isolates has been associated with increased use of disinfectants [22]. In dairy farms, this association is of particular concern, due to the necessity for increased and frequent use of disinfectants, as part of the routine for parlour cleaning post-milking. This also increases the chances for resistant bacterial isolates to enter into the chain of milk production, as was seen in this study. Cross-resistance of disinfectants with antibiotics has been shown in various bacteria [23,24], and wide use of benzalkonium-type disinfectants can promote antibiotic resistance due to co-selection. Further, according to some studies, there is a linkage between antibiotic and disinfectant resistance, which is either genetic (i.e., co-localisation of responsible genes in plasmid elements [25]) or functional [26], and the strains carrying both traits appear to have a strong selective advantage, due to their positive selection from the intense selective pressures, leading to the prevalence of multidrug resistance species. Various studies have revealed the genes and genetic networks responsible for the development of resistance mechanisms; their dissemination across strains and species is enhanced by specific mechanisms, while horizontal gene transfer figures are at the top of the list of the exchange of genetic elements. Resistance to antibiotics and disinfectants has been found to be highly associated in various bacterial species (e.g., resistance genes *qacF*, *qacE*Δ*1*, *tet*, *sul* [27]), underlying the possibility that common mechanisms are governing the resistance mechanisms to multiple substances. Moreover, staphylococcal isolates can harbour multiple plasmids responsible for resistance to antibiotics, heavy metals, antiseptics, and disinfectants [28–30], which can explain the strong association between increased frequency of systemic disinfections and antibiotic resistance. Some of these genes can also encode for resistance to antibiotics, and it is possible that the use of disinfectants could lead to the elimination of susceptible isolates, thus contributing to the increased prevalence of multidrug-resistant isolates. These pose serious threats to both human and animal populations, leading to the development of alternative approaches to control bacterial growth [31], which will enhance the levels of biosecurity and the avoidance of threats for public health.

The presence of working staff in a farm was seen more often in herds with intensive management (78% of herds with intensive management in this study), where practices found to be associated with recovery of resistant isolates are often performed; working staff would be necessary for such time-consuming tasks, e.g., administration of antibiotics to newborns, frequent disinfections etc., etc. In their majority (in 32 of 36 herds, 89%; Lianou unpublished data) the working staff were of non-Greek ethnicity and possibly did not speak the local language well; therefore, one may postulate that they might not have fully assimilated the campaigns for preventing antibiotic resistance, thus following practices that might have contributed to that. Moreover, a study in the United States indicated that farmworkers could be healthy carriers of antibiotic-resistant bacterial strains [32]. Hence, they could have disseminated these within their farm or even to other farms if they changed their workplace.

4. Materials and Methods

4.1. Goat Herds and Sampling

A cross-sectional study involving 119 herds was performed from April 2019 to July 2020 and covered all the 13 administrative regions of Greece (Figure 3). Herds were included in the study on a convenience basis (willingness of goatherds to accept a visit by university personnel for interview and sample collection), as detailed before [5]. The principal investigators (D.T.L. and G.C.F.), accompanied by other investigators, visited all the herds for sample collection.

Initially, the management practices applied in the herds were recorded during an interview of the goatherd by means of a detailed questionnaire [33]. Bulk-tank milk samples were taken aseptically from each herd for somatic cell counting and milk composition evaluation and for bacteriological examinations. Samples were packed at 0.0 to 4.0 °C and transported for laboratory examinations [5].

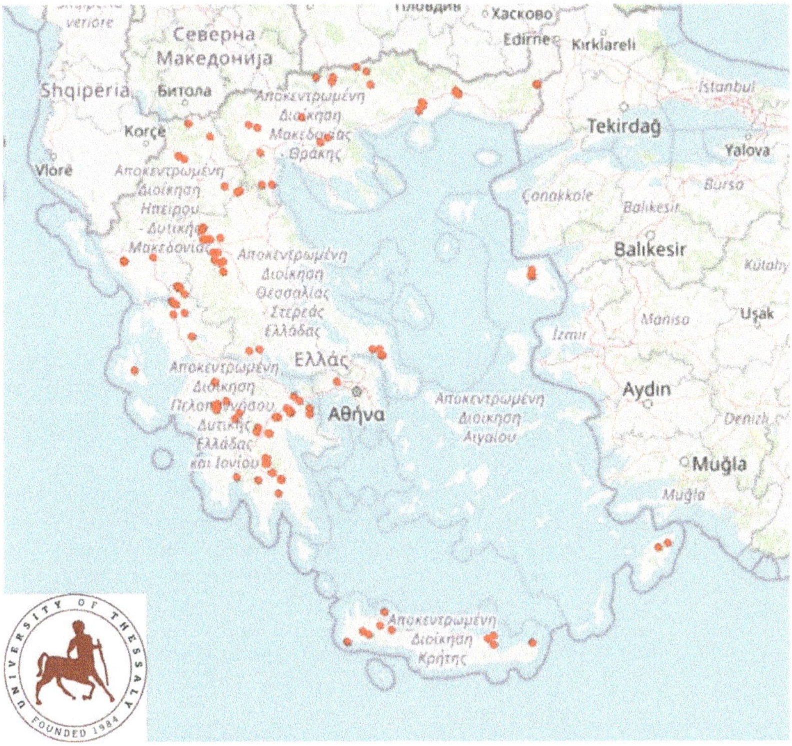

Figure 3. Location of 119 goat herds around Greece, which were visited for bulk-tank milk sampling.

4.2. Laboratory Examinations

Two milk samples from each bulk tank were used for somatic cell counts (SCC) and milk composition measurement; the other two were used for the bacteriological examinations. Two sub-samples were created and processed from each of the four samples so that each separate test was performed four times (each one in different sub-samples).

Somatic cell counting and milk content measurement were performed within 4 h of collection, whilst bacteriological examinations started within 24 h after collection of samples [Lianou et al. 2021]. Bacteriological examinations from each of the four relevant sub-samples included total bacterial counts (TBC), performed by employing the standardised procedures described by Laird et al. [34] and culturing on Staphylococcus selective medium (Mannitol salt agar; BioPrepare Microbiology, Athens, Greece) for aerobic incubation at 37 °C for 48 h; if there was no growth, media were reincubated for a further 24 h. After completion of sample aliquot withdrawal for microbiological examination, the temperature of the respective samples was measured and was never found to exceed 3.8 °C.

Bacterial isolation and initial identification by means of Gram staining and evaluation of catalase production were performed using standard methods [35,36]. Definite identification of the staphylococcal isolates to species level was performed by using matrix-assisted laser desorption/ionisation time-of-flight mass spectrometry (VITEK MS; BioMerieux, Marcy-l'-Étoile, France).

Then, in vitro biofilm formation by the staphylococcal isolates was evaluated. This was performed by using the combination of (a) the culture appearance on Congo Red agar plates and (b) the results of a microplate adhesion test. The procedures were detailed by Vasileiou et al. [37] for staphylococcal isolates recovered from milk.

Finally, the susceptibility testing to 20 antibiotics (amikacin, ampicillin, ceftaroline, ciprofloxacin, clindamycin, erythromycin, fosfomycin, fusidic acid, gentamicin, linezolid, moxifloxacin, mupirocin, mupirocin high level, oxacillin, penicillin G, rifampin, teicoplanin, tetracycline, tobramycin, trimethoprim–sulfamethoxazole) was performed by means of the automated system BD Phoenix™ M50 (BD Diagnostic Systems, Sparks, MD, USA). The interpretation of the results was based on the criteria of the European Committee on Antimicrobial Susceptibility Testing (EUCAST) (http://www.eucast.org (accessed on 17 September 2021)).

4.3. Data Management and Analysis

4.3.1. Data Management

The presence of staphylococci in bulk-tank milk was defined by the isolation of $\geq$3 staphylococcal colonies on at least one agar plate of the four that were cultured with a sub-sample from each bulk-tank milk from a herd.

Biofilm formation by the staphylococcal isolates was indicated by a combination of the results of the two methods (culture appearance on Congo Red agar and microplate adhesion) [37] and staphylococcal strains were then characterised as biofilm-forming or non-biofilm-forming.

Based on the results of susceptibility/resistance testing, isolates were classified as susceptible, susceptible increased exposure, or resistant to each antibiotic according to the EUCAST criteria. As no 'susceptible increased exposure' isolates were found, this possible result was omitted from the analyses. Multidrug-resistant isolates were those found resistant to at least three different classes of antibiotics [38].

During cell counting, total bacterial counting, and milk content measurement for each bulk-tank milk sample, the results of the two sub-samples from each sample were averaged, and then the two means were again averaged for the final result regarding each bulk-tank milk.

SCCs were transformed to somatic cell scores (SCS) [39,40] by using the following formula: $SCS = \log_2(SCC/100) + 3$, and TBCs were transformed to $\log_{10}$; for both parameters, the transformed data were used in the analyses. For the presentation of results, the transformed findings were back-transformed as follows: $100 \times 2^{(SCS-3)}$ for SCC and $10^{\log}$ for TBC data.

4.3.2. Statistical Analysis

Data were entered into Microsoft Excel and analysed using SPSS v. 21 (IBM Analytics, Armonk, NY, USA). Basic descriptive analysis was performed. Exact binomial confidence intervals (CI) were obtained.

The country was divided into four parts: central part, islands, northern part, and southern part, and herds were allocated to the appropriate one according to their geographical location. Pearson's chi-squared test was employed to compare between the four parts of the country, the proportions of herds in each one, in which staphylococcal isolates were recovered.

In total, 25 variables were evaluated for potential association with the recovery of staphylococcal isolates resistant to antibiotics from bulk-tank milk of these herds (Appendix A); these were either taken directly from the answers of the interview performed at the start of the visit or calculated based on these answers. For each of these variables, categories were created according to the answers of the farmers.

The outcomes of 'isolation of oxacillin-resistant staphylococcal isolates from bulk-tank milk' and 'isolation of resistant staphylococcal isolates from bulk-tank milk' (i.e., isolates resistant to any (at least one) antibiotic) were considered. Exact binomial CIs were obtained. Initially, the importance of predictors was assessed by using cross-tabulation with Pearson's chi-squared test and with simple logistic regression. Subsequently, multivariable models were created, initially offering to the model all variables, which achieved a significance of $p < 0.2$ in the univariable analysis. Variables were removed from the initial model by backward elimination. The p value of removal of a variable was assessed by the likelihood ratio test, and for those with a p value of >0.2, the variable with the largest probability was removed. This process was repeated until no variable could be removed with a p value of >0.2. The variables required for the final multivariable models are shown in Table S5.

Subsequently, the outcome of 'isolation of multi-resistant staphylococcal isolates from bulk-tank milk' was considered. Only the variables that achieved $p < 0.2$ in the analysis for isolation of resistant staphylococci were evaluated, and the same procedures as above (i.e., univariable and multivariable analyses) were performed. The variables required for the final multivariable model are shown in Table S5.

Finally, the potential association of isolation of a resistant staphylococcal isolate with SCC, TBC, and composition of bulk-tank milk was assessed by using a one-way analysis of variance.

In all analyses, statistical significance was defined at $p \leq 0.05$.

5. Conclusions

The recovery of resistant staphylococci in bulk-tank milk in goat farms, which is intended for human consumption, raises concerns within the 'one health' concept. Potentially, the genetic material of these resistant staphylococci, which is not destroyed during the thermal processing of milk, might possibly be transferred to humans [41,42]. These genes could be incorporated into other bacteria, which constitute a part of the normal flora of humans. Thus, further dissemination of resistance genes can occur. Resistant staphylococcal isolates in raw milk from goats act as 'containers' of resistance genes and the dairy products as the means for their dissemination. This indicates the need for limiting the staphylococcal presence in the milk and for preventing resistance development in dairy goat herds, finally reducing the relevant public health concerns.

The current findings focused on identifying variables and factors in goat herds that can be related to the presence of resistant isolates in raw milk. These findings should act as a guide to allow the application of good practices, thus contributing to preventing the development of resistance and supporting the 'one health' concept.

As a future prospect, modern genetics and genomics techniques, such as multi-locus sequence typing (MLST) or whole-genome sequencing (WGS), can be applied, in order to study the origin of such resistant isolates (e.g., from people or other animals in the farms). Thus, further measures can be applied to minimise the risk of cross-species transmission events and to reduce the prevalence of staphylococcal species in milk and dairy products.

Supplementary Materials: The following are available online at https://www.mdpi.com/article/10.3390/antibiotics10101225/s1, Table S1: Frequency of susceptibility/resistance to individual antibiotics of staphylococcal isolates recovered from bulk-tank milk of 119 goat herds in Greece, Table S2: Details of associations of antibiotic resistance with biofilm formation by staphylococcal isolates from bulk-tank milk of 119 goat herds in Greece, Table S3: Details of associations of milk quality with isolation of resistant or multi-resistant staphylococcal isolates from bulk-tank milk of 119 goat herds in Greece, Table S4: Results of univariable analysis for association with isolation of oxacillin-resistant staphylococcal isolates from bulk-tank milk of 119 goat herds in Greece, Table S5: Details of multivariable models employed for the evaluation of the isolation of resistant staphylococcal isolates from bulk-tank milk of 119 goat herds in Greece, Table S6: Results of univariable analysis for association with isolation of staphylococcal isolates resistant to at least one antibiotic from bulk-tank milk of 119 goat herds in Greece, Table S7: Results of univariable analysis for association with isolation of multi-resistant staphylococcal isolates from bulk-tank milk of 119 goat herds in Greece.

Author Contributions: Conceptualisation, D.T.L. and G.C.F.; methodology, D.T.L., E.P., P.J.C., C.V. and G.C.F.; formal analysis, D.T.L., P.J.C. and D.A.G.; investigation, D.T.L., C.K.M., K.T., A.S., A.I.K., N.G.C.V., E.I.K., C.V. and G.C.F.; resources, D.T.L. and G.C.F.; data curation, D.T.L.; writing—original draft preparation, D.T.L. and G.C.F.; writing—review and editing, E.P., T.G., V.S.M., M.C. and G.C.F.; visualisation, D.T.L.; supervision, E.P., V.S.M., M.C. and G.C.F.; project administration, E.P. and G.C.F.; funding acquisition, E.P. and G.C.F. All authors have read and agreed to the published version of the manuscript.

Funding: This research received no external funding.

Institutional Review Board Statement: The protocols of the study were approved by the academic board of the Veterinary Faculty of the University of Thessaly, Meeting 34/03.04.19.

Informed Consent Statement: Not applicable.

Data Availability Statement: Most data presented in this study are in the Supplementary Materials. The remaining data are available on request from the corresponding author. The data are not publicly available as they form part of the PhD thesis of the first author, which has not yet been examined, approved, and uploaded in the official depository of PhD theses from Greek Universities.

Acknowledgments: The help received by the veterinarians, who selected the herds and arranged the visits to these for sample collection, is gratefully acknowledged.

Conflicts of Interest: The authors declare no conflict of interest.

Appendix A

Table A1. Variables (n = 25) evaluated for potential association with the presence of antibiotic resistance in staphylococci isolated from bulk-tank milk of 119 goat herds in Greece.

Management system applied in the herd (description according to EFSA classification) [EFSA 2014]
Month into the lactation period at sampling (month)
Machine- or hand-milking (description)
No. of does in the herd (no.)
Total milk quantity per doe obtained during the preceding milking period (litres)
Average number of kids born per doe (no.)
Collaboration with a veterinarian (yes/no)
Total visits made annually by veterinarians to the herd during the preceding season (no.)
Clinical mastitis annual incidence risk in the herd (%)
Age of kid removal from their dams (days)
Daily number of milking sessions (no.)
Duration of the dry period (months)
Means of calculating live bodyweight for the administration of pharmaceutical products (weighing/estimation)
Routine overdosing (compared to the dose prescribed) of pharmaceuticals (yes/no)
Annual frequency of systemic disinfections in the farm (no. of occasions)
Routine administration of antimicrobials in newborns (yes/no)
Vaccination against mastitis (yes/no)
Administration of 'dry-ewe' treatment at the end of the lactation period (yes/no)
Use of teat disinfection after milking (yes/no)
Age of the farmer (years)
Length of previous animal farming experience of the farmer (years)
Education of the farmer (description)
Farmer by profession (yes/no)
Family tradition in farming (yes/no)
Presence of working staff in the herd (yes/no)

References

1. Hellenic Agricultural Organisation—Demeter (2020). Deliveries of Ovine and Caprine Milk by Region and Regional Authority and Average Milk Price—Calendar Year 2019. Cumulative Data Updated. Available online: https://www.elgo.gr/images/ELOGAK_files/Statistics/2020/AIGO_%CE%A0%CE%B1%CF%81%CE%B1%CE%B4%CF%8C%CF%83%CE%B5%CE%B9%CF%82_%CE%A0%CF%81%CF%8C%CE%B2%CE%B5%CE%B9%CE%BF%CF%85_%CE%BA%CE%B1%CE%B9_%CE%93%CE%AF%CE%B4%CE%B9%CE%BD%CE%BF%CF%85_%CE%93%CE%AC%CE%BB%CE%B1%CE%BA%CF%84%CE%BF%CF%82_2019.pdf (accessed on 20 December 2020).
2. Pulina, G.; Milan, M.J.; Lavin, M.P.; Theodoridis, A.; Morin, E.; Capote, J.; Thomas, D.L.; Francesconi, A.H.D.; Caja, G. Current production trends, farm structures, and economics of the dairy sheep and goat sector. *J. Dairy Sci.* **2018**, *101*, 6715–6729. [CrossRef]
3. Muehlherr, J.E.; Zweifel, C.; Corti, S.; Blanco, J.E.; Stephan, R. Microbiological quality of raw goat's and ewe's bulk-tank milk in Switzerland. *J. Dairy Sci.* **2003**, *86*, 3849–3856. [CrossRef]

4. Rola, J.G.; Sosnowski, M.; Ostrowska, M.; Osek, J. Prevalence and antimicrobial resistance of coagulase-positive staphylococci isolated from raw goat milk. *Small Rumin. Res.* **2015**, *123*, 124–128. [CrossRef]
5. Lianou, D.T.; Michael, C.K.; Vasileiou, N.G.C.; Petinaki, E.; Cripps, P.J.; Tsilipounidaki, K.; Katsafadou, A.I.; Politis, A.P.; Kordalis, N.G.; Ioannidi, K.S.; et al. Extensive countrywide field investigation of somatic cell counts and total bacterial counts in bulk tank raw milk in goat herds in Greece. *J. Dairy Res.* **2021**, *88*, 307–313. [CrossRef]
6. Altaf, M.; Ijaz, M.; Iqbal, M.K.; Rehman, A.; Avais, M.; Ghaffar, A.; Ayyub, R.M. Molecular characterization of methicillin resistant *Staphylococcus aureus* (MRSA) and associated risk factors with the occurrence of goat mastitis. *Pak. Vet. J.* **2020**, *40*, 1–6.
7. Caruso, M.; Latorre, L.; Santagada, G.; Fraccalvieri, R.; Miccolupo, A.; Sottili, R.; Palazzo, L.; Parisi, A. Methicillin-resistant *Staphylococcus aureus* (MRSA) in sheep and goat bulk tank milk from Southern Italy. *Small Rumin. Res.* **2016**, *135*, 26–31. [CrossRef]
8. Lira, M.C.; Givisiez, P.E.N.; de Sousa, F.G.C.; Magnani, M.; de Souza, E.L.; Spricigo, D.A.; Gebreyes, W.A.; Wondwossen, A.; de Oliveira, C.J.B. Biofilm-forming and antimicrobial resistance traits of staphylococci isolated from goat dairy plants. *J. Inf. Dev. Ctries* **2016**, *10*, 932–938. [CrossRef] [PubMed]
9. Obaidat, M.M.; Roess, A.A.; Mahasneh, A.A.; Al-Hakimi, R.A. Antibiotic-resistance, enterotoxin gene profiles and farm-level prevalence of *Staphylococcus aureus* in cow, sheep and goat bulk tank milk in Jordan. *Int. Dairy J.* **2018**, *81*, 28–34. [CrossRef]
10. European Union. Regulation (EC) No. 853/2004 of the European Parliament and of the Council of 29 April 2004 laying down specific hygiene rules foron the hygiene of foodstuffs. *Off. J. Eur. Union* **2004**, *L 139/55*.
11. Andreoletti, O.; Baggesen, D.L.; Bolton, D.; Butaye, P.; Cook, P.; Davies, R.; Escamez, P.S.F.; Griffin, J.; Hald, T.; Havellar, A.; et al. Scientific opinion on the public health risks related to the consumption of raw drinking milk. *EFSA J* **2015**, *13*, 3940.
12. Virdis, S.; Scarano, C.; Cossu, F.; Spanu, V.; Spanu, C.; De Santis, E.P.L. Antibiotic Resistance in *Staphylococcus aureus* and coagulase negative staphylococci isolated from goats with subclinical mastitis. *Vet. Med. Int.* **2010**, *2010*, 517060. [CrossRef]
13. Koop, G.; De Visscher, A.; Collar, C.A.; Bacon, D.A.C.; Maga, E.A.; Murray, J.D.; Supre, K.; De Vliegher, S.; Haesebrouck, F.; Rowe, J.D.; et al. Identification of coagulase-negative staphylococcus species from goat milk with the API Staph identification test and with transfer RNA-intergenic spacer PCR combined with capillary electrophoresis. *J. Dairy Sci.* **2012**, *95*, 7200–7205. [CrossRef]
14. Michael, C.K.; Lianou, D.T.; Vasileiou, N.G.C.; Tsilipounidaki, K.; Katsafadou, A.I.; Politis, A.I.; Kordalis, N.G.; Ioannidi, K.S.; Gougoulis, D.A.; Trikalinou, C.; et al. Association of staphylococcal populations on teatcups of milking rarlours with vaccination against staphylococcal mastitis in sheep and goat farms. *Pathogens* **2021**, *10*, 385. [CrossRef]
15. Anderson, K.L.; Kearns, R.; Lyman, R.; Correa, M.T. Staphylococci in dairy goats and human milkers, and the relationship with herd management practices. *Small Rumin. Res.* **2019**, *171*, 13–22. [CrossRef]
16. Verhoeven, P.O.; Gagnaire, J.; Botelho-Nevers, E.; Grattard, F.; Carricajo, A.; Lucht, F.; Pozzetto, B.; Berthelot, P. Detection and clinical relevance of *Staphylococcus aureus* nasal carriage: An update. *Expert Rev. Anti-Infect. Ther.* **2014**, *12*, 75–89. [CrossRef]
17. Vasileiou, N.G.C.; Sarrou, S.; Papagiannitsis, C.; Chatzopoulos, D.C.; Malli, E.; Mavrogianni, V.S.; Petinaki, E.; Fthenakis, G.C. Antimicrobial agent susceptibility and typing of staphylococcal isolates from subclinical mastitis in ewes. *Microb. Drug. Res.* **2019**, *25*, 1099–1110. [CrossRef]
18. Mavrogianni, V.S.; Menzies, P.I.; Fragkou, I.A.; Fthenakis, G.C. Principles of mastitis treatment in sheep and goats. *Vet. Clin. N. Am. Food Anim. Pract.* **2011**, *27*, 115–120. [CrossRef]
19. Koulenti, D.; Fragkou, P.C.; Tsiodras, S. Editorial for Special Issue 'Multidrug-Resistant Pathogens'. *Microorganisms* **2020**, *8*, 1383. [CrossRef]
20. Hellenic Veterinary Association. European Day for Information and Awareness for the Use of Antibiotics. Press release (ref. 1631, 15 Nov. 2018), Athens, 2018.
21. Wassenaar, T.M.; Ussery, D.; Nielsen, L.N.; Ingmer, H. Review and phylogenetic analysis of *qac* genes that reduce susceptibility to quaternary ammonium compounds in *Staphylococcus* species. *Eur. J. Microbiol. Immunol.* **2015**, *5*, 44–61. [CrossRef]
22. Slifierz, M.J.; Friendship, R.M.; Weese, J.S. Methicillin-resistant *Staphylococcus aureus* in commercial swine herds is associated with disinfectant and zinc usage. *Appl. Environ. Microbiol.* **2015**, *81*, 2690–2695. [CrossRef]
23. Templeton, M.R.; Oddy, F.; Leung, W.K.; Rogers, M. Chlorine and UV disinfection of ampicillin-resistant and trimetoprim-resistant *Escherichia coli*. *Can. J. Civ. Eng.* **2009**, *36*, 889–894. [CrossRef]
24. Khan, S.; Beattie, T.; Knapp, C. Relationship between antibiotic- and disinfectant-resistance profiles in bacteria harvested from tap water. *Chemosphere* **2016**, *152*, 132–141. [CrossRef]
25. Sidhu, M.S.; Heir, E.; Leegaard, T.; Wiger, K.; Holck, A. Frequency of disinfectant resistance genes and genetic linkage with beta-lactamase transposon *Tn552* among clinical staphylococci. *Antimicrobal Agents Chemother.* **2002**, *46*, 2797–2803. [CrossRef]
26. Russell, A.D. Do biocides select for antibiotic resistance? *J. Pharm. Pharmacol.* **2000**, *52*, 227–233. [CrossRef]
27. Deng, W.; Quan, Y.; Yang, S.Z.; Guo, L.J.; Zhang, X.L.; Liu, S.L.; Chen, S.J.; Zhou, K.; He, L.; Li, B.; et al. Antibiotic resistance in salmonella from retail foods of animal origin and its association with disinfectant and heavy metal resistance. *Microb. Drug Res.* **2018**, *24*, 782–791. [CrossRef]
28. Yarwood, J.M.; McCormick, J.K.; Paustian, M.L.; Kapur, V.; Schlievert, P.M. Repression of the *Staphylococcus aureus* accessory gene regulator in serum and in vivo. *J. Bacteriol.* **2002**, *184*, 1095–1101. [CrossRef]
29. Malachowa, N.; DeLeo, F.R. Mobile genetic elements of *Staphylococcus aureus*. *Cell. Mol. Life Sci.* **2010**, *18*, 3057–3071. [CrossRef]
30. Shearer, J.E.S.; Wireman, J.; Hostetler, J.; Forberger, H.; Borman, J.; Gill, J.; Sanchez, S.; Mankin, A.; LaMarre, J.; Lindsay, J.A.; et al. Major families of multiresistant plasmids from geographically and epidemiologically diverse staphylococci. *Gen. Genom. Genet.* **2011**, *1*, 581–591. [CrossRef]

31. Allen, H.K.; Trachsel, J.; Looft, T.; Casey, T.A. Finding alternatives to antibiotics. *Antimicrob. Ther. Rev. Inf. Dis. Curr. Emerg. Conc.* **2014**, *1323*, 91–100. [CrossRef]
32. Heinz, D. Farm workers contracting drug-resistant bacteria, study shows. *Healthline* **2013**. Available online: https://www.healthline.com/health-news/public-farmhands-develop-antibiotic-resistance-070613 (accessed on 26 August 2021).
33. Lianou, D.T.; Chatziprodromidou, I.P.; Vasileiou, N.G.C.; Michael, C.K.; Mavrogianni, V.S.; Politis, A.P.; Kordalis, N.G.; Billinis, C.; Giannakopoulos, A.; Papadopoulos, E.; et al. A detailed questionnaire for the evaluation of health management in dairy sheep and goats. *Animals* **2020**, *10*, 1489. [CrossRef] [PubMed]
34. Laird, D.T.; Gambrel-Lenarz, S.A.; Scher, F.M.; Graham, T.E.; Reddy, R. Microbiological Count Methods. In *Standard Methods for the Examination of Dairy Products*, 17th ed.; Wehr, H.M., Frank, J.F., Eds.; APHA Press: Washington, DC, USA, 2004; pp. 153–186.
35. Barrow, G.I.; Feltham, R.K.A. *Manual for the Identification of Medical Bacteria*, 3rd ed.; Cambridge University Press: Cambridge, UK, 1993.
36. Euzeby, J.P. List of bacterial names with standing in nomenclature: A folder available on the Internet. *Int. J. Syst. Bacteriol.* **1997**, *47*, 590–592. [CrossRef] [PubMed]
37. Vasileiou, N.G.C.; Chatzopoulos, D.C.; Gougoulis, D.A.; Sarrou, S.; Katsafadou, A.I.; Spyrou, V.; Mavrogianni, V.S.; Petinaki, E.; Fthenakis, G.C. Slime-producing staphylococci as causal agents of subclinical mastitis in sheep. *Vet. Microbiol.* **2018**, *224*, 93–99. [CrossRef]
38. Magiorakos, A.P.; Srinivasan, A.; Carey, R.B.; Carmeli, Y.; Falagas, M.E.; Giske, C.G.; Harbarth, S.; Hindler, J.F.; Kahlmeter, G.; Olsson-Liljequist, B.; et al. Multidrug-resistant, extensively drug-resistant and pandrug-resistant bacteria: An international expert proposal for interim standard definitions for acquired resistance. *Clin. Microbiol. Infect.* **2012**, *18*, 268–281. [CrossRef] [PubMed]
39. Wiggans, G.R.; Shook, G.E. A lactation measure of somatic cell count. *J. Dairy Sci.* **1987**, *70* (Suppl. 13), 2666–2672. [CrossRef]
40. Franzoi, M.; Manuelian, C.L.; Penasa, M.; De Marchi, M. Effects of somatic cell score on milk yield and mid-infrared predicted composition and technological traits of Brown Swiss, Holstein Friesian, and Simmental cattle breeds. *J. Dairy Sci.* **2020**, *103*, 791–804. [CrossRef]
41. Wang, H.; McEntire, J.C.; Zhang, L.; Li, X.; Doyle, M. The transfer of antibiotic resistance from food to humans: Facts, implications and future directions. *Rev. Sci. Tech. (Int. Off. Epizoot.)* **2012**, *31*, 249–260. [CrossRef]
42. Schwarz, S.; Loeffler, A.; Kadlec, K. Bacterial resistance to antimicrobial agents and its impact on veterinary and human medicine. *Vet. Dermatol.* **2017**, *28*, 82-e19. [CrossRef]

antibiotics

Article

Concomitant Effect of Quercetin- and Magnesium-Doped Calcium Silicate on the Osteogenic and Antibacterial Activity of Scaffolds for Bone Regeneration

Arul Murugan Preethi [1] and Jayesh R. Bellare [1,2,*]

[1] Department of Chemical Engineering, Indian Institute of Technology Bombay, Mumbai 400076, Maharashtra, India; 174020006@iitb.ac.in
[2] Wadhwani Research Center for Bioengineering (WRCB), Indian Institute of Technology Bombay, Mumbai 400076, Maharashtra, India
* Correspondence: jb@iitb.ac.in

Abstract: Quercetin is a bioflavonoid which has a broad spectrum of biological activity. Due to its lower chemical stability, it is usually encapsulated, or a metal–quercetin complex is formed to enhance its biological activity at a lower concentration. Here, our novel approach was to form a quercetin complex to magnesium-doped calcium silicate (CMS) ceramics through a coprecipitation technique so as to take advantage of quercetin's antibacterial activity within the antibacterial and osteogenic potential of the silicate. Due to quercetin's inherent metal-chelating ability, (Ca+Mg)/Si increased with quercetin concentration. Quercetin in magnesium-doped calcium silicate ceramic showed concentration-dependent pro-oxidant and antioxidant activity in SaOS-2 with respect to quercetin concentration. By optimizing the relative concentration, we were able to achieve 3-fold higher proliferation and 1.6-fold higher total collagen at day 14, and a 1.7-fold higher alkaline phosphatase production at day 7 with respect to polycaprolactone/polyvinylpyrrolidone (PCL/PVP) scaffold. Quercetin is effective against Gram-positive bacteria such as *S. aureus*. Quercetin is coupled with CMS provided similar effect with lower quercetin concentration than quercetin alone. Quercetin reduced bacterial adhesion, proliferation and biofilm formation. Therefore, quercetin-coupled magnesium-doped calcium silicate not only enhanced osteogenic potential, but also reduced bacterial adhesion and proliferation.

Keywords: quercetin; magnesium-doped calcium silicate; osteogenic activity; antibacterial activity; bone regeneration and nanofiber scaffold

Citation: Preethi, A.M.; Bellare, J.R. Concomitant Effect of Quercetin- and Magnesium-Doped Calcium Silicate on the Osteogenic and Antibacterial Activity of Scaffolds for Bone Regeneration. *Antibiotics* **2021**, *10*, 1170. https://doi.org/10.3390/antibiotics10101170

Academic Editor: Helena Felgueiras

Received: 30 July 2021
Accepted: 18 September 2021
Published: 27 September 2021

1. Introduction

Designing resorbable scaffolds for bone tissue engineering is a multifactorial design problem. The current design aspect of scaffold design requires it to reduce/prevent microbial adhesion and growth and, if possible, kill the microbes, as well as aid in successful bone regeneration. Currently, many synthetic polymers such as polycaprolactone (PCL) do not possess inherent antibacterial property. Passive resistance against bacteria can be provided by making the scaffold hydrophilic. This can be achieved by including polyvinylpyrrolidone (PVP). Other routes to incorporate antibacterial properties into scaffold can be through the addition of nanoparticle and/or through antibiotics [1]. However, the excessive use of antibiotics leads to the development of antibiotic-resistant microbes. Therefore, one section of research focuses on identifying biomolecules that can offer properties such as those of antibiotics and also support tissue regeneration.

Quercetin (Q), a phenolic bioflavonoid which is predominantly found in vegetables such as onion, has antioxidant, anti-inflammatory, antibacterial and anti-viral properties [2]. Based on the cell type, quercetin can exhibit pro-oxidant or antioxidant effects [3]. Foundational requirements for successful bone regeneration are osteoblastogenesis and angiogenesis. When bone-marrow-derived mesenchymal stem cells (MSCs) were treated with 0.1 to 10 μM of quercetin, MSCs differentiated into osteoblast lineage by upregulating osteoblast-specific gene expression. Quercetin inhibits osteoclasts by reducing cell proliferation and resorption pits. Additionally, quercetin enhances angiogenesis by activating vascular endothelial growth factor signaling, upregulating angiogenin-1 [4]. Antibacterial mechanisms of flavonoids are different from those of conventional antibiotics. Quercetin exhibits antibacterial activity by decreasing bilayer thickness, opposing bacterial cell–cell signaling, inhibiting the biofilm of *E. coli* EAEC 042, inhibiting DNA gyrase, and preventing ATP hydrolysis [5]. The viability of *E. coli* and *S. aureus* when treated with 2 μg/mL of quercetin for 24 h was 40% and 60%. This reveals that quercetin did not offer complete bacterial growth inhibition. The efficacy was enhanced by cadmium complexing with N–N bidentate ligands [6].

Even though quercetin has a broad spectrum of biological activity, its chemical stability depends on pH, temperature, light and the oxidative environment. To enhance the chemical stability, thereby, bioavailability, suitable delivery systems have been designed. Their advantages and disadvantages are discussed elsewhere [7]. The sole purpose of many drug delivery system or vehicles is to release the bioflavonoid without affecting its chemical stability. However, many vehicles mostly do not possess inherent properties essential for osteoblast activity. Fabricating bioactive nanoparticles as delivery vehicles for bioflavonoids will enhance the overall biological performance.

Calcium-silicate-based ceramic nanoparticles demonstrate excellent bioactivity. Their degradation rate can be fine-tuned by doping elements such as magnesium. This inherently upregulates osteoblast activity. There are various synthesis techniques for magnesium-doped calcium silicate (CMS) ceramics [8]. Commonly used techniques such as coprecipitation are flexible to accommodate bioflavonoids without compromising their chemical stability. The objective of this article is to investigate the effect of quercetin–CMS systems on their ability to enhance osteoblast activity using human osteosarcoma (SaOS-2) cell lines and on their ability to resist bacterial adhesion and proliferation.

2. Results

This section discusses nanoparticle and scaffold characterization under two different subsections.

2.1. Nanoparticle Characterization

Magnesium-doped calcium silicate (CMS) ceramics prepared through coprecipitation technique rendered them as nano-plate-like structures, as shown in Figure 1. The structure did not change upon quercetin addition. Incorporation of quercetin increased the Mg/Ca ratio in the nanoparticle, and (Ca+Mg)/Si was also found to be higher for the CMSQ10 nanoparticle (Table 1). FTIR spectra (Figure 2A) of the CMS nanoparticle exhibited Si–O–Si antisymmetric stretching at ~1080 to 1095 cm^{-1} and symmetric stretching at ~465 cm^{-1}. FTIR spectra of quercetin show C=C stretching in the aromatic ring at 1560 cm^{-1} and –OH (phenolic group) at 1379 cm^{-1}. These quercetin functional groups were detected in CMSQ5, CMSQ10 and CMSQ20 nanoparticles, confirming the presence of quercetin in its structure [9]. XRD patterns of all the nanoparticles (Figure 2B) showed that nanoparticles are amorphous in nature, and peaks at around 29° showed the characteristic peak of calcium silicate [10]. Peaks of $CaCO_3$ appeared because the nanoparticles were prepared in an ambient environment.

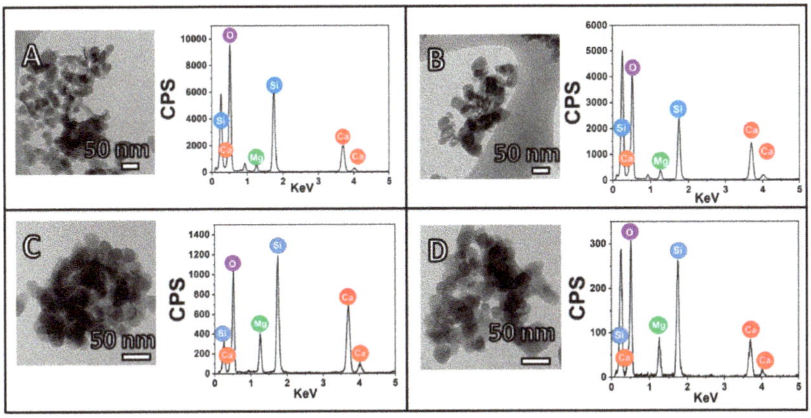

Figure 1. TEM and EDX of (**A**) CMS, (**B**) CMSQ5, (**C**) CMSQ10 and (**D**) CMSQ20 nanoparticles. The shapes of all nanoparticles are nano-plate. EDX confirmed the presence of calcium, magnesium and silicate ions.

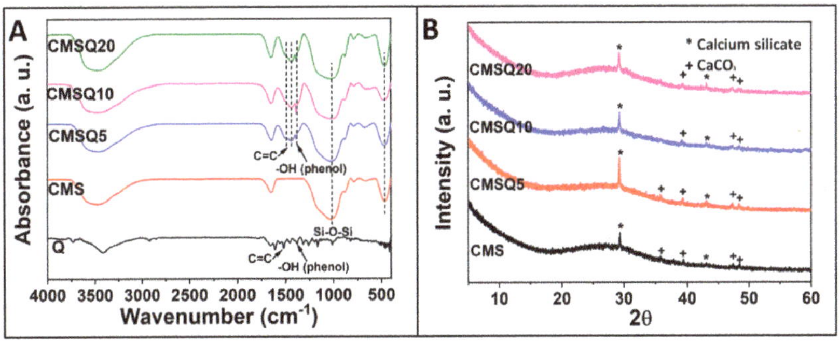

Figure 2. (**A**) FTIR and (**B**) XRD of CMS, CMSQ5, CMSQ10, and CMSQ20 nanoparticles. FTIR confirmed the presence of quercetin in its structure. XRD showed the presence of calcium silicate and $CaCO_3$ peaks.

2.2. Scaffold Characterization

The scaffold notation PCMSQx (where x = 0, 5, 10 and 20 mg of quercetin per 100 mL of total nanoparticle precursor solution) indicates the electrospun scaffold using PCL/PVP as a polymer that had a quercetin-coupled CMS nanoparticle. Electrospinning parameters for the scaffold are tabulated in Table 2. Addition of the nanoparticle onto the polymer solution altered solution viscosity and conductivity, which, in turn, required a higher flow rate which affected the nanofiber diameter and nanofiber orientation, followed by scaffold surface roughness (Figure 3). PCMSQ20 had the smallest nanofiber diameter that affected the roughness of the scaffold (Figure 4B). A protein adsorption study was performed to evaluate the scaffold's ability to attract blood protein upon insertion, thereby starting the cascade of the bone regeneration process. From Figure 4B, it can be observed that with the increasing concentration of quercetin in CMS, protein adsorption reduced. This is due to the hydrophobic nature of quercetin and its strong affinity to BSA protein [11]. With increasing concentrations of quercetin in CMS, more quercetin will be released, which will then bind to a hydrophobic BSA protein, preventing it from further adsorption on to the scaffold surface (Figure 4). From the ion release study (Figure 5), it was revealed that the amorphous nature of nanoparticles supported ion release. Additionally, quercetin interacted with all the ions effectively. With the increase in quercetin concentration, the sustained release of silicate ion was observed, because quercetin bonded with silicon.

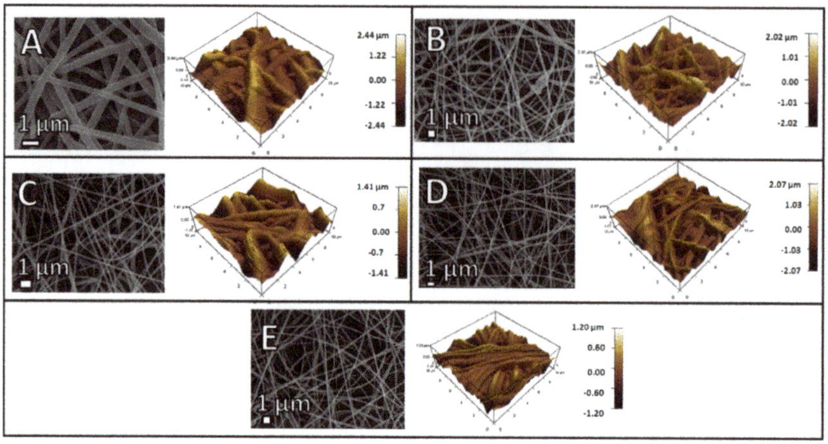

Figure 3. SEM and AFM images of (**A**) P (**B**) PCMS, (**C**) PCMSQ5, (**D**) PCMSQ10 and (**E**) PCMSQ20 scaffolds. Incorporation of a biomolecule loaded and unloaded with CMS nanoparticles significantly changed the nanofiber diameter and scaffold roughness.

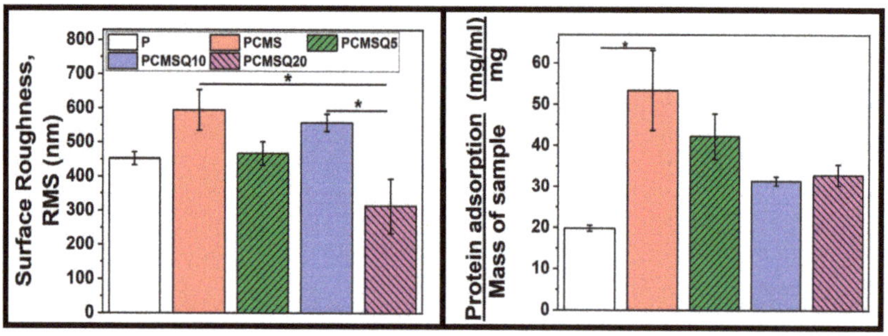

A

B

Figure 4. (**A**) Surface roughness and (**B**) protein adsorption of the scaffold. Nanofiber arrangement altered scaffold roughness. The presence of quercetin affected BSA adsorption. * stand for $p < 0.05$.

To study the mechanical property of the scaffold, the tensile stress, extension at break and modulus was analyzed. It was observed that the tensile stress and modulus of the scaffold increased with the addition of CMS. The presence of CMS-based nanoparticle into the scaffold significantly enhanced the load-bearing ability of the scaffold by restricting the polymer elongation (Figure 6).

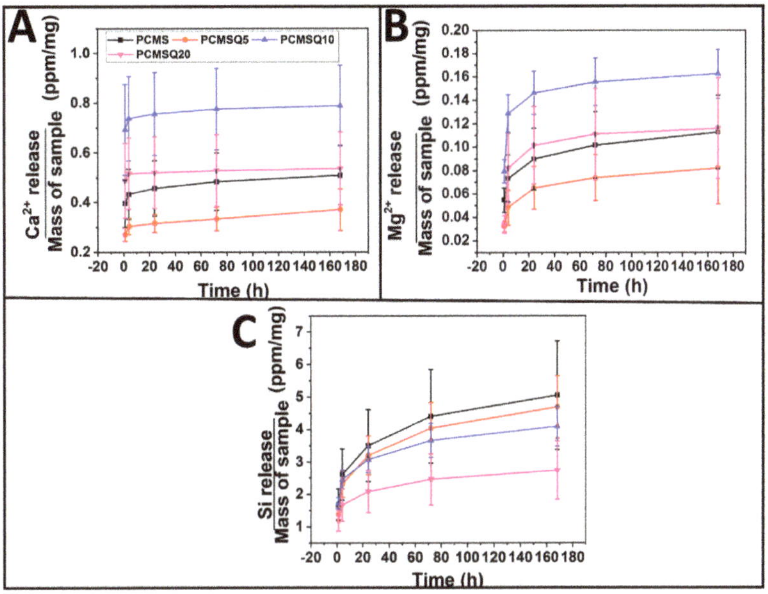

Figure 5. Ion release from the scaffold upon immersion in DI water. (**A**) Calcium ion release, (**B**) magnesium ion release, and (**C**) silicon ion release from the scaffold. Release of calcium and magnesium ion was similar across all the scaffolds, but silicon ion release decreased with increasing quercetin into the nanoparticle.

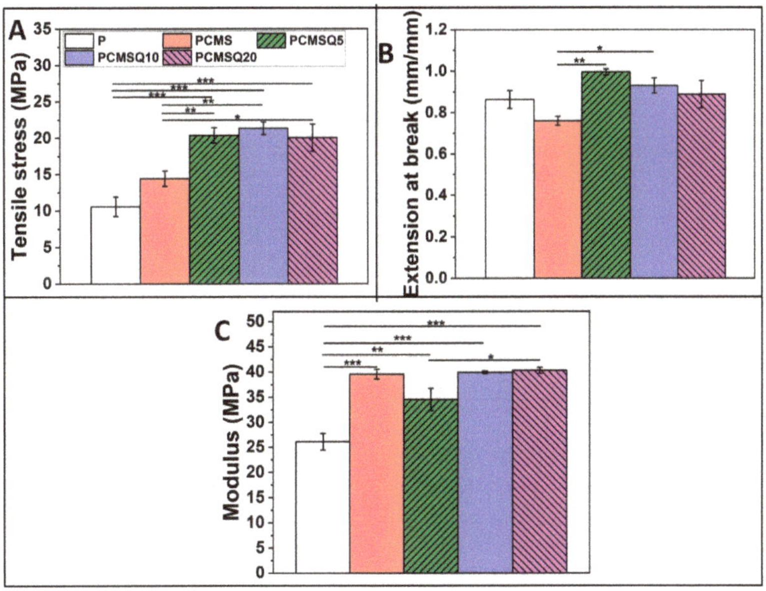

Figure 6. (**A**) Tensile stress, (**B**) extension at break, and (**C**) modulus of P, PCMS, PCMSQ5, PCMSQ10 and PCMSQ20 scaffolds. Presence of the nanoparticle improved strength of the scaffold, followed by the modulus. *, ** and *** stand for $p < 0.05$, 0.01 and 0.001.

The osteogenic potential of the scaffold was tested with the MTT assay (Figure 7A), DNA quantification (Figure 7B), ALP quantification (Figure 7C), ROS generation

(Figure 7D) and total collagen synthesis (Figure 7E) using the SaOS-2 cell line. An in vitro study of quercetin and the CMS system in the PCL/PVP scaffold revealed that the presence of quercetin did not affect the osteogenic potential of CMS. The maximum osteogenic potential in the form of higher proliferation, ALP and collagen synthesis was observed for the PCMSQ10 scaffold. With further increases in quercetin concentration, intercellular reactive oxygen species (ROS) production was increased, which affected the osteogenic potential of the scaffold. The in vitro data were corroborated with confocal images, as shown in Figure 8.

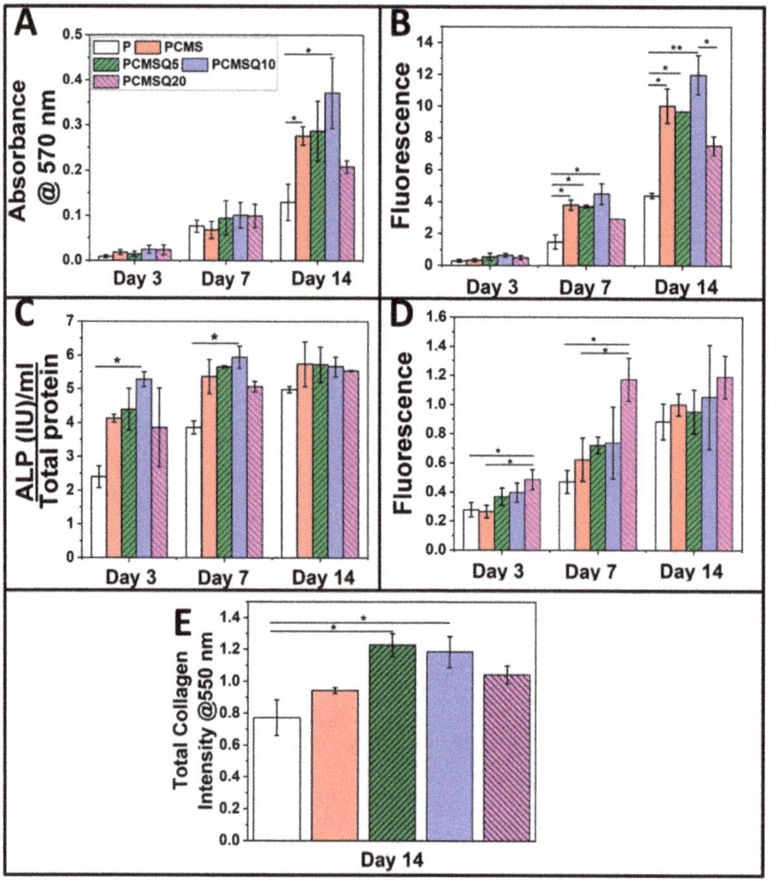

Figure 7. Osteogenic potential assessment (**A–E**). (**A**) MTT assay, (**B**) DNA quantification, (**C**) ALP (alkaline phosphatase), (**D**) ROS production, and (**E**) total collagen quantification of SaOS-2. Quercetin coupled with CMS increased the osteogenic activity by enhancing osteogenic markers such as ALP and collagen production. The maximum acceptable quercetin in the system that exhibited osteogenic properties is PCMSQ10. * and ** stand for $p < 0.05$ and 0.01.

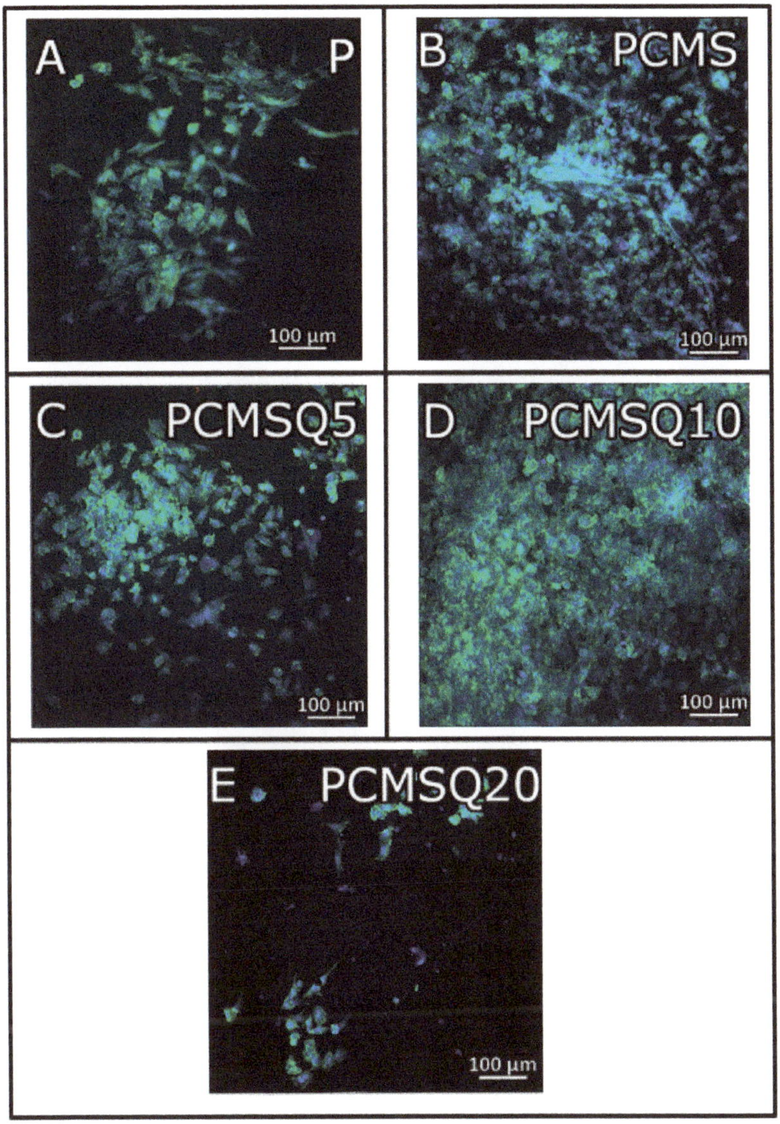

Figure 8. Confocal image of (**A**) P, (**B**) PCMS, (**C**) PCMSQ5, (**D**) PCMSQ10 and (**E**) PCMSQ20 scaffolds at day 14 confirms that PCMSQ10 had enhanced osteogenic propertied. The confocal images corroborated the MTT and DNA quantification analyses.

The antibacterial activity of the scaffold was analyzed by using *E. coli* and *S. aureus*. The scaffold was placed in an environment that supported bacterial proliferation (Figure 9). It was observed that the presence of CMS alone in the scaffold reduced *E. coli* adhesion by 1 log factor, whereas for quercetin alone, it required 10% loading on PCL/PVP (PQ10) to provide a similar effect. When quercetin was coupled with CMS, with reduced quercetin loading, bacterial adhesion was reduced by 1 log factor, which was mainly due to CMS but did not reduce the biofilm formation significantly.

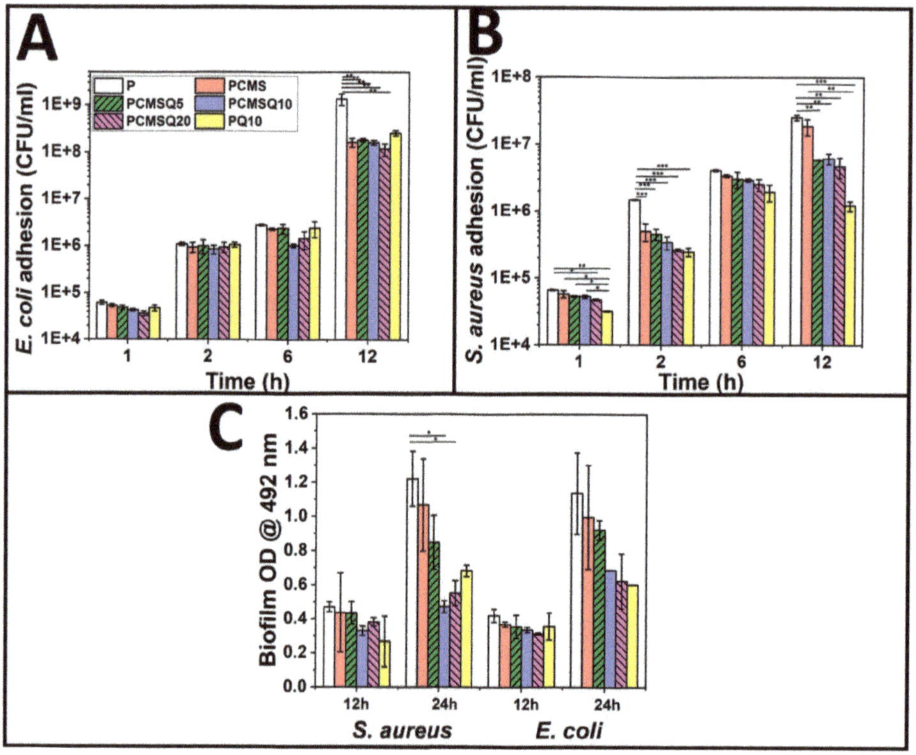

Figure 9. Antibacterial potential assessment of the scaffold. Kinetic study of adhered bacteria (**A**) *E. coli* and (**B**) *S. aureus* on the scaffold. (**C**) Biofilm quantification on the scaffold at 12 h and 24 h. Quercetin is effective against *S. aureus*. Coupling magnesium-doped calcium silicate and quercetin reduced *S. aureus* adhesion and biofilm formation at lower quercetin concentrations. *, ** and *** stand for $p < 0.05$, 0.01 and 0.001.

However, quercetin is effective against Gram-positive bacteria and significantly reduced the proliferation and biofilm formation in *S. aureus* (Figure 9B). The coupling effect of CMS and quercetin in the PCMSQ10 scaffold reduced biofilm formation by 2.4-fold compared to scaffold P at 24 h. The SEM of the scaffold with *S. aureus* (Figure 10) corroborated the result, as shown in Figure 9E.

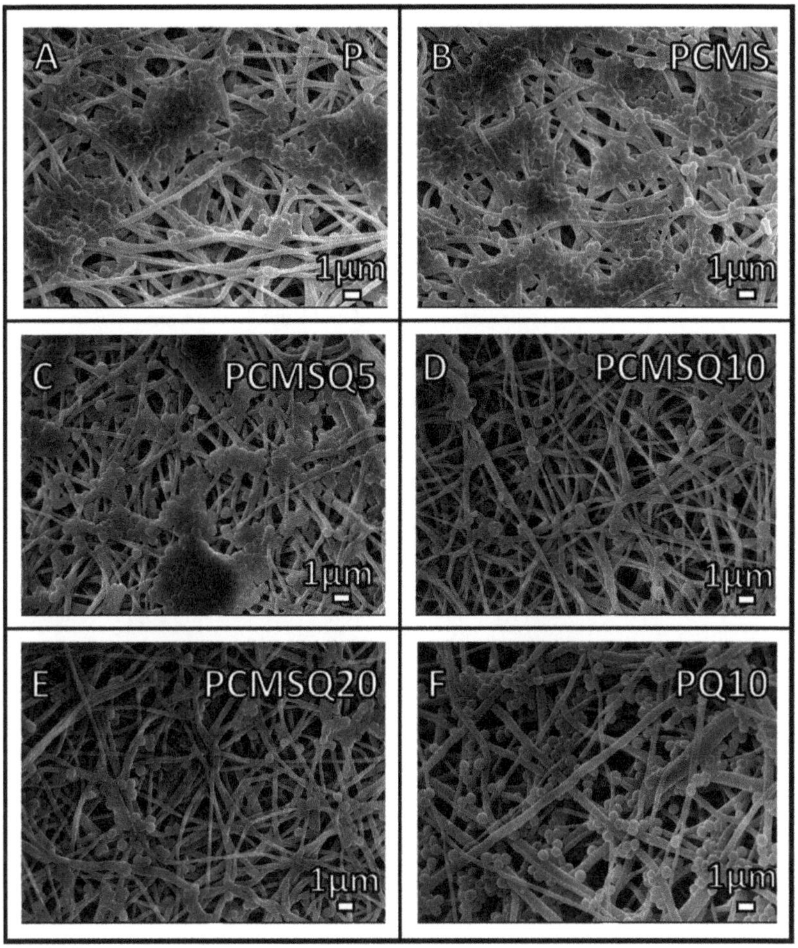

Figure 10. SEM images of *S. aureus* on (**A**) P, (**B**) PCMS, (**C**) PCMSQ5, (**D**) PCMSQ10, (**E**) PCMSQ20 and (**F**) PQ10 scaffolds at 24 h. The PCMSQ10 scaffold had the fewest adhered bacteria compared to the other scaffold. The SEM images correlated well with the OD of the biofilm.

3. Discussion

Scaffold design for bone tissue regeneration along with local antibiotic therapy is an important research area that aims to avoid post-operative infection leading to osteomyelitis. Conventional antibiotic-loaded scaffold eliminates microbes at the cost of developing antibiotic-resistant bacteria, and it also requires additional compounds that impart osteogenic potential to the scaffold [1]. The research gap can be bridged by finding a suitable scaffold system that reduces bacterial adhesion along with improving the osteogenic activity.

Synthetic polymer scaffolds made out of PCL in general do not possess antibacterial properties [1]. They are either blended or modified with a polymer that can provide at least passive resistance to bacterial adhesion. Polymers such as polyamides, polyethylene glycol, etc., provide antibiofouling effects through passive resistance [1]. PVP is also one such polymer that exhibits antibiofouling effects, whose incorporation increases hydrophilicity to the scaffold that not only improves osteoblast adhesion, but also decreases bacterial adhesion. Their solubility in water provides a suitable platform for the enhanced availability of molecules for drug-delivery-based scaffolds [12].

Flavonoids such as quercetin are known to exhibit a spectrum of biological activity. They are synthesized by plants in response to microbial attack. Quercetin has found its foothold in nerve [13], skin tissue engineering applications [14] and also in cancer treatment [15]. Recently, studies on quercetin-based scaffolds in bone tissue engineering are gaining attention among researchers because of quercetin's multifaceted properties. The dose-dependent activity of quercetin is cell-line-specific. Quercetin at a lower concentration supports cell proliferation in nerve [13], skin [14] and bone scaffolds, but at higher concentrations, quercetin acts as an anticancer agent [15]. Therefore, it is important to administer appropriate dosages to gain the potential of quercetin-based scaffolds.

Bone-marrow-derived MSCs cultured on quercetin inlaid silk hydroxyapatite scaffolds revealed that the lowest quercetin concentration, i.e., 0.03 wt.%, had the highest ALP production and COL-I and Runx2 gene expression in vitro. In vivo studies on rat calvaria also confirmed that, at 0.03 wt.%, the bone mineral density, bone volume and fraction were found to be higher [16]. When MC3T3-E1 cells were cultured on a 3D-printed polydopamine-poly (l-lactide) scaffold, it was revealed that osteogenic activity such as cell proliferation, ALP and mineralization was found to be higher for coating concentrations up to 200 μM. However, the osteogenic activity was lower for coating concentrations of 400 μM [17]. Similarly, a poly (l-lactide) chitosan scaffold coated with polydopamine and 200 μM of quercetin exhibited higher cell proliferation, ALP and mineralization by MC3T3-E1 cells [18]. The presence of –OH groups in quercetin helps them effectively chelate with metal ions. A zinc (quercetin)(phenanthroline) complex in PCL/gelatin scaffold enhanced angiogenic and osteogenic activity [19]. Similar effects were found in a copper (quercetin)(phenanthroline) complex and copper (quercetin)(neocuproine) complex [20]. From the above metal–quercetin complex study, it can be understood that MG-63 cells treated with quercetin concentrations above 80 μM show cytotoxic effect. However, the cytotoxic limit was reduced to 60 μM.

Quercetin exhibits better antibacterial activity towards Gram-positive bacteria. Due to their poor water solubility and low chemical stability, they are chemically modified to improve their antibacterial performance [21,22]. To enhance the quercetin's antibacterial activity, it needs to be complexed with metal ions. Quercetin complexed with Mn^{2+}, Hg^{2+}, Co^{2+} and Cd^{2+} showed antibacterial activity against *S. aureus*, *Bacillus cereus*, *P. aeruginosa*, *E. coli*, and *Klebsiella pneumonia* than quercetin at similar concentrations [5].

Thus far, to the best of our knowledge, no studies have focused on the dual properties (i.e., osteogenic and antibacterial activity) of quercetin in bone tissue engineering. Quercetin expresses both pro-oxidant and antioxidant effects [3]. Therefore, optimizing quercetin concentration that provides the scaffold with dual property has been the aim of this article.

In our study, the osteogenic potential of quercetin showed dose-dependent behavior. The coupling of CMS and quercetin increased the scaffold's osteogenic activity up to the PCMSQ10 scaffold, i.e., the proliferation and total collagen production were 3-fold and 1.6-fold higher than PCL/PVP at day 14, respectively. With any further increase in quercetin concentration in the scaffold, the scaffold started showing signs of reduced cell viability and osteogenic potential by increasing the ROS production. Similar effects were found in scaffolds used for neural repair [13]. We were able to achieve higher osteogenic potential at the lowest quercetin concentration compared to the concentration reported in the literature. This was due to the presence of calcium, magnesium and silicon ions along with quercetin in the scaffold, which provided favorable outcomes in osteoblast activity.

The antibacterial potential of the scaffold was evaluated using *E. coli* and *S. aureus*. CMS quercetin system showed better antibacterial potential towards *S. aureus* from the start of the experiment than *E. coli*. This reveals that Gram-positive bacteria are susceptible to quercetin even at the lowest concentration than Gram-negative bacteria because quercetin affects the cell membrane permeability and integrity of *S. aureus* [23]. At lower quercetin concentrations, antibacterial activity against *E. coli* comes from CMS alone. This may be because the concentration of quercetin inside the scaffold is too low to provide any antibacterial activity against *E. coli*. Our data corroborate the literature which conveys that the minimum inhibition concentration of quercetin towards *S. aureus* is much lower than that of *E. coli* [20]. The mode of antibacterial activity in *S. aureus* can be due to outbursts of reactive oxygen species and decreases in the proton-motive force in *S. aureus* that affects the membrane permeability [18].

Therefore, our study addressed the important aspect of bridging the anti-microbial research gap by formulating a biomolecule-based scaffold and demonstrating that, it has both osteogenic and antibacterial activity.

4. Experimental

4.1. Materials

Polycaprolactone (PCL, M.W. 80,000 Da), sodium silicate solution (Extra pure), 3-(4,5-dimethylthiazol-2-yl)-2,5-diphenyltetrazolium bromide (MTT) and Direct Red 80 was purchased from Sigma-Aldrich, India. Polyvinylpyrrolidone (PVP, M.W. 40,000 Da), magnesium nitrate hexahydrate (98% purity), McCoy's 5A media with L-glutamine, fetal bovine serum (FBS, gamma-irradiated, sterile-filtered, South American) and Antibiotic Antimycotic Solution 100X Liquid (w/10,000 U penicillin, 10 mg streptomycin and 25 μg amphoteric B per ml in 0.9% normal saline) was purchased from Himedia, India. Calcium nitrate tetrahydrate (99% purity) was purchased from S D fine-Chem limited, India. GlutaMAX^{TM}-1(100X) was purchased from Thermofisher Scientific, India. Picric acid extrapure AR, 99.8% was purchased from SRL Pvt. Ltd., Mumbai, India. All chemicals were used as purchased.

4.2. Sample Preparation

4.2.1. One-Pot Synthesis of Quercetin in Calcium Magnesium Silicate

Solution A containing 0.09 M calcium nitrate tetrahydrate and 0.01 M magnesium nitrate hexahydrate was adjusted to pH 11, before it was mixed with solution B containing 0.1 M sodium silicate. The entire solution was mixed for 30 min. The precipitate was washed and dried overnight. For the quercetin loading, 5, 10, and 20 mg of quercetin per 100 mL of total solution was added to solution B and was then mixed with solution A. Nanoparticles with 0, 5, 10, and 20 g of quercetin/mL of total solution were named as CMS, CMSQ5, CMSQ10 and CMSQ20, respectively. Elemental compositions of nanoparticles are given in Table 1.

Table 1. Elemental composition of nanoparticles as per TEM.

Sl. No.	Sample Code	Elements	(Ca+Mg)/Si	Mg/Ca
1	CMS	Ca, Mg, Si	0.44 ± 0.09	0.28 ± 0.07
2	CMSQ5	Ca, Mg, Si	0.65 ± 0.13	0.28 ± 0.14
3	CMSQ10	Ca, Mg, Si	1.06 ± 0.06	0.48 ± 0.05
4	CMSQ20	Ca, Mg, Si	0.61 ± 0.04	0.69 ± 0.28

4.2.2. Electrospinning Solution Preparation and Nanofiber Fabrication

The solution for electrospinning consisted of a solvent comprising 2.5 mL dichlorometh ane and 1 mL methanol, and the polymer comprised 0.25 g of PCL and 0.05 g of PVP. The solution was vigorously mixed for 1 h. The nanofiber mat was prepared using a 2ml syringe and 23 G blunt needle (BD Discardit^{TM} II syringe, India) in an electrospinning machine (ESPIN NANO, India) and is denoted as "P". To prepare nanoparticle-incorporated nanofiber mats, 5 wt.% of nanoparticles with respect to PCL was added to the above solution and the scaffolds were named as PCMS, PCMS5Q, PCMS10Q and PCMS20Q, respectively. All the scaffolds were vacuum-dried at room temperature in a desiccator; the parameters for electrospinning are given in Table 2.

Table 2. Optimized electrospinning parameters of the scaffolds and their fiber diameter.

Sl. No.	Sample Code	Flowrate (mL/h)	Voltage (KV)	Distance (cm)	Fiber Diameter (nm)
1	P	0.5	25	23	0.56 ± 0.14
2	PCMS	1.2	19	21	0.31 ± 0.07
3	PCMS5Q	1.2	17	17	0.35 ± 0.11
4	PCMS10Q	1.2	19	17	0.24 ± 0.06
5	PCMS20Q	1.2	21	21	0.29 ± 0.06

4.3. *Characterization*

4.3.1. Scanning Electron Microscopy (SEM)

Parameters for electrospinning were optimized with the help of field emission gun scanning electron microscopy (JEOL JSM-7600F FEGSEM). All the samples were sputter-coated with a 10 nm thickness of platinum before analysis.

4.3.2. Transmission Electron Microscopy (TEM)

Morphology and elemental analyses of the nanoparticles were performed with JEOL, JEM 2100F and energy-dispersive X-ray spectroscopy in combination with TEM. To prepare the sample for analysis, a few milligrams of nanoparticles were added to isopropanol and sonicated for 30 min. Then, a few droplets of the above solution were drop-casted on top of the carbon-coated copper grid and dried.

4.3.3. Atomic Force Microscopy (AFM)

AFM (MFP3D Origin, Asylum/Oxford Instruments) was used to analyze the surface roughness of the scaffold. The scan range was 10 × 10 μm^2 with a frequency of 0.5/Hz.

4.3.4. Fourier-Transfer Infrared Spectroscopy (FTIR)

The nanoparticle functional groups were analyzed using a 3000 Hyperion Microscope with Vertex 80 FTIR system (Bruker, Germany) in the range of 4000–400 cm^{-1}.

4.3.5. X-ray Diffraction (XRD)

The phase and crystallinity of nanoparticles were analyzed using a Rigaku Smartlab X-ray diffractometer with a 3 kW X-ray generator Cu tube. The analysis was performed between 2θ of 5° to 60° at room temperature with a scan rate of 0.05°/s.

4.3.6. Ion Release Study

The scaffold was pre-weighed and immersed in 5 mL deionized water at 37 °C (DI water). This scaffold was re-immersed into DI water for every time point. The liquid samples were then analyzed using inductively coupled plasma–atomic emission spectroscopy, ICP-AES (ARCOS, Simultaneous ICP Spectrometer, SPECTRO Analytical Instruments GmbH, Kleve, Germany).

4.3.7. Quantification of Protein Adsorption on the Scaffold

This analysis was performed to understand the effect of quercetin on the scaffold's ability to adsorb bovine serum albumin (BSA). The scaffolds of size of 1 × 1 cm^2 were immersed in a 1ml solution containing 5 g/dL of BSA and were incubated for 2 h at 37 °C. Next, the scaffold after incubation was immersed in 1% sodium dodecyl sulfate solution (SDS) for 2 h to strip adsorbed BSA away. Later, the BSA protein in SDS was quantified using Micro BCA Protein Assay Kit 23235 (ThermoFisher Scientific, Mumbai, India), as per the manufacturer's protocol.

4.3.8. Tensile Test

Uniaxial tensile testing of the scaffolds was performed using an Instron 2519 series using a 5 kN load cell at room temperature with a strain rate of 5 mm/min. Analysis was performed according to ASTM D882 standards.

4.4. In Vitro Assessment of Scaffold Using SaOS-2

The human osteosarcoma SaOS-2 cell line was purchased from NCCS, Pune, India, and was cultured using McCoy's 5A media containing L-glutamine containing 1% GlutaMAX^{TM}-1(100X), 1% antibiotic and antimycotic solution. The cells were maintained in a humidified incubator kept at 37 °C with 5% carbon dioxide (CO_2). For the assays, the scaffolds were placed in non-tissue-culture-treated 24-well plate (Eppendorf USA), and sterilized using 70% ethanol and UV for 1 h each. The scaffolds were preconditioned using cell culture media for 1 h each. Cells were seeded at a density of 4×10^4 cells per cm^2 and incubated for 4 h at 37 °C with 5% CO_2. Afterwards, 0.4 mL media were added to all the wells, and replenished every 3 days.

Cell viability on the scaffold was evaluated using (3-(4,5-Dimethylthiazol-2-yl)-2,5-Diphenyltetrazolium Bromide) solution (MTT, 1 mg/mL in PBS). After culturing cells until a predetermined time point, the scaffolds were washed with PBS and then incubated in 200 μL of MTT solution for 4 h, followed by adding 800 μL of DMSO to dissolve the formazan crystals. The optical density at 470 nm was measured using MultiskanSkyHigh Microplate Spectrophotometer (Thermo-Fischer Scientific, Mumbai, India).

Cell proliferation on the scaffold was assessed using a Quant-iT Pico Green DNA assay kit. After culturing cells to a predetermined time point, the scaffolds were washed with PBS and then freeze–thawed twice in 500 μL of autoclaved deionized water. The solution was then centrifuged at 10,621× *g* for 10 min; then, 100 μL of cell lysate supernatant was mixed with 100 μL of Picogreen working solution and incubated for 5 min, as per the manufacturer's protocol. Fluorescence intensity was measured using a Varioskan LUX Multimode Microplate Reader at 490/538 nm, respectively.

To measure the earlier marker for osteogenic maturation (alkaline phosphatase), a Sensolyte® pNPP Alkaline Phosphatase Assay colorimetric kit was used. The assay was performed as per the manufacturer's protocol.

SaOS-2 cells majorly produce collagen type-I, which is also a marker for osteoblast differentiation. To economically quantify total collagen, picosirius red dye is used. In this study, 1×10^5 cells were seeded on top of the 1.5×1.5 cm^2 scaffold in 12-well plate for 14 days. After culturing cells for 14 days, cells were lysed using 0.2% Triton X-100 prepared in autoclaved deionized water, followed by freeze–thawing and centrifugation (4 °C at 2500 rpm for 10 min). To 100 μL of cell lysate supernatant, 900 μL of Sirius red solution (0.1% direct red dye 80 in saturated picric acid) was mixed for 30 min followed by centrifugation (10 min at 14,000 rpm). The supernatant was discarded, and 500 μL of 0.5 N NaOH was added to the pellet and then vortexed for 10 min followed by measuring the optical density at 550 nm.

Cells on the scaffold were imaged using spinning disc confocal microscopy (Yokogawa Electric Corporation, CSU-X1). Cells in the scaffolds were permeabilized using 0.2% Triton-X 100. Actin filaments were stained using 2 units/mL of FITC-phallodin, and the nucleus was stained using 10 μg/mL of DAPI. Later, images were processed through Zen software (Zeiss).

4.5. In Vitro Adhesion Assessment of E. coli *and* S. aureus *on Scaffold*

Microorganisms (*E. coli* K12 or *S. aureus* MTCC 96) at 0.1 optical density (at 600 nm) in LB broth were added to the scaffold and incubated at 37 °C for 1 h, 2 h, 6 h and 12 h. Later, the scaffold was dipped in 1 mL PBS, sonicated for 10 min, and vortexed for 1 min to detach the adhered microorganism from scaffold and was diluted with PBS. After diluting several times, the bacteria were grown on agar plates and the colony-forming units per ml were counted. One set of adhered bacteria on the scaffold was dehydrated by serially increasing the concentration of ethanol and dried at 37 °C for 12 h and imaged under SEM.

4.6. Biofilm Formation on the Scaffold

Biofilm formation on the scaffold was quantified by the tissue culture plate method [24]. Scaffolds were placed in LB broth for 12 h and 24 h. Later, the microorganisms on the scaffolds were fixed using glutaraldehyde (2.5%) at 4 °C for 30 min and dried at 60 °C for 1 h. The biofilms were stained using crystal violet (500 µL, 0.1%) solution at room temperature for 20 min, followed by rinsing with PBS and drying at 37 °C. Stained biofilms on the scaffold were dissolved in 500 µL of 2% acetic acid for 15 min under gentle agitation. The OD at 492 nm was measured using a microplate spectrophotometer.

4.7. Statistical Analysis

Data presented in this article are the result of at least triplicates of every experiment, expressed as the mean ± standard deviation, and analyzed using one-way analysis of variance (ANOVA). Significant differences were calculated using Tukey's test and are represented as *, ** and *** for $p < 0.05$, 0.01 and 0.001, respectively.

5. Conclusions

In our study, quercetin-coupled CMS nanoparticles were prepared through the co-precipitation technique. Quercetin chelated well with ions by increasing the (Ca+Mg)/Si ratio. Nanoparticles were incorporated in the PCL/PVP matrix and electrospun to produce a nanofibrous scaffold. Incorporation of this nanoparticle improved the tensile stress and modulus of the scaffold. The effect of quercetin-coupled CMS was optimized to provide improved osteogenic activity by enhancing the proliferation of SaOS-2, ALP and collagen synthesis, and inhibiting the proliferation of both *E. coli* and *S. aureus* on the scaffold with reduced quercetin loading, making it an attractive material for studies in bone tissue engineering.

Author Contributions: A.M.P., conceptualization, methodology, investigation and writing—original draft preparation. J.R.B., conceptualization, experimental guidance, writing—review and editing and supervision. All authors have read and agreed to the published version of the manuscript.

Funding: This research received no external funding.

Institutional Review Board Statement: Not applicable.

Informed Consent Statement: Not applicable.

Data Availability Statement: The data can be available on request to the corresponding author.

Acknowledgments: We thank Sophisticated Analytical Instrument Facility, IIT Bombay and Industrial Research and Consultancy Centre, IIT Bombay for providing us with the high-end facility for scaffold characterization. We also thank Rajdip Bandyopadhyaya and Archana Kumari, Department of Chemical Engineering, IIT Bombay, for providing us with the MultiskanSkyHigh Microplate Spectrophotometer (Thermo-Fischer Scientific, Mumbai, India) for analysis.

Conflicts of Interest: The authors declare no conflict of interest.

References

1. Preethi, A.; Bellare, J.R. Tailoring scaffolds for orthopedic application with anti-microbial properties: Current scenario and future prospects. *Front. Mater.* **2020**, *7*, 452. [CrossRef]
2. David, A.V.; Arulmoli, R.; Parasuraman, S. Overviews of biological importance of quercetin: A bioactive flavonoid. *Pharmacogn. Rev.* **2016**, *10*, 84. [CrossRef]
3. Kim, S.Y.; Jeong, H.C.; Hong, S.K.; Lee, M.O.; Cho, S.J.; Cha, H.J. Quercetin induced ROS production triggers mitochondrial cell death of human embryonic stem cells. *Oncotarget* **2017**, *8*, 64964. [CrossRef] [PubMed]
4. Wong, S.K.; Chin, K.Y.; Ima-Nirwana, S. Quercetin as an agent for protecting the bone: A review of the current evidence. *Int. J. Mol. Sci.* **2020**, *21*, 6448. [CrossRef]
5. Górniak, I.; Bartoszewski, R.; Króliczewski, J. Comprehensive review of antimicrobial activities of plant flavonoids. *Phytochem. Rev.* **2019**, *18*, 241–272. [CrossRef]

6. Srivastava, T.; Mishra, S.K.; Tiwari, O.P.; Sonkar, A.K.; Tiwari, K.N.; Kumar, P.; Dixit, J.; Kumar, J.; Singh, A.K.; Verma, P.; et al. Synthesis, characterization, antimicrobial and cytotoxicity evaluation of quaternary cadmium (II)-quercetin complexes with 1, 10-phenanthroline or 2, 2′-bipyridine ligands. *Biotechnol. Biotechnol. Equip.* **2020**, *34*, 999–1012. [CrossRef]
7. Wang, W.; Sun, C.; Mao, L.; Ma, P.; Liu, F.; Yang, J.; Gao, Y. The biological activities, chemical stability, metabolism and delivery systems of quercetin: A review. *Trends Food Sci. Technol.* **2016**, *56*, 21–38. [CrossRef]
8. Chen, C.C.; Ho, C.C.; Lin, S.Y.; Ding, S.J. Green synthesis of calcium silicate bioceramic powders. *Ceram. Int.* **2015**, *41*, 5445–5453. [CrossRef]
9. Catauro, M.; Papale, F.; Bollino, F.; Piccolella, S.; Marciano, S.; Nocera, P.; Pacifico, S. Silica/quercetin sol–gel hybrids as antioxidant dental implant materials. *Sci. Technol. Adv. Mater.* **2015**, *16*, 035001. [CrossRef]
10. Wang, Y.; Zhao, Q.; Zhou, S.; Wang, S. Effect of C/S Ratio on Microstructure of Calcium Silicate Hydrates Synthesised By Solution Reaction Method. In *IOP Conference Series: Materials Science and Engineering*; IOP Publishing: Bristol, UK, 2019; Volume 472, p. 012003. [CrossRef]
11. Papadopoulou, A.; Green, R.J.; Frazier, R.A. Interaction of flavonoids with bovine serum albumin: A fluorescence quenching study. *J. Agric. Food Chem.* **2005**, *53*, 158–163. [CrossRef]
12. Kurakula, M.; Koteswara Rao, G.S. Moving polyvinyl pyrrolidone electrospun nanofibers and bioprinted scaffolds toward multidisciplinary biomedical applications. *Eur. Polym. J.* **2020**, *136*, 109919. [CrossRef]
13. Jang, S.R.; Kim, J.I.; Park, C.H.; Kim, C.S. The controlled design of electrospun PCL/silk/quercetin fibrous tubular scaffold using a modified wound coil collector and L-shaped ground design for neural repair. *Mater. Sci. Eng. C* **2020**, *111*, 110776. [CrossRef] [PubMed]
14. Ajmal, G.; Bonde, G.V.; Mittal, P.; Khan, G.; Pandey, V.K.; Bakade, B.V.; Mishra, B. Biomimetic PCL-gelatin based nanofibers loaded with ciprofloxacin hydrochloride and quercetin: A potential antibacterial and anti-oxidant dressing material for accelerated healing of a full thickness wound. *Int. J. Pharm.* **2019**, *567*, 118480. [CrossRef] [PubMed]
15. Zhang, H.; Zhang, M.; Yu, L.; Zhao, Y.; He, N.; Yang, X. Antitumor activities of quercetin and quercetin-5′, 8-disulfonate in human colon and breast cancer cell lines. *Food Chem. Toxicol.* **2012**, *50*, 1589–1599. [CrossRef] [PubMed]
16. Song, J.E.; Tripathy, N.; Lee, D.H.; Park, J.H.; Khang, G. Quercetin inlaid silk fibroin/hydroxyapatite scaffold promotes enhanced osteogenesis. *ACS Appl. Mater. Interfaces* **2018**, *10*, 32955–32964. [CrossRef] [PubMed]
17. Chen, S.; Zhu, L.; Wen, W.; Lu, L.; Zhou, C.; Luo, B. Fabrication and evaluation of 3D printed poly (L-lactide) scaffold functionalized with quercetin-polydopamine for bone tissue engineering. *ACS Biomater. Sci. Eng.* **2019**, *5*, 2506–2518. [CrossRef]
18. Zhu, L.; Chen, S.; Liu, K.; Wen, W.; Lu, L.; Ding, S.; Zhou, C.; Luo, B. 3D poly (L-lactide)/chitosan micro/nano fibrous scaffolds functionalized with quercetin-polydopamine for enhanced osteogenic and anti-inflammatory activities. *Chem. Eng. J.* **2020**, *391*, 123524. [CrossRef]
19. Preeth, D.R.; Saravanan, S.; Shairam, M.; Selvakumar, N.; Raja, I.S.; Dhanasekaran, A.; Vimalraj, S.; Rajalakshmi, S. Bioactive Zinc (II) complex incorporated PCL/gelatin electrospun nanofiber enhanced bone tissue regeneration. *Eur. J. Pharm. Sci.* **2021**, *160*, 105768. [CrossRef]
20. Vimalraj, S.; Rajalakshmi, S.; Preeth, D.R.; Kumar, S.V.; Deepak, T.; Gopinath, V.; Murugan, K.; Chatterjee, S. Mixed-ligand copper (II) complex of quercetin regulate osteogenesis and angiogenesis. *Mater. Sci. Eng. C* **2018**, *83*, 187–194. [CrossRef]
21. Kho, W.; Kim, M.K.; Jung, M.; Chong, Y.P.; Kim, Y.S.; Park, K.H.; Chong, Y. Strain-specific anti-biofilm and antibiotic-potentiating activity of 3′, 4′-difluoroquercetin. *Sci. Rep.* **2020**, *10*, 14162. [CrossRef]
22. Osonga, F.J.; Akgul, A.; Miller, R.M.; Eshun, G.B.; Yazgan, I.; Akgul, A.; Sadik, O.A. Antimicrobial activity of a new class of phosphorylated and modified flavonoids. *ACS Omega* **2019**, *4*, 12865–12871. [CrossRef] [PubMed]
23. Wang, S.; Yao, J.; Zhou, B.; Yang, J.; Chaudry, M.T.; Wang, M.; Xiao, F.; Li, Y.; Yin, W. Bacteriostatic effect of quercetin as an antibiotic alternative in vivo and its antibacterial mechanism in vitro. *J. Food Prot.* **2018**, *81*, 68–78. [CrossRef] [PubMed]
24. Ma, R.; Lai, Y.X.; Li, L.; Tan, H.L.; Wang, J.L.; Li, Y.; Tang, T.T.; Qin, L. Bacterial inhibition potential of 3D rapid-prototyped magnesium-based porous composite scaffolds–An in vitro efficacy study. *Sci. Rep.* **2015**, *5*, 13775. [CrossRef] [PubMed]

antibiotics

Article

Live Biosensors for Ultrahigh-Throughput Screening of Antimicrobial Activity against Gram-Negative Bacteria

Margarita N. Baranova [1], Polina A. Babikova [1], Arsen M. Kudzhaev [1], Yuliana A. Mokrushina [1,2], Olga A. Belozerova [1], Maxim A. Yunin [1], Sergey Kovalchuk [1], Alexander G. Gabibov [1,2,*], Ivan V. Smirnov [1,2,*] and Stanislav S. Terekhov [1,2,*]

[1] Shemyakin-Ovchinnikov Institute of Bioorganic Chemistry of the Russian Academy of Sciences, 117997 Moscow, Russia; baranova@ibch.ru (M.N.B.); babikova.pa@phystech.edu (P.A.B.); kudzhaev_arsen@mail.ru (A.M.K.); yuliana256@mail.ru (Y.A.M.); o.belozyorova@gmail.com (O.A.B.); yuninma@gmail.com (M.A.Y.); xerx222@gmail.com (S.K.)

[2] Department of Chemistry, Lomonosov Moscow State University, 119991 Moscow, Russia

* Correspondence: gabibov@ibch.ru (A.G.G.); smirnov@ibch.ru (I.V.S.); sterekhoff@gmail.com (S.S.T.)

Abstract: Gram-negative pathogens represent an urgent threat due to their intrinsic and acquired antibiotic resistance. Many recent drug candidates display prominent antimicrobial activity against Gram-positive bacteria being inefficient against Gram-negative pathogens. Ultrahigh-throughput, microfluidics-based screening techniques represent a new paradigm for deep profiling of antibacterial activity and antibiotic discovery. A key stage of this technology is based on single-cell cocultivation of microbiome biodiversity together with reporter fluorescent pathogen in emulsion, followed by the selection of reporter-free droplets using fluorescence-activated cell sorting. Here, a panel of reporter strains of Gram-negative bacteria *Escherichia coli* was developed to provide live biosensors for precise monitoring of antimicrobial activity. We optimized cell morphology, fluorescent protein, and selected the most efficient promoters for stable, homogeneous, high-level production of green fluorescent protein (GFP) in *E. coli*. Two alternative strategies based on highly efficient constitutive promoter pJ23119 or T7 promoter leakage enabled sensitive fluorescent detection of bacterial growth and killing. The developed live biosensors were applied for isolating potent *E. coli*-killing *Paenibacillus polymyxa* P4 strain by the ultrahigh-throughput screening of soil microbiome. The multi-omics approach revealed antibiotic colistin (polymyxin E) and its biosynthetic gene cluster, mediating antibiotic activity. Live biosensors may be efficiently implemented for antibiotic/probiotic discovery, environmental monitoring, and synthetic biology.

Keywords: ultrahigh-throughput screening; live biosensors; antibiotic discovery; gram-negative pathogens; microfluidic droplet cocultivation; efficient promoters; polymyxins; colistin biosynthetic gene cluster; single cell; multi-omics

Citation: Baranova, M.N.; Babikova, P.A.; Kudzhaev, A.M.; Mokrushina, Y.A.; Belozerova, O.A.; Yunin, M.A.; Kovalchuk, S.; Gabibov, A.G.; Smirnov, I.V.; Terekhov, S.S. Live Biosensors for Ultrahigh-Throughput Screening of Antimicrobial Activity against Gram-Negative Bacteria. *Antibiotics* **2021**, *10*, 1161. https://doi.org/10.3390/antibiotics10101161

Academic Editor: Helena Felgueiras

Received: 3 September 2021
Accepted: 22 September 2021
Published: 24 September 2021

1. Introduction

Global use of antimicrobials provokes intensive antimicrobial resistance (AMR) selection. AMR represents a threat to sustainable development, leading to 11 million deaths annually [1,2]. The recent COVID-19 pandemic resulted in a significant increase in antibiotic sales [3] and extensive antibiotic use without proper clinical indication [4]. Hence, the overuse of antibiotics lays the foundations for further resistome propagation and multi-resistance evolution. Further deterioration in this field threatens the emergence of epidemics caused by multiresistant pathogens and their subsequent persistence in the population under selection pressure.

Gram-negative pathogens represent a particularly dangerous cohort, including three of five urgent threats highlighted by the Centers for Disease Control and Prevention (CDC) [5]. New antibiotics targeting resistant Gram-negatives have been approved, but most of them belong to existing classes of antibiotics, and resistance to them has already emerged [6]. Gram-negative bacteria have an outer membrane, a protective and unique feature that distinguishes them from Gram-positive bacteria. This shield provides an efficient barrier for a vast variety of antimicrobials. Together with acquired resistance mechanisms, like mutations in chromosomal genes or mobile genetic elements carrying resistance genes, this provides a challenge to medication, often unresolvable [7].

Despite the urgent antibiotic rediscovery problem [8], classical antibiotic-producing species still provide a source for new drug candidates [9]. However, exotic microbial communities represent a more promising reservoir for the isolation of new antibiotics [10]. Recently, we developed an ultrahigh-throughput microfluidic platform for biodiversity screening [11]. This technology is based on single-cell cultivation of microorganisms in isolated microcompartments of double water-in-oil-in-water emulsion with subsequent isolating phenotypes of interest by fluorescence-activated cell sorting (FACS). More than 10,000 single bacterial clones may be screened for antibiotic activity in a second to isolate the most efficient antibiotic producers [12] or resistant strains [13]. This productivity enables deep functional profiling of microbiota communities [12] and the discovery of new molecular mechanisms of resistance [14]. The critical step of this technique is a coencapsulation of a highly fluorescent reporter GFP-producing bacterial strain together with single cells from the microbiome followed by their cocultivation in droplet compartments. Efficient bacterial killers are subsequently selected with FACS by a low GFP fluorescence level in a minor subpopulation of droplets. Previously, this platform was implemented for deep profiling of anti-*S. aureus* activity [11–13]. In this study, cell morphology, fluorescent protein nature, and promoter efficiency were optimized to adopt this strategy for extensive anti-Gram-negative screening based on model bacteria *E. coli*. Common laboratory *E. coli* strains, including Rosetta, BL21(DE3), TG1, XL-1, and SHuffle T7, were investigated to maximize GFP fluorescence and homogeneity. Two different green fluorescent proteins, i.e., TagGFP2 [15] and sfGFP [16], were examined as reporters in live biosensors. Moreover, the efficiency of GFP production under the control of different promoters was compared, including highly efficient constitutive *E. coli* promoters, i.e., pEm7 [17], pglpT [18], pJ23119 [19], OXB20 [20], and leaking T7 promoter.

We obtained that both highly efficient constitutive promoter pJ23119 and T7 promoter leakage enable sensitive fluorescent detection of bacterial growth and killing. Live biosensor based on BL21(DE3) strain, producing sfGFP via leaking T7 promoter, outperformed pJ23119 in terms of fluorescence level, while the fluorescence distribution of T7-based reporters was higher than pJ23119. Finally, pJ23119-sfGFP BL21(DE3) reporter cells were applied for a proof-of-concept soil microbiome screening. In a single round of screening, a potent *E. coli*-killing *Paenibacillus polymyxa* P4 strain was isolated and analyzed by complex multi-omics strategy, including activity-based metabolomics and genomics. Colistin (polymyxin E) was determined as a key metabolite mediating anti-Gram-negative antibiotic activity. The identified biosynthetic gene cluster (BGC) of colistin displayed close similarity to BGCs of polymyxin A [21], D-Dab$_3$-polymyxin B [22], and polymyxin E [23]. However, it did not contain the epimerization domain in module 3, unlike all previously published BGCs of polymyxins. We believe that the developed live biosensors may be efficiently implemented for ultrahigh-throughput screening of antimicrobial activity against gram-negative bacteria for antibiotic/probiotic discovery, environmental monitoring, and synthetic biology.

2. Results

2.1. General Requirements for Live Biosensors Applied in Ultrahigh-Throughput Screening

Ultrahigh-throughput screening of antimicrobial activity is based on a single-cell encapsulation of microbiome representatives together with fluorescent protein-producing reporter bacteria followed by isolation of droplets with inhibited growth of reporter bacteria using FACS (Figure 1).

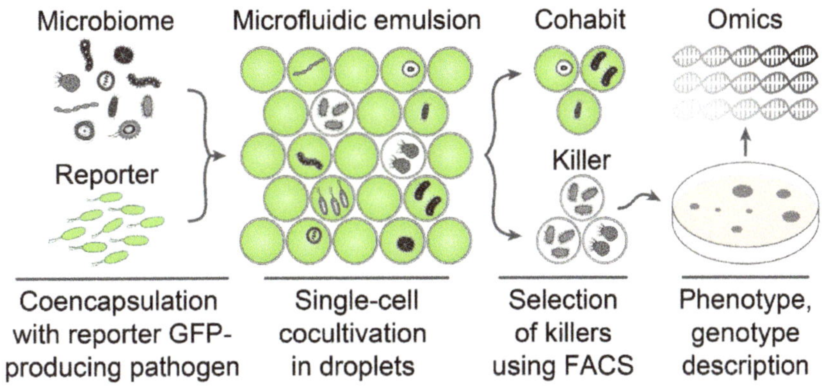

Figure 1. The general pipeline of ultrahigh-throughput screening of antimicrobial activity. The bacterial community is encapsulated with reporter GFP-producing pathogen in biocompatible droplets of microfluidic double water-in-oil-in-water emulsion. Cocultivation of bacterial community with reporter bacteria in droplets results in two distinct populations containing bacterial cohabits and killers. The latter is selected by a low level of GFP fluorescence by FACS. The selected droplets are plated on agar to regenerate culturable killers analyzed by activity-guided metabolomics and genomics. Detailed phenotype and genotype description enable identifying antibiotics and their biosynthetic gene clusters.

The critical component of this platform is a reporter pathogen strain. It must follow certain criteria, essential for efficient screening: (1) Cells must have regular morphology; aggregates or big non-uniform cells are undesirable; (2) production of fluorescent protein should be constitutive and homogeneous in population; and (3) a high level of cell culture fluorescence is required for precise detection of antimicrobial activity. A model Gram-negative bacteria *E. coli* was optimized following these criteria to provide efficient, live biosensors for ultrahigh-throughput screening and sensitive antimicrobial activity detection.

2.2. Selection of GFP-Producing Strain

Cell morphology plays an important role for reporter strain selection since cell aggregate clot microfluidic channels, while big and irregular cells tend to sediment in fluidics. Moreover, cell aggregates and non-uniformity may influence regular droplet occupancy. Hence, common laboratory *E. coli* strains including Rosetta (DE3), BL21(DE3), TG1, XL-1, and SHuffle T7 were transformed with pYTK047 plasmid for constitutive production of GFP [24], and cell morphology was visualized by fluorescence microscopy (Figure 2).

BL21(DE3) and TG1 strains of *E. coli* were suitable as a template for the creation of live biosensors since they provided homogeneous cell cultures with a high level of cell fluorescence. Other strains were inappropriate as a reporter. Rosetta (DE3) had a mediocre fluorescence. Xl-1 had a stretched morphology with a high number of odd rod cells. SHuffle T7 formed cell aggregates. Further, *E. coli* BL21(DE3) was used for live biosensors' engineering.

2.3. Stable and Homogeneous Production of GFP in E. coli

Different fluorescent proteins and promoters were compared to maximize the fluorescence of live *E. coli* culture (Figure 3).

While TagGFP2 was declared non-toxic to the host [15], we observed dramatically decreased fluorescence of cell cultures in *E. coli* transformed with plasmids under control of T7 promoter compared with the same constructs coding sfGFP fluorescent protein (Figure 4A).

Moreover, TagGFP2-producing plasmids based on T7 promoter tend to be lost under induction, resulting in a highly heterogeneous population with varying fluorescence of colonies (Figure 4B). Hence, sfGFP was used as a reporter fluorescent protein.

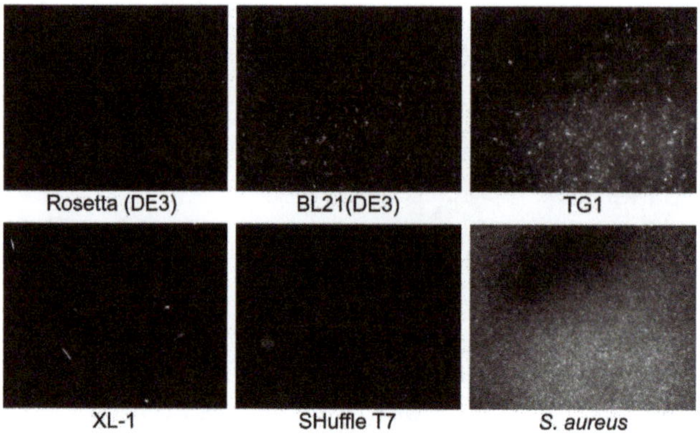

Figure 2. Cell morphology of different *E. coli* strains visualized by fluorescence microscopy. GFP-producing reporter *S. aureus* cells were used as a control.

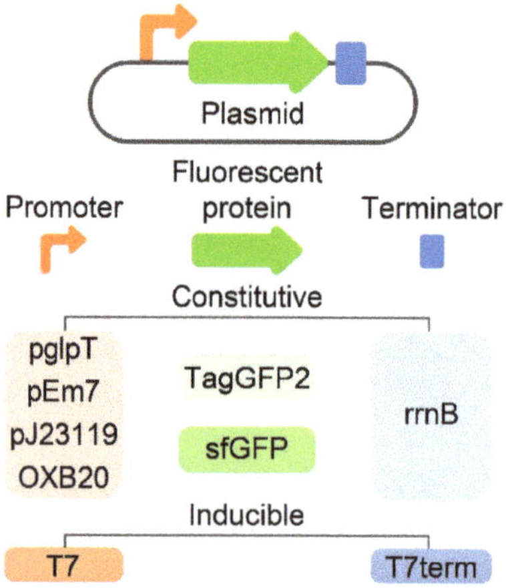

Figure 3. A panel of plasmids that were used for the optimization of *E. coli*-based live biosensors. All genetic constructs were constructed on the same high-copy number template vector. Two different fluorescent proteins, i.e., TagGFP2 and sfGFP, were used. Constitutive (pglpT, pEm7, pj23119, and OXB20) and inducible (T7) promoters were compared in terms of efficiency, homogeneity of cell fluorescence, and stability.

The efficiencies of different promoters were compared to maximize GFP fluorescence in *E. coli*. Brain Heart Infusion (BHI) was used as a basal medium since it enables culturing a variety of microorganisms, which is preferred for subsequent ultrahigh-throughput screening of antimicrobial activity. Surprisingly, efficient T7 leakage was observed in *E. coli* BL21(DE3) (Figure 5A). Highly efficient constitutive *E. coli* promoters, i.e., pEm7, pglpT, pJ23119, and OXB20, were compared with leaking T7 in agar plates (Figure 5A), culture medium (Figure 5B), and flow cytometry (Figure 5C). Leaking T7 results in 2.3–8.9 times higher fluorescence of bacterial cultures in comparison with constitutive *E. coli* promoters. The pJ23119 was the strongest constitutive promoter that enabled stable and homogeneous fluorescence of cell cultures, similar to GFP-producing reporter *S. aureus* cells used previously (Figure 5B). While live biosensors based on leaking T7 promoter outperformed pJ23119 in cell cultures, the cell fluorescence distribution of T7-based reporters was higher (Figure 5C). The fluorescence levels of cell cultures were 1.3–1.6 times higher with the TB medium. However, we suggest that BHI is more preferred to maintain broad biodiversity in emulsion culture.

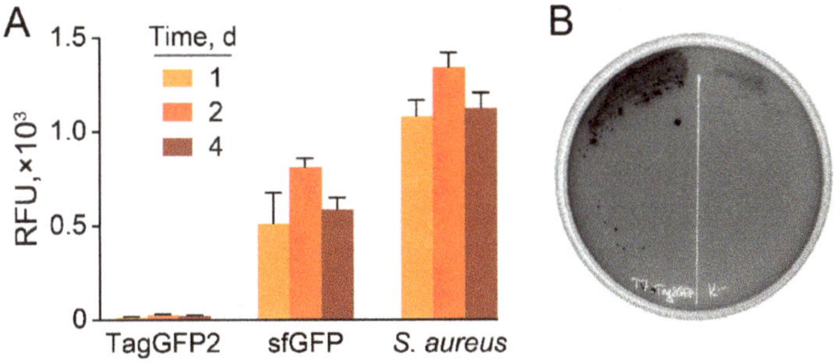

Figure 4. Hyperproduction of TagGFP2 fluorescent protein results in plasmid loss. (**A**) Fluorescence of cell cultures transformed with synonymous plasmids encoding TagGFP2 and sfGFP fluorescent proteins under the control of T7 promoter, induced by the addition of 1 mM IPTG. GFP-producing reporter *S. aureus* cells were used as a control. Data represent the mean of three biological replicates ± SD. (**B**) A representative plate with *E. coli*-producing TagGFP2 under control of T7 promoter, induced by 1 mM IPTG.

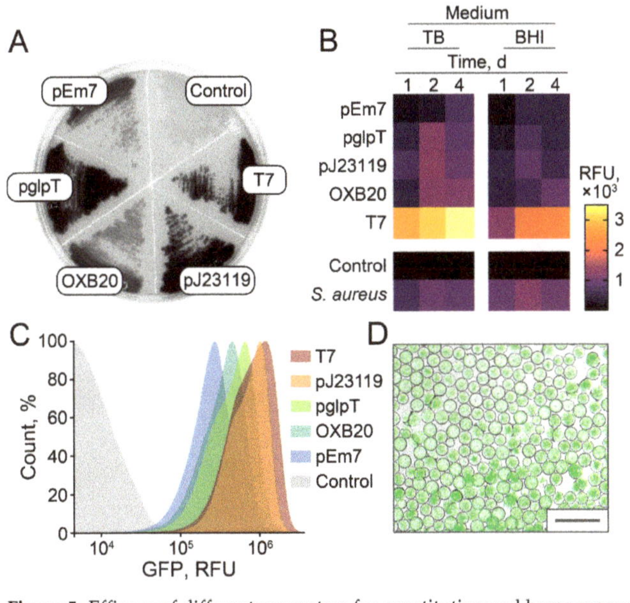

Figure 5. Efficacy of different promoters for constitutive and homogeneous production of GFP in *E. coli*. (**A**) A representative BHI-agar plate with *E. coli*, producing sfGFP under control of various promoters. Constitutive *E. coli* promoters, i.e., pEm7, pglpT, pJ23119, and OXB20, were compared with leaking T7. *E. coli* cells transformed with empty vector without sfGFP insert were used as a negative control. (**B**) Fluorescence of bacterial cultures obtained after 1, 2, and 4 days of cultivation in TB or BHI medium. Relative fluorescence units (RFU) are presented as a heatmap indicating bulk fluorescence of cell cultures. GFP-producing reporter *S. aureus* cells were used as a positive control. Data represent the mean of three biological replicates. (**C**) Flow cytometry of bacterial cultures producing sfGFP obtained after 2 days of cultivation in BHI medium. (**D**) Live biosensors producing sfGFP under control of pJ23119 promoter after 1 day of cultivation in droplets of microfluidic double water-in-oil-in-water emulsion. Scale bar: 100 µm.

Hence, we propose that alternative strategies based on highly efficient constitutive promoter pJ23119 or T7 promoter leakage enabled sensitive fluorescent detection of bacterial growth and killing. Live biosensors producing sfGFP under control of pJ23119 promoter were encapsulated in biocompatible droplets of microfluidic double water-in-oil-in-water emulsion with occupancy of ~5 *E. coli* cells per droplet. Cultivation of reporters in emulsion resulted in efficient bacterial growth, providing highly fluorescent droplet compartments (Figure 5D) suitable for ultrahigh-throughput screening of antimicrobial activity.

2.4. Ultrahigh-Throughput Screening of Antimicrobial Activity

A model ultrahigh-throughput screening of antimicrobial activity was performed to demonstrate the efficiency of the developed live biosensors. Soil microbiome isolated in the Moscow region was used as a source of bacterial biodiversity. GFP-producing live biosensors were coencapsulated with ~10^6 soil microbiome bacteria, followed by cocultivation, selection, and regeneration of culturable anti-*E. coli* bacteria. Potent *E. coli*-killing *Paenibacillus polymyxa* P4 strain was isolated in one round of selection. Metabolomic analysis revealed that polymyxin E (colistin) is the major secondary metabolite active against Gram-negative bacteria. Polymyxins represent closely related lipopeptide antibiotics having a high number of positively charged 2,4-diaminobutyric acid (Dab) residues and hydrophobic residues of Leu and Phe (Figure 6A). Similar to previously identified *Paenibacillus alvei* B-LR [23], *P. polymyxa* P4 produced two analogous polymyxins E_1 and E_2 that differ by 6-methyloctanoic acid and 6-methylheptanoic acid moieties, respectively (Figure 6B).

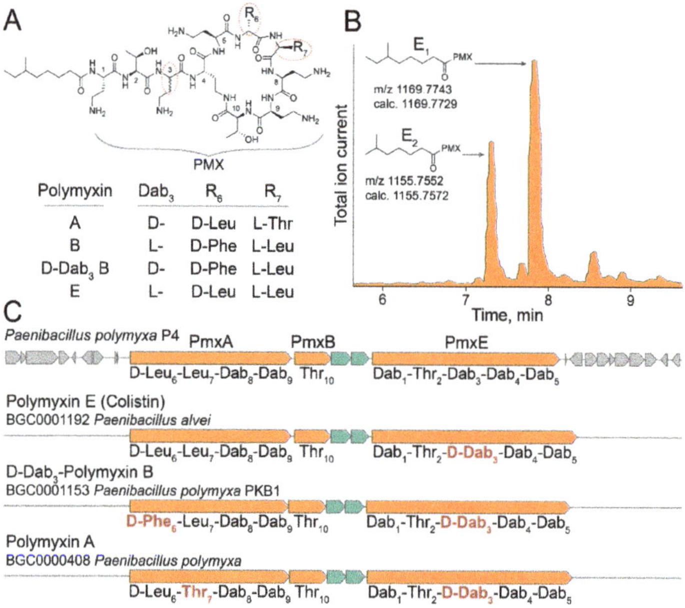

Figure 6. Multi-omic characterization of *Paenibacillus polymyxa* P4 strain selected by ultrahigh-throughput screening of anti-Gram-negative antibiotic activity using the developed live biosensor. (**A**) Polymyxin E (colistin) was identified as a major secondary metabolite of *P. polymyxa* P4 active against Gram-negative bacteria. The chemical structures of polymyxin E and related polymyxins A, B, and D-Dab_3 B produced by distinct *Paenibacillus* are presented. PMX—colistin peptide backbone. (**B**) LC-MS chromatogram of active fraction of *P. polymyxa* P4 metabolites. Specific peaks of polymyxin E_1 and polymyxin E_2 are presented with their experimental and calculated $[M+H]^+$ molecular ion masses. (**C**) BGC of polymyxin E identified in the genome of *P. polymyxa* P4. Core NRPSs (PmxA, PmxB, and PmxE) and ABC transporters are colored with orange and aquamarine, respectively. Predicted amino acid specificity of NRPS modules are presented. Related BGCs of polymyxin A [21], D-Dab_3-polymyxin B [22], and polymyxin E [23] are presented with their predicted modular specificities. Distinct modular specificities are highlighted with red.

Whole genome sequencing of *P. polymyxa* P4 enabled identifying the biosynthetic gene cluster (BGC) of polymyxin E (Figure 6C). *P. polymyxa* P4 polymyxin E BGC has the same architecture as all polymyxin BGCs mediating the production of polymyxin A [21], D-Dab_3-polymyxin B [22], and polymyxin E [23] identified previously. Polymyxin E BGC encodes D-Leu instead of D-Phe in module 6 of D-Dab_3-polymyxin B, Leu instead of Thr in module 7 of polymyxin A, and Dab instead of D-Dab in module 3 of all known polymyxins. While modules 6 and 7 encode amino acid residues varying between polymyxins, module 3 does not have an epimerization domain. Hence, we predicted that the identified polymyxin E produced by *P. polymyxa* P4 has natural L-stereochemistry. It was recently shown that the epimerization domain of module 3 may be functional, at least in the case of *P. polymyxa* PKB1 strain producing D-Dab_3-polymyxin B [22]. Therefore, the stereochemistry of Dab_3 is questionable for some polymyxins. However, it is unambiguous for the identified polymyxin E produced by *P. polymyxa* P4.

3. Discussion

Estimates indicate that antibiotics not yet discovered are likely to be produced at frequencies as low as $\leq$1 in 10^7 in fermentation broths from random actinomycetes [25]. Hence, deep profiling of antimicrobial activity of microbiomes on a single-cell level provides a new perspective to antibiotic discovery. The miniaturization of antibiotic activity assays is an essential step forward to the next-generation screening platforms. Microfluidic technologies enable single-cell bacterial culturing [26], enzymatic activity screening [27], and antimicrobial activity profiling [28]. Biocompatible droplet microcompartments allow transitioning from classical 2D culture on the surface of agar plates to 3D emulsion culture. This transition results in a dramatic increase in explored diversity since ~10^6–10^9 unique bacterial clones may be cultured in 1 mL of 100–10 μm emulsion droplets instead of ~10^2–10^3 clones on a single agar plate.

Here, we described how ultrahigh-throughput technologies could be applied for antimicrobial activity screening against Gram-negative bacteria. Live biosensors based on engineered GFP-producing *E. coli* enable detecting bacterial antagonism of individual bacterial clones cultured in droplet microcompartments. Different *E. coli* strains, GFPs, and promoters were tested to optimize cell morphology and maximize cell fluorescence. T7 promoter leakage enables sensitive fluorescent detection of bacterial growth and killing regardless of IPTG or lactose induction using common laboratory strain BL21(DE3) and high-copy number plasmid. Highly efficient constitutive promoter pJ23119 may be an alternative with a slightly reduced fluorescence level but increased homogeneity of fluorescence. Finally, the efficiency of engineered live biosensors was illustrated by the ultrahigh-throughput screening of *E. coli*-killing bacteria. *P. polymyxa* P4 strain producing potent anti-Gram-negative antibiotic polymyxin E was isolated using a single round of selection. The biosynthetic gene cluster (BGC) of polymyxin E has the same architecture as polymyxin A, D-Dab_3-polymyxin B, and polymyxin E BGCs identified previously. The unique feature of the identified polymyxin E BGC is that its module 3 does not have an epimerization domain confirming the L-stereochemistry of Dab_3 residue.

Engineered live biosensors provide a simple, efficient, and highly sensitive tool for precise monitoring of antimicrobial activity. Basic principles of their construction may be transferred to different Gram-negative bacteria. The implementation of ultrahigh-throughput technologies in antibiotic discovery enables deep profiling of antimicrobial activity, accelerating hit identification, and expanding biodiversity coverage. While a number of problems regarding the cultivation of unculturable microorganisms should be resolved to amplify the power of this technique, microfluidic droplet platforms already outperform classical cultivation strategies in some applications [26]. Another option is a search for specific potentiating agents targeting antibiotic resistance. In this case, using an AMR reporter strain supplemented with a conventional antimicrobial may be a target if the antibiotic-producing microorganism is resistant. It may be achieved using naturally resistant bacterial killers like fungi or engineered strains having improved efflux or mutation providing resistance. The application field of live biosensors is not restricted to microfluidics-based technologies like ultrahigh-throughput screening. Live biosensors may provide sensitive detection of antimicrobial activity in a broad sense, including such applications as routine antibiotic/probiotic screening, pollution monitoring, detection of antibiotic contamination, and more sophisticated fields based on synthetic biology principles.

4. Materials and Methods

Genetic constructs and strains. All genetic constructs were based on high-copy vector plasmid PURExpress Control DHFR Plasmid (NEB, Ipswich, MA, USA). Multiple cloning sites including *Xba*I, *Xho*I, and *Xma*I restriction sites flanked by *Nhe*I/*Hind*III sites were inserted to replace the T7 promoter-DHFR-T7 terminator region, resulting in pIvi-MCS vector. Promoter sequences were obtained by PCR assembly and cloned into pIvi-MCS digested with *Xba*I and *Xho*I. The pglpT is a strong constitutive promoter [18]. OXB20 is the strongest RecA promoter derivative with an ablated repressor binding site to enable constitutive expression (PSF-OXB20, OGS50, Sigma). The pJ23119 is the strongest promoter in a family of constitutive promoters isolated from a combinational library (PMID: 23560087). The pEm7 is a constitutive synthetic derivative of a T7 promoter (part Doulix biofundry, part ENW51Y). TagGFP2 and sfGFP genes were PCR amplified from pTagGFP2-N (Evrogen, Moscow, Russia) and pYTK047 plasmids, respectively, and cloned with *Xho*I/*Xma*I restriction sites. The pYTK047 was a gift from John Dueber (Addgene plasmid # 65154; http://n2t.net/addgene:65154; RRID:Addgene_65154, accessed on: 1 May 2018). The terminator region containing rrnB1 and T7 terminators was PCR amplified from pYTK047 and cloned with *Xma*I/*Hind*III restriction sites. The following *E. coli* strains were used: Rosetta (DE3) (Novagen, Madison, WI, USA), BL21(DE3) (Invitrogen, Waltham, MA, USA), TG1 (Lucigen, Middleton, WI, USA), XL-1 (Agilent, Santa Clara, CA, USA), and SHuffle T7 (NEB, Ipswich, MA, USA). Control GFP-producing reporter *S. aureus* cells were described previously [11–13].

Fluorescence measurements. *E. coli* cultures were grown overnight using 2YT medium (16 g/L tryptone, 10 g/L yeast extract, 5 g/L NaCl) supplemented with 100 µg/mL ampicillin in shaking flasks at 37 °C and 250 rpm. Brain Heart Infusion (BHI) medium (BD, Franklin Lakes, NJ, USA) or TB medium (12 g/L tryptone, 24 g/L yeast extract, 4 g/L glycerol) was inoculated in 1:100 ratio and cultivated at 30 °C for 1, 2, and 4 days. Fluorescence measurements were made using Varioskan Flash Multimode plate reader (Thermo Fisher Scientific, Waltham, MA, USA) with $\lambda_{ex}/\lambda_{em}$ = 488/513 nm and NovoCyte Flow Cytometer (Agilent, Santa Clara, CA, USA). GFP-producing *E. coli* were visualized using an Eclipse Ti inverted fluorescence microscope (Nikon, Tokyo, Japan) with a standard FITC filter. Bacterial colonies grown on agar plates were analyzed by GFP fluorescence using VersaDoc (Bio-Rad, Hercules, CA, USA).

Encapsulation of *E. coli* in droplets. BL21(DE3) *E. coli*-producing sfGFP under control of pJ23119 promoter was cultured in BHI medium in shaking flasks at 37 °C and 250 rpm until early logarithmic growth phase. Subsequently, liquid cultures were filtered using 40-µm cell strainers (Greiner Bio-One) and 20-µm solvent filters (A-313, IDEX, Northbrook, IL, USA) and then diluted to reach OD_{600} = 0.3 (occupancy (λ) ~ 5 *E. coli* cells per a droplet). *E. coli* cells were encapsulated in droplets of microfluidic double emulsion (MDE), using 20-µm microfluidic chips produced via soft lithography, as was described previously [11]. MDE droplets with encapsulated bacterial cells were cultured at 30 °C in a water vapor saturated incubator. MDE droplets were loaded into a hemocytometer and were visualized using an Eclipse Ti inverted fluorescence microscope (Nikon) with a standard FITC filter.

Ultrahigh-throughput screening of anti-Gram-negative antibiotic activity. The selection of bacteria displaying antibacterial activity was described in detail previously [11–13]. Briefly, sfGFP-producing *E. coli* cells were vitally stained with sulfo-Cyanine5 NHS (Lumiprobe, Moscow, Russia), washed, and filtered using 20-µm solvent filters (A-313, IDEX, Northbrook, IL, USA). The soil microbiome was isolated in the Moscow region. Microbiome samples were unfrozen directly before encapsulation, resuspended in BHI broth (BD, Franklin

Lakes, NJ, USA), and filtered through 40-µm cell strainers (Greiner Bio-One, Monroe, NC, USA). The sfGFP-producing live biosensors were co-encapsulated with a soil microbiome suspension in droplets of MDE. After overnight incubation at 35 °C, Calcein Violet AM (Thermo Fisher Scientific, Waltham, MA, USA) was added to the droplet emulsion to the final concentration of 10 µM. Subsequently, the droplets with simultaneous $sCy5^{high}$, GFP^{low}, and Calcein $Violet^{high}$ fluorescence were sorted using a FACSAria III cell sorter (BD, Franklin Lakes, NJ, USA). Bacterial colonies were regenerated after plating on BHI–agar (BD, Franklin Lakes, NJ, USA) and tested for antibiotic activity against *E. coli* using the agar overlay assay.

***P. polymyxa* cultivation.** *P. polymyxa* P4 was cultivated in SYC medium containing 40 g/L sucrose, 5 g/L yeast extract, 4 g/L $CaCO_3$, 1.5 g/L K_2HPO_4, 2 g/L glucose, 2 g/L NaCl, 1.5 g/L $MgSO_4$, 2 g/L $(NH_4)_2SO_4$, 0.01 g/L $FeSO_4$, and 0.01 g/L $MnCl_2$ for 24 h at 30 °C. *P. polymyxa* P4 was inoculated from overnight culture using 1:100 dilution and cultivated using 750-mL flasks in 100 mL with 250 rpm shaking for 4 days.

Antimicrobial activity. Inhibition of bacterial cell growth was measured by a doubling dilution of *P. polymyxa* P4 medium and C18 HPLC fractions in 2YT medium inoculated with *E. coli* OD_{600} = 0.002. After overnight incubation at 30 °C, *E. coli* growth was analyzed by GFP fluorescence ($\lambda_{ex}/\lambda_{em}$ = 488/513 nm) and OD_{600} using a Varioskan Flash Multimode Reader (Thermo Fisher Scientific).

Whole-genome sequencing and bioinformatic analysis. Total DNA was isolated using the QIAamp DNA Investigator Kit (Qiagen, Germantown, MD, USA). Genomic DNA was disrupted into 400–550-bp fragments by Covaris S220 System (Covaris, Woburn, MA, USA). Fragment libraries were prepared using the NEBNext® DNA Library Prep Reagent Set for Illumina and the NEBNext® Multiplex Oligos for Illumina® (96 Index Primers) (Illumina, San Diego, CA, USA) according to the manufacturer's instructions. Sequencing of libraries was performed using the genetic analyzer HiSeq2500, the HiSeq® PE Cluster Kit v4–cBot™, and the HiSeq® SBS Kit v4 (250 cycles) (Illumina, San Diego, CA, USA) according to the manufacturer's instructions. Genome assemblies were performed using SPAdes 3.9.0 [29]. Genomes were annotated with prokka [30]. Identification of biosynthetic gene clusters and NRPS modular organization was performed with antiSMASH 6.0 [31]. Comparative analysis of homologous gene clusters was provided by MultiGeneBlast [32] based on the MIBiG database [33].

Active metabolite extraction and metabolomic analysis. The culture medium of *P. polymyxa* P4 was centrifuged at 10,000× *g* for 10 min. Active metabolites were extracted by solid-phase extraction with LPS-500 sorbent (Technosorbent, Moscow, Russia) using buffer A (10 mM NH_4OAc pH 6.0, 20% ACN) for sorbent wash and buffer B (10 mM NH_4OAc pH 6.0, 80% ACN) for elution. LC-MS analysis was carried out on an Ultimate 3000 RSLCnano HPLC system connected to an Orbitrap Fusion Lumos mass spectrometer (ThermoFisher Scientific) with the loading pump used for analytical flow gradient delivery. Samples were separated on Luna Omega C18 1.6 µm 100 Å column 100 × 2.1 mm at a 200 µL/min flow rate. Separation was done by a gradient of 99.9% ACN, 10 mM ammonium formate, 0.1% FA (Buffer B) in 99.9% H_2O, 10 mM ammonium formate, 0.1% FA (Buffer A): 5% B at 0 min, 5% B at 5 min, 99% B at 20 min, followed by 5 min wash at 99% B and 10 min equilibration at 5% B before the next run. UV data were collected at 260 and 315 nm. MS1 spectra were collected in Positive ion mode at 30 K Orbitrap resolution in profile mode with 200–2000 a.e.m mass range and RF lens 30%. For the rest of the MS1 parameters as well as for the ESI parameters, the default values suggested by Xcalibur software ver. 4.3.73.11 were taken. MS2 precursors were selected based on MS1 intensity: Intensity threshold was 5×10^4 with the dynamic exclusion set to 10 s after two selections with the mass tolerance of 10 ppm and isotope exclusion. MS2 spectra were collected at 15 K resolution in centroid mode. The isolation window was set to 1/6 m/z with no offset and Quadrupole isolation mode. Fragmentation was done by HCD with a stepped CE of 20, 35, and 50%. The rest of the MS2 parameters were taken as default values. The total MS1-MS2 cycle time was selected to 1 sec. LC-MS/MS raw data were analyzed in Compound Discoverer 3.2 (Thermo Fisher Scientific). Peak annotation was performed with

ChemSpider, Natural Product Atlas 2020, and MzCloud databases using MS1 and MS1-MS2 information correspondingly with 5 ppm mass accuracy, isotopic distribution $\geq$ 50%, and match score $\geq$ 85%.

Author Contributions: M.N.B., I.V.S., A.G.G. and S.S.T. designed the research; M.N.B., P.A.B., A.M.K., Y.A.M., O.A.B. and M.A.Y. performed the research; O.A.B. and S.K. contributed new analytic tools; M.N.B., S.K., Y.A.M., S.S.T., I.V.S. and A.G.G. analyzed the data; M.N.B., I.V.S., A.G.G. and S.S.T. wrote the paper. All authors have read and agreed to the published version of the manuscript.

Funding: This work was supported by Grant 21-14-00357 from the Russian Science Foundation and personal scholarships from the Council for Grants of the President of the Russian Federation СП-3370.2019.4 (Y.A.M.) and СП-2911.2019.4 (S.S.T.).

Institutional Review Board Statement: Not applicable.

Informed Consent Statement: Not applicable.

Data Availability Statement: Data is contained within the article. Additional data are freely available on request from the corresponding author.

Conflicts of Interest: The authors declare no conflict of interest.

References

1. Fleischmann, M.C.; Scherag, A.; Adhikari, N.K.J.; Hartog, C.S.; Tsaganos, T.; Schlattmann, P.; Angus, D.C.; Reinhart, K. Assessment of Global Incidence and Mortality of Hospital-treated Sepsis. Current Estimates and Limitations. *Am. J. Respir. Crit. Care Med.* **2016**, *193*, 259–272. [CrossRef]
2. Rudd, K.E.; Johnson, S.C.; Agesa, K.M.; Shackelford, K.A.; Tsoi, D.; Kievlan, D.R.; Colombara, D.V.; Ikuta, K.S.; Kissoon, N.; Finfer, S.; et al. Global, regional, and national sepsis incidence and mortality, 1990–2017: Analysis for the Global Burden of Disease Study. *Lancet* **2020**, *395*, 200–211. [CrossRef]
3. Sulis, G.; Batomen, B.; Kotwani, A.; Pai, M.; Gandra, S. Sales of antibiotics and hydroxychloroquine in India during the COVID-19 epidemic: An interrupted time series analysis. *PLoS Med.* **2021**, *18*, e1003682. [CrossRef] [PubMed]
4. Elsayed, A.A.; Darwish, S.F.; Zewail, M.B.; Mohammed, M.; Saeed, H.; Rabea, H. Antibiotic misuse and compliance with infection control measures during COVID-19 pandemic in community pharmacies in Egypt. *Int. J. Clin. Pract.* **2021**, *75*, e14081. [CrossRef]
5. Centers for Disease Control and Prevention. Antibiotic Resistance Threats in the United States. 2019. Available online: https://www.cdc.gov/drugresistance/pdf/threatsreport/2019-ar-threats-report-508.pdf (accessed on 21 February 2020).
6. Fitzpatrick, M.A. Real-world antibiotic needs for resistant Gram-negative infections. *Lancet Infect. Dis.* **2020**, *20*, 1108–1109. [CrossRef]
7. Breijyeh, Z.; Jubeh, B.; Karaman, R. Resistance of Gram-Negative Bacteria to Current Antibacterial Agents and Approaches to Resolve It. *Molecules* **2020**, *25*, 1340. [CrossRef] [PubMed]
8. Culp, E.J.; Waglechner, N.; Wang, W.; Fiebig-Comyn, A.A.; Hsu, Y.-P.; Koteva, K.; Sychantha, D.; Coombes, B.K.; Van Nieuwenhze, M.S.; Brun, Y.V.; et al. Evolution-guided discovery of antibiotics that inhibit peptidoglycan remodelling. *Nat. Cell Biol.* **2020**, *578*, 582–587. [CrossRef]
9. Genilloud, O. Actinomycetes: Still a source of novel antibiotics. *Nat. Prod. Rep.* **2017**, *34*, 1203–1232. [CrossRef]
10. Imai, Y.; Meyer, K.J.; Iinishi, A.; Favre-Godal, Q.; Green, R.; Manuse, S.; Caboni, M.; Mori, M.; Niles, S.; Ghiglieri, M.; et al. A new antibiotic selectively kills Gram-negative pathogens. *Nature* **2019**, *576*, 459–464. [CrossRef]
11. Terekhov, S.; Smirnov, I.; Stepanova, A.V.; Bobik, T.V.; Mokrushina, Y.; Ponomarenko, N.A.; Belogurov, A.A., Jr.; Rubtsova, M.P.; Kartseva, O.; Gomzikova, M.O.; et al. Microfluidic droplet platform for ultrahigh-throughput single-cell screening of biodiversity. *Proc. Natl. Acad. Sci. USA* **2017**, *114*, 2550–2555. [CrossRef]
12. Terekhov, S.; Smirnov, I.; Malakhova, M.V.; Samoilov, A.; Manolov, A.I.; Nazarov, A.S.; Danilov, D.V.; Dubiley, S.A.; Osterman, I.; Rubtsova, M.P.; et al. Ultrahigh-throughput functional profiling of microbiota communities. *Proc. Natl. Acad. Sci. USA* **2018**, *115*, 9551–9556. [CrossRef]
13. Terekhov, S.S.; Nazarov, A.S.; Mokrushina, Y.A.; Baranova, M.N.; Potapova, N.A.; Malakhova, M.V.; Ilina, E.N.; Smirnov, I.V.; Gabibov, A.G. Deep Functional Profiling Facilitates the Evaluation of the Antibacterial Potential of the Antibiotic Amicoumacin. *Antibiotics* **2020**, *9*, 157. [CrossRef] [PubMed]
14. Terekhov, S.S.; Mokrushina, Y.A.; Nazarov, A.S.; Zlobin, A.; Zalevsky, A.; Bourenkov, G.; Golovin, A.; Belogurov, A., Jr.; Osterman, I.A.; Kulikova, A.A.; et al. A kinase bioscavenger provides antibiotic resistance by extremely tight substrate binding. *Sci. Adv.* **2020**, *6*, eaaz9861. [CrossRef] [PubMed]
15. Subach, O.M.; Gundorov, I.S.; Yoshimura, M.; Subach, F.V.; Zhang, J.; Grüenwald, D.; Souslova, E.A.; Chudakov, D.; Verkhusha, V.V. Conversion of Red Fluorescent Protein into a Bright Blue Probe. *Chem. Biol.* **2008**, *15*, 1116–1124. [CrossRef] [PubMed]
16. Pédelacq, J.-D.; Cabantous, S.; Tran, T.; Terwilliger, T.; Waldo, G.S. Engineering and characterization of a superfolder green fluorescent protein. *Nat. Biotechnol.* **2005**, *24*, 79–88. [CrossRef] [PubMed]

17. Lane, M.C.; Alteri, C.J.; Smith, S.N.; Mobley, H.L.T. Expression of flagella is coincident with uropathogenic Escherichia coli ascension to the upper urinary tract. *Proc. Natl. Acad. Sci. USA* **2007**, *104*, 16669–16674. [CrossRef] [PubMed]
18. Liu, X.; Yuk, H.; Lin, S.; Parada, G.A.; Tang, T.-C.; Tham, E.; de la Fuente-Nunez, C.; Lu, T.K.; Zhao, X. 3D Printing of Living Responsive Materials and Devices. *Adv. Mater.* **2018**, *30*, 1704821. [CrossRef] [PubMed]
19. Yan, Q.; Fong, S.S. Study of in vitro transcriptional binding effects and noise using constitutive promoters combined with UP element sequences in Escherichia coli. *J. Biol. Eng.* **2017**, *11*, 33. [CrossRef]
20. Zhu, Y.; Hua, Y.; Zhang, B.; Sun, L.; Li, W.; Kong, X.; Hong, J. Metabolic engineering of indole pyruvic acid biosynthesis in Escherichia coli with tdiD. *Microb. Cell Factories* **2017**, *16*, 1–15. [CrossRef]
21. Choi, S.-K.; Park, S.-Y.; Kim, R.; Kim, S.-B.; Lee, C.-H.; Kim, J.F.; Park, S.-H. Identification of a Polymyxin Synthetase Gene Cluster of Paenibacillus polymyxa and Heterologous Expression of the Gene in Bacillus subtilis. *J. Bacteriol.* **2009**, *191*, 3350–3358. [CrossRef]
22. Shaheen, M.; Li, J.; Ross, A.C.; Vederas, J.; Jensen, S.E. Paenibacillus polymyxa PKB1 Produces Variants of Polymyxin B-Type Antibiotics. *Chem. Biol.* **2011**, *18*, 1640–1648. [CrossRef] [PubMed]
23. Tambadou, F.; Caradec, T.; Gagez, A.-L.; Bonnet, A.; Sopéna, V.; Bridiau, N.; Thiery, V.; Didelot, S.; Barthélémy, C.; Chevrot, R. Characterization of the colistin (polymyxin E1 and E2) biosynthetic gene cluster. *Arch. Microbiol.* **2015**, *197*, 521–532. [CrossRef] [PubMed]
24. Lee, M.E.; DeLoache, W.C.; Cervantes, B.; Dueber, J.E. A Highly Characterized Yeast Toolkit for Modular, Multipart Assembly. *ACS Synth. Biol.* **2015**, *4*, 975–986. [CrossRef]
25. Baltz, R.H. Renaissance in antibacterial discovery from actinomycetes. *Curr. Opin. Pharmacol.* **2008**, *8*, 557–563. [CrossRef] [PubMed]
26. Watterson, W.J.; Tanyeri, M.; Watson, A.R.; Cham, C.M.; Shan, Y.; Chang, E.B.; Eren, A.M.; Tay, S. Droplet-based high-throughput cultivation for accurate screening of antibiotic resistant gut microbes. *eLife* **2020**, *9*. [CrossRef]
27. Saito, K.; Ota, Y.; Tourlousse, D.M.; Matsukura, S.; Fujitani, H.; Morita, M.; Tsuneda, S.; Noda, N. Microdroplet-based system for culturing of environmental microorganisms using FNAP-sort. *Sci. Rep.* **2021**, *11*, 1–9. [CrossRef]
28. Mahler, L.; Niehs, S.P.; Martin, K.; Weber, T.; Scherlach, K.; Hertweck, C.; Roth, M.; Rosenbaum, M.A. Highly parallelized droplet cultivation and prioritization of antibiotic producers from natural microbial communities. *eLife* **2021**, *10*, 64774. [CrossRef]
29. Bankevich, A.; Nurk, S.; Antipov, D.; Gurevich, A.A.; Dvorkin, M.; Kulikov, A.S.; Lesin, V.M.; Nikolenko, S.I.; Pham, S.; Prjibelski, A.D.; et al. SPAdes: A New Genome Assembly Algorithm and Its Applications to Single-Cell Sequencing. *J. Comput. Biol.* **2012**, *19*, 455–477. [CrossRef]
30. Seemann, T. Prokka: Rapid Prokaryotic Genome Annotation. *Bioinformatics* **2014**, *30*, 2068–2069. [CrossRef]
31. Blin, K.; Shaw, S.; Kloosterman, A.M.; Charlop-Powers, Z.; van Wezel, G.P.; Medema, M.H.; Weber, T. antiSMASH 6.0: Improving cluster detection and comparison capabilities. *Nucleic Acids Res.* **2021**, *49*, W29–W35. [CrossRef] [PubMed]
32. Medema, M.H.; Takano, E.; Breitling, R. Detecting Sequence Homology at the Gene Cluster Level with MultiGeneBlast. *Mol. Biol. Evol.* **2013**, *30*, 1218–1223. [CrossRef] [PubMed]
33. Kautsar, S.A.; Blin, K.; Shaw, S.; Navarro-Muñoz, J.C.; Terlouw, B.R.; Van Der Hooft, J.J.J.; Van Santen, J.A.; Tracanna, V.; Duran, H.G.S.; Andreu, V.P.; et al. MIBiG 2.0: A repository for biosynthetic gene clusters of known function. *Nucleic Acids Res.* **2019**, *48*, D454–D458. [CrossRef] [PubMed]

antibiotics

MDPI

Article

Aerosolized Hypertonic Saline Hinders Biofilm Formation to Enhance Antibiotic Susceptibility of Multidrug-Resistant *Acinetobacter baumannii*

Hui-Ling Lin [1,2,3], Chen-En Chiang [2], Mei-Chun Lin [4], Mei-Lan Kau [4], Yun-Tzu Lin [1] and Chi-Shuo Chen [1,*]

1 Department of Biomedical Engineering and Environmental Sciences, National Tsing Hua University, Hsinchu 300044, Taiwan; huiling@cgu.edu.tw (H.-L.L.); wendy19951208@gmail.com (Y.-T.L.)
2 Department of Respiratory Therapy, Chang Gung University, Taoyuan 33323, Taiwan; paulz60610@gmail.com
3 Department of Respiratory Care, Chang Gung University of Science and Technology, Chiayi 61363, Taiwan
4 Department of Respiratory Therapy, Linkou Chang Gung Memorial Hospital, Taoyuan 33305, Taiwan; lmc0819@gmail.com (M.-C.L.); himeilan@gmail.com (M.-L.K.)
* Correspondence: chen.cs@mx.nthu.edu.tw; Tel.: +886-3-574-2680; Fax: +886-3-571-8649

Abstract: Limited therapeutic options are available for multidrug-resistant *Acinetobacter baumannii* (MDR-AB), and the development of effective treatments is urgently needed. The efficacy of four aerosolized antibiotics (gentamicin, amikacin, imipenem, and meropenem) on three different MDR-AB strains was evaluated using hypertonic saline (HS, 7 g/100 mL) as the aerosol carrier. HS aerosol effectively hindered biofilm formation by specific MDR-AB strains. It could also interrupt the swarming dynamics of MDR-AB and the production of extracellular polymeric substances, which are essential for biofilm progression. Biofilms protect the microorganisms from antibiotics. The use of HS aerosol as a carrier resulted in a decreased tolerance to gentamicin and amikacin in the biofilm-rich MDR-AB. Moreover, we tested the aerosol characteristics of antibiotics mixed with HS and saline, and results showed that HS enhanced the inhaled delivery dose with a smaller particle size distribution of the four antibiotics. Our findings demonstrate the potential of using "old" antibiotics with our "new" aerosol carrier, and potentiate an alternative therapeutic strategy to eliminate MDR-AB infections from a biofilm-disruption perspective.

Keywords: multidrug-resistant *Acinetobacter baumannii* (MDR-AB); hypertonic saline; antibiotics; biofilm; aerosol delivery

Citation: Lin, H.-L.; Chiang, C.-E.; Lin, M.-C.; Kau, M.-L.; Lin, Y.-T.; Chen, C.-S. Aerosolized Hypertonic Saline Hinders Biofilm Formation to Enhance Antibiotic Susceptibility of Multidrug-Resistant *Acinetobacter baumannii*. *Antibiotics* **2021**, *10*, 1115. https://doi.org/10.3390/antibiotics10091115

Academic Editor: Helena Felgueiras

Received: 24 July 2021
Accepted: 12 September 2021
Published: 15 September 2021

1. Introduction

Hospital-acquired pneumonia is most commonly caused by multidrug resistant Gram-negative bacteria, such as *Acinetobacter baumannii*, *P. aeruginosa*, and *K. pneumonia*. Among these, *A. baumannii* is one of the most common causative pathogens [1]. *A. baumannii*, a Gram-negative coccobacillus, is a leading cause of severe nosocomial infections in the current health system [2]. *A. baumannii* is the primary agent associated with pneumonia, septicemia, endocarditis, meningitis, and urinary tract infections [3]. *A. baumannii* can be intrinsically resistant to many commonly used antibiotics, such as aminopenicillins, first-generation and second-generation cephalosporins. The increasing prevalence of multidrug-resistant *A. baumannii* (MDR-AB) infection has emerged worldwide due to prolonged hospital stays [4,5]. A few mechanisms are suspected in the development of MDR-AB, including altered membrane permeability, mutations in efflux pumps and aminoglycoside-modifying enzymes, and the expression of β-lactamases [3]. With the high prevalence of MDR-AB, combination therapy is frequently used to decrease the risk of resistance and improve patient outcomes [6].

Inhaled antibiotics allow rapid and direct delivery to the lungs at a high concentration [7]. To treat bacterial pneumonia effectively, antibiotics must reach the minimum inhibitory concentration in the region of the infected site. However, with drugs administered systemically, the drug concentration in the lungs depends on the drug's ability to penetrate the alveolar capillaries. For example, fluoroquinolones can highly penetrate the lungs compared to other β-lactams or colistin, as colistin has low penetrance through the capillaries [8–10]. Routinely inhaled antibiotics have been the standard treatment for patients diagnosed with cystic fibrosis infected with *P. aeruginosa* [11]. Previous studies have illustrated that adjunct aerosolized colistin to treat patients with MDR-AB had better eradication and cure rates than intravenous administration alone [12,13].

Biofilm formation may alter the responses of the microbial community to antibiotic agents, and contribute to drug resistance challenges [14–16]. The formation of biofilm is composed of several steps: First, through the secreted extracellular polymeric substances (EPSs) on the cell surface, bacteria attach to the solid surface. Under proper conditions, the attached bacteria cluster together as a complex multicellular community with an EPS matrix. In addition to providing anchorage for bacteria, the biofilm matrix provides a microenvironment with a unique nutrient gradient and oxygen conditions, which may stimulate various physiological functions of the bacteria, such as dormancy and intercellular communication in biofilms [16]. Although various mechanisms have been proposed to interpret the altered properties of bacteria in biofilms, it is widely recognized that the biofilm matrix can enhance the survival of bacteria to antimicrobials.

MDR of *A. baumannii* is highly associated with biofilm formation [14]. Studies have shown that biofilms prompt adherence to the host and abiotic surfaces and enhance the survival rate of bacteria to antibiotics. For *A. baumannii*, biofilms can shield bacteria from therapeutic agents and stimulate intercellular communication for colonization [17]. Since the efficacy of antimicrobial agents against microbes is highly dependent on the integrity of the biofilm matrix [15,16], interfering with the biofilm structure is a promising approach to eliminate the protection of the matrix from antibiotics. Different pharmacological approaches and engineering methods have been proposed to disrupt biofilms and eliminate microbial MDR [18]. However, due to the complicated composition of biofilms, such as EPS polymers, proteins, and DNA fragments [15,19], an effective approach for biofilm destruction remains challenging in the biomedical field.

This study aimed to eliminate biofilm formation of *A. baumannii* to recover the therapeutic efficacy of antibiotic agents. We speculated that the delivery of aerosolized hypertonic saline (950 mM sodium chloride) can modulate the ionic concentration of the bacterial microenvironment, and we explored the potency of hypertonic saline for MDR-AB therapy. By replacing the divalent ions within the biofilm matrix [15], high concentrations of mono-ions are expected to interrupt the biofilm of MDR-AB on abiotic surfaces. Four antibiotics that are commonly used in combinational therapies for *A. baumannii* infections were selected: imipenem, meropenem, amikacin, and gentamicin [6]. In addition to the direct impact on the biofilm structure and microbial colonization, we further evaluated the influence of aerosol hypertonic saline on the extracellular secretion of MDR-AB during the colonization process. By regulating the microenvironment of MDR-AB using aerosol hypertonic saline, our approach should provide an alternative perspective for current therapeutic agents to overcome MDR *A. baumannii* and its related diseases.

2. Materials and Methods

2.1. Bacteria Culture and Drug Resistance Test

Three MDR-AB strains were used in this study. MDR-AB isolates (14B0087, 14B0091, and 14B0094) were purchased from the Bioresource Collection and Research Center, Taiwan, following the biosafety protocol.

Bacterial colonies were routinely subcultured with Difco™ Tryptic Soy agar (TSA) plates. Cells were inoculated in 3 mL liquid culture, using Difco™ Tryptic Soy Broth (TSB), and grown at 37 °C in a shaking incubator overnight (14–16 h). The overnight liquid cultures with optical density (OD_{600}) exceeding 1.0 were used for subsequent experiments.

Four antibiotics agents were used to evaluate the drug response of MDR-AB: Imipenem/Cilastatin (500 mg/500 mg, Facta Farmaceutici, Italy), Meropenem (250 mg, Sumitomo Dainippon Pharma Co., Ltd., Japan), acemycin (Amikacin 125 mg/mL, Yung Shin Pharmaceutical Ind. Co. LTD, Taichung, Taiwan), and gentamicin (40 mg/mL, Tai Yu Chemical & Pharmaceutical Co., LTD, Hsinhsu, Taiwan)]. The chemical structures of the four antibiotics listed are presented in Figure 1. Antibiotic agents were aerosolized with either regular saline (135 mM NaCl) or hypertonic saline (950 mM). The resistance tests were revised according to a previous study. In brief, 2 μL of overnight liquid culture (OD_{600} = 1.0) was dripped onto TSA. Thereafter, 4 mL of antibiotic at the desired concentration was aerosolized and deposited onto the specimens. Approximately 0.2 μL of antibiotic solution was deposited on the bacteria culture. After aerosol treatment, the agar plate was incubated at 37 °C overnight (14–16 h). MDR-AB grew into visible colonies after overnight incubation. Selected colonies were scooped into 1 mL of 1× phosphate-buffered saline (PBS); the colony was dispersed and further diluted to 1×10^5–10^9 in 1× PBS. The diluted cells (20 μL) were spread onto TSA agar plates and incubated overnight for colony formation unit quantification. The survival rate of MDR-AB was determined by quantifying the number of recovered colonies on the plates, and normalized with aerosolized saline treatment for each independent experiment.

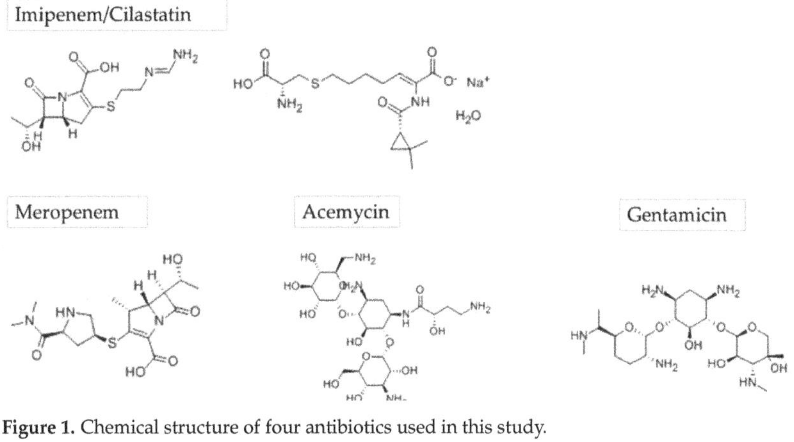

Figure 1. Chemical structure of four antibiotics used in this study.

2.2. *Aerosol Generation and Aerosol Particle Size Distribution*

A 2.5 L closed aerosol delivery chamber was designed, and the culture dishes were placed in the middle of the chamber. Antibiotic selection by the Bioresource Collection and Research Center, Taiwan, was based on sensitivity and susceptibility, and the dose was determined as the maximum inhibition of bacterial motility. Imipenem (7.81 mg), meropenem (31.25 mg), acemycin (7.81 mg), and gentamicin (10 mg) were used. A pneumatic jet nebulizer (Besmed Inc., Taipei, Taiwan) powered by a 50 psi compressed oxygen flow at 8 L/min was filled with 4 mL antibiotics mixed with 0.9% saline or 7% hypertonic saline. Nebulization was stopped by sputtering, and the culture dish was removed for testing 30 s later (n = 5).

Aerosol characteristics were determined by a cascade impaction, according to the United States and European Pharmacopeia recommendations. A Next-Generation Impactor (Copley Scientific Limited, Nottingham, United Kingdom) was assembled with internal and external filters and placed in a temperature-controlled chamber at 4 °C. The impactor was calibrated at 15 L/min using a mass flow meter (TSI Cooperation, Shoreview, Minnesota). The mass median aerodynamic diameter (MMAD), geometric standard deviation (GSD), and fine-particle fractions (percentage of particles < 5 mm) were calculated using the CITDAS 3.1 software (Copley Scientific, Nottingham, United Kingdom). The dry weight of the nebulizers was taken after loading 4 mL of the selected antibiotic mixture, and after the completion of nebulization. The emitted dose of the nebulizer was calculated as the difference between the loaded and post-nebulization weights.

2.3. Biofilm Quantitative Measurement and Scanning Electron Microscopy

To evaluate the influence of the hypertonic saline on biofilm formation, overnight cultures were diluted to OD_{600} = 0.01, with the TSB containing either 135 nM NaCl or 950 mM and deposited in 96-well plates at 200 μL/well. After incubation at 37 °C for 48 h, the biofilm was gently washed with 1× PBS to remove excessive suspended cells. Thereafter, the specimens were stained with 0.5% crystal violet (*w*/*v*) for 10 min. The stained biofilm was dissolved in 95% ethanol, and biofilm formation was quantified by measuring OD_{550} with a spectrometer.

A 12 × 12 mm glass circle coverslip was set at an angle of 30° to 50° in a flat-bottom 24-well plate. Diluted overnight liquid cultures at 1:100 in TSB were carefully added at 300 μL/well. The cells were incubated for 48 h. After 48 h, the circle coverslips were carefully moved from the well, and the cells were prepared for visualization using scanning electron microscope (SEM). Biofilms were first fixed in 4% glutaraldehyde for 20 min, and then serially diluted with ethanol. Critical point drying was performed before coating 2 nm of gold onto the specimen surface. The prepared specimens were imaged using SEM.

2.4. The Spatial Distribution of Protein and Carbohydrate in Biofilm

MDR-AB colonies were prepared as described above. The prepared colonies were treated with experimental aerosols and incubated at 37 °C for 4 h. To identify the protein/carbohydrate distribution, WGA (Wheat Germ Agglutinin, 1 mg/mL) stained carbohydrates, and SYPRO™ Ruby Biofilm Matrix Stain (used as manufacturer's suggestion), stained proteins in the biofilm, were applied. Stained biofilms were observed using laser scanning confocal microscopy at 20× magnification.

2.5. The Dynamic of Bacteria Swarming

Bacterial swarming assays were performed on a substrate containing 0.3% agarose (semisolid surface) in 3 μL of TSB overnight culture (OD_{600} = 0.3). MDR-AB was dripped onto the surface of 0.3% agar. Bacterial swarming was monitored for 10 h at 37 °C using time-lapse microscopy (interval = 1 image/30 min).

2.6. Statistical Analysis

All data are presented as the mean± standard deviation (SD). Comparisons among groups were conducted using one-way analysis of variance (ANOVA) with post hoc Bonferroni correction. A Student's two-tailed *t*-test was used to determine the significance of the difference between the mixture of 7% hypertonic saline or 0.9% saline, and the results are indicated as * $p < 0.05$, ** $p < 0.01$, and *** $p < 0.001$.

3. Results and Discussion

3.1. Hypertonic Saline Hinders the Biofilm Formation of A. baumannii

Biofilms provide protection from antibiotic agents to the microbial community. The stickiness of EPS plays an essential role in the structure formation of the microbial community. A previous study showed that the stickiness of EPS of Sagutula can be altered by ionic strength in the surrounding microenvironment [20]. As a critical substance for bacteria to adhere to the surface, the influence of ionic strength on biofilm formation by *A. baumannii* has not yet been fully explored. We first tested whether the treatment of hypertonic saline aerosol could eliminate biofilm formation on the solid surface with three MDR *A. baumannii* strains. First, we cultured *A. baumannii* in a medium containing 950 mM sodium chloride to recapture high ionic strength in the microenvironment. After 48 h of culture, the biofilm was labeled with crystal violet staining, and different biofilm patterns were observed over these three MDR strains (Figure 2a). An abundant biofilm was formed with MDR-087, and there was almost no biofilm formation with MDR-091. After culturing in a medium containing 950 mM NaCl, MDR-094 showed approximately 54% reduced biofilm formation, and the biofilm of MDR-087 also showed a slight decrease (Figure 2b). The results indicated that a high concentration of NaCl could help to limit *A. baumannii* biofilm formation.

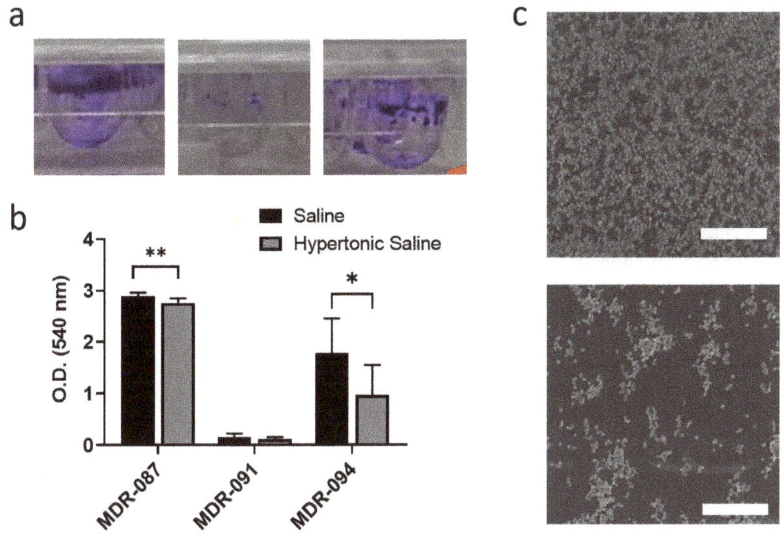

Figure 2. The biofilm of *A. baumannii*: (**a**) images of crystal violet staining to show the biofilm formed by MDR-AB; (**b**) quantitative measurement of biofilm formation using a spectrometer; (**c**) SEM images of colonized MDR-087 at the air–liquid interface with aerosolized saline (top) and aerosolized hypertonic saline (bottom). ** $p < 0.05$; * $p < 0.001$.

Furthermore, SEM was used to examine the microstructures of the biofilm. From the images, we observed a more fractural biofilm structure after treatment with the hypertonic aerosol. *A. baumannii* was separated into small clusters, rather than colonizing together (Figure 2c). Combining the alteration of the biofilm microstructure and quantitative biofilm assay at the macroscale, our data demonstrated that hypertonic saline aerosol hinders biofilm formation and disperses microbial colonization. The biofilm matrix is an important abiotic factor that influences the antibiotic resistance of microbes [14,16]. In comparison to dense biofilms, antibiotic agents can easily penetrate the fractal matrix and kill bacteria within it. Although the dosage of hypertonic saline is not enough to eliminate bacterial growth through osmotic stress, our data implied that the abolishment of dense biofilm formation may enhance the efficacy of antibiotic agents.

3.2. Hypertonic Saline Stimulates Bacterial Swarming and Alters the Distribution of EPS

We examined the potential mechanisms underlying the decrease in biofilm formation. A previous study illustrated a negative correlation between bacterial motility and biofilm formation [20]; as the first step of biofilm formation, microbes slow down and adhere to the substrate. Thus, we speculated that hypertonic saline can stimulate the movement of bacteria and decrease the adhesion of bacteria to the substrate. The inhibition of motility promotes biofilm formation. The observed increasing motility of *A. baumannii* implies an unstable adherence between bacteria and substrate, which can contribute to the loss of biofilm formation [21]. The results of the swarming assay showed that the swarming motility of all three MDR strains significantly increased after the aerosol treatments, either with saline or with hypertonic saline (Figure 3a). To further determine the difference between aerosolized saline and aerosolized hypertonic saline treatment, we measured the swarming dynamics of *A. baumannii* using time-lapse microscopy. Under microscopy, active bacterial twitching in the transparent leading-edge surrounding the colony was observed (Figure 3b).

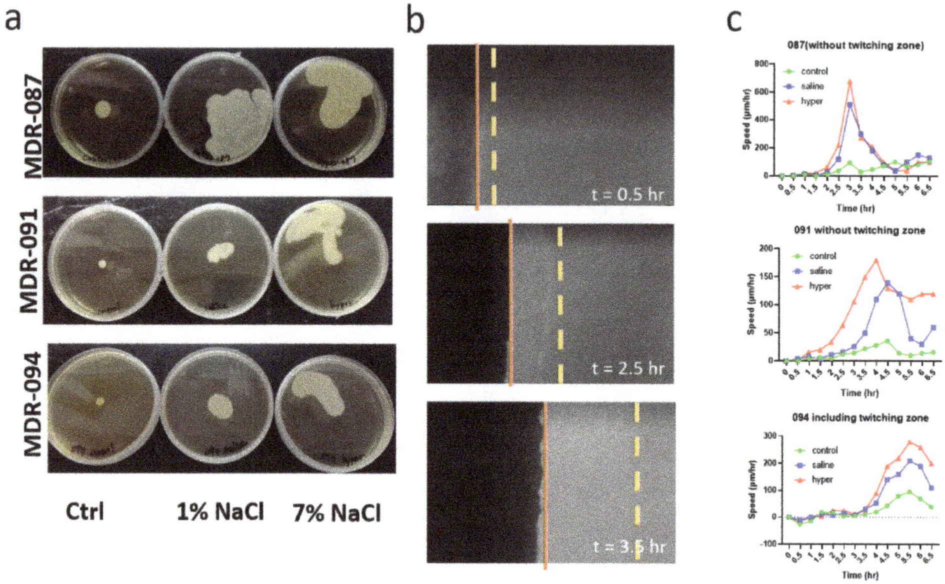

Figure 3. The swarming dynamics of MDR-AB: (**a**) pictures of MDR-AB strains swarming on soft agar plated after 72 h incubation; (**b**) time-lapse microscopy images of active twitching movement of MDR-AB; (yellow dashed line: front edge of the twitching layer; orange line: back edge of the twitching layer); (**c**) quantitative analysis of MDR-AB swarming under various experimental conditions.

Following the rapid expansion of the lead edge, a three-dimensional colonized bacterial community formed gradually, which was shown to expand the opaque portion under phase microscopy (Figure 3b). In the presence of hypertonic saline aerosol, we observed an increasing swarming movement of *A. baumannii* (Figure 3c). For instance, for the MDR-091 group at t = 3.5 h after seeding, the data showed that the velocity of swarming velocity increased from 22 to 50 μm/h with saline treatment and further increased to 150 μm/h with hypertonic saline treatment.

The EPSs, serving as the fundamental material of biofilm, critically influence the adhesion of bacteria to the surroundings [22]. Previous studies have shown that increasing the mono-ionic concentration enhances the stickiness of EPSs extracted from *E. Huxieyi* and *Amphora* sp. [20]. Our data on unstable adhesion and high motility suggested that the high concentration of monotonic ions may cover the negative surface charge of EPS and reduce the entanglement of *A. baumannii* EPSs. On the other hand, a further increase in salt concentration can lead to decreased motility. Studies have also shown the limited motility of *A. baumannii*, due to the increased surface hydrophobicity under high salt conditions (300 mM in 0.5% agar); excessive hypertonic saline aerosol may also lead to undesired physiological responses of patients, such as coughing. More detailed experiments are required for dose optimization before clinical respiratory therapy.

The hypertonic saline aerosol may directly reduce the entanglement of the EPS matrix and change the EPS secretion of bacteria [23]. It is known that microorganisms produce different EPSs under different environmental stresses. In contrast to the salt concentration (~400 mM) reported in other osmotic stress studies, our experimental deposited NaCl dosage (approximately 150 mM) may not lead to significant osmotic stress in *A. baumannii*.

However, aerosolized hypertonic saline can locally alter the ionic concentration at the deposition sites [24] and potentially regulate the EPS secretion of *A. baumannii*.

By applying laser scanning confocal microscopy with protein/carbohydrate labeling assays [15,25], we reconstructed the spatial distribution of protein/carbohydrate in the fast-progressing colony edges to evaluate the influence of aerosol treatment on EPS production. The results showed different compositions at the colony edge of the three MDR strains (Figure 4). MDR-087 showed the lowest protein content compared to the other two MDR strains. A remarkable protein/carbohydrate segregated distribution was observed in MDR-091 and MDR-094, and a 50 μm-thick distinguished carbohydrate layer was found at the edge of the MDR-094 colony. When treated with hypertonic saline aerosol, all three strains seemed to express more carbohydrate-rich EPS (as shown in the insets). A more segregated protein/carbohydrate distribution was observed in MDR-091 and MDR-094, and a thin layer of proteins was present in the EPS layer at the edge of MRD-091 colony.

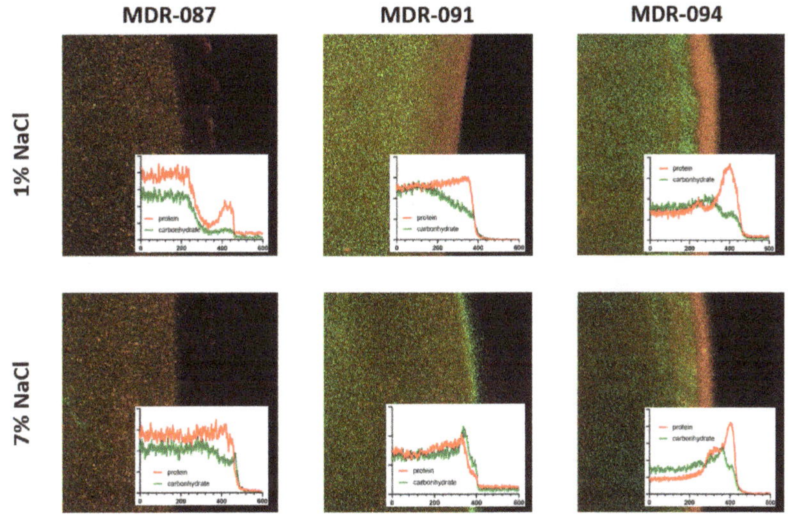

Figure 4. The spatial distribution of protein/carbohydrate composition in biofilm matrix. Represented confocal images of colony edge under different treatments. Proteins (red) and carbohydrate were labeled with fluorescein. Insets: Intensity profiles of protein staining (red) and carbohydrate labeling (green) cross the colony edge.

Our data showed that the deposited hypertonic saline aerosol could regulate the EPSs produced by *A. baumannii*. Extracellular proteins and carbohydrates are known to play important roles in the maintenance of biofilm matrices. It has also been shown that a lack of protein is expressed on the cell surface, and *A. baumannii* cannot colonize the epithelium of the respiratory airway. In this study, high carbohydrate expression implied a lower colonizing capacity of *A. baumannii* after aerosolized hypertonic saline treatment. Although we evaluated the composition using bacterial colonies on soft agar surfaces, the lower protein/carbohydrate ratio may also support the formation of fractured colonies at the liquid–air interface (Figure 2c). Moreover, the hydrophobic interactions between proteins can contribute to the stability of the biofilm matrix, and the sticky EPSs are associated with a higher protein to carbohydrate ratio of EPSs [20,25]. The observed alteration of protein/carbohydrate in the biofilm matrix implied lower adhesion for the bacteria within the matrix, showing higher motility.

Since biofilm formation can contribute to the antibiotic resistance of microorganisms, after identifying the impact of hypertonic saline aerosol on biofilm formation, we aimed to study the influences of aerosol hypertonic saline on the antibiotic resistance of MDR-

ABs. First, we observed the enhancing efficacy of gentamicin and acemycin on MDR-087, which is known to show intermediate resistance to gentamicin (Figure 5a,b). For MDR-094, which is resistant to gentamicin, a similar effect of hypertonic saline aerosol for decreasing antibiotic resistance was observed (Figure 5a). However, for MDR-091, which is resistant to imipenem and meropenem, aerosolized hypertonic saline showed no significant influence on suppressing the bacterial survival rate under antibiotic treatments (Figure 5c,d). Together with the biofilm quantification measurement, we observed that MDR-091 produced the lowest biofilm under both experimental conditions compared to MDR-087 and MDR-094. Thus, biofilm formation does not seem to contribute to the drug resistance of MDR- 091, and the interruption of biofilm formation showed no impact on MDR-091.

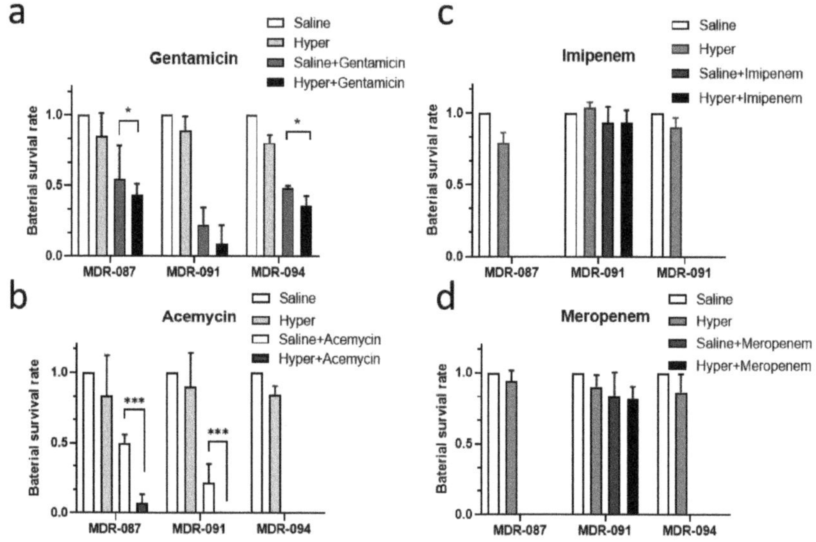

Figure 5. The antibiotic response of MDR-AB. (**a**–**d**) Different antibiotics were aerosolized with either saline or hypertonic saline and were deposited on MDR-AB strains. * $p < 0.05$; *** $p < 0.001$.

3.3. *Influence of Hypertonic Saline to Aerosol Characteristics and Delivered Dose*

Changing the diluent in aerosol treatment may change the characteristics of aerosols and lead to alterations in the inhaled dosage [26]. An impactor was used to simulate physiological inhalation/exhalation to determine the aerosol characteristics. Our study showed that hypertonic saline as a diluent for antibiotics altered the emitted dose and particle size distribution (Figure 5). Compared to normal saline, the emitted doses with hypertonic saline–antibiotic mixtures were significantly greater (Figure 6a), indicating that hypertonic saline might carry higher antibiotic doses to the lungs. Furthermore, the smaller MMAD and larger fine particle fraction would facilitate antibiotics in the peripheral regions of the lungs where pneumonia is most likely to occur (Figure 6b,c). Previous studies have proven the safety of hypertonic saline, and nebulized hypertonic saline alone for patients with airway hypersecretions, such as cystic fibrosis and COPD [27]. Additionally, hypertonic saline reduces inflammation in the respiratory systems [28]. Our study demonstrated that using hypertonic saline as a diluent of antibiotics before nebulization facilitates greater drug delivery to the peripheral regions, and further studies of drug deposition confirmed by radiolabeled or clinical outcomes are warranted. Moreover, considering the interactions between drug molecules and solvent, more detail studies are required to determine pharmacological characteristics, such as degradation and hydrolysis, while applying hypertonic saline with specific drug molecules.

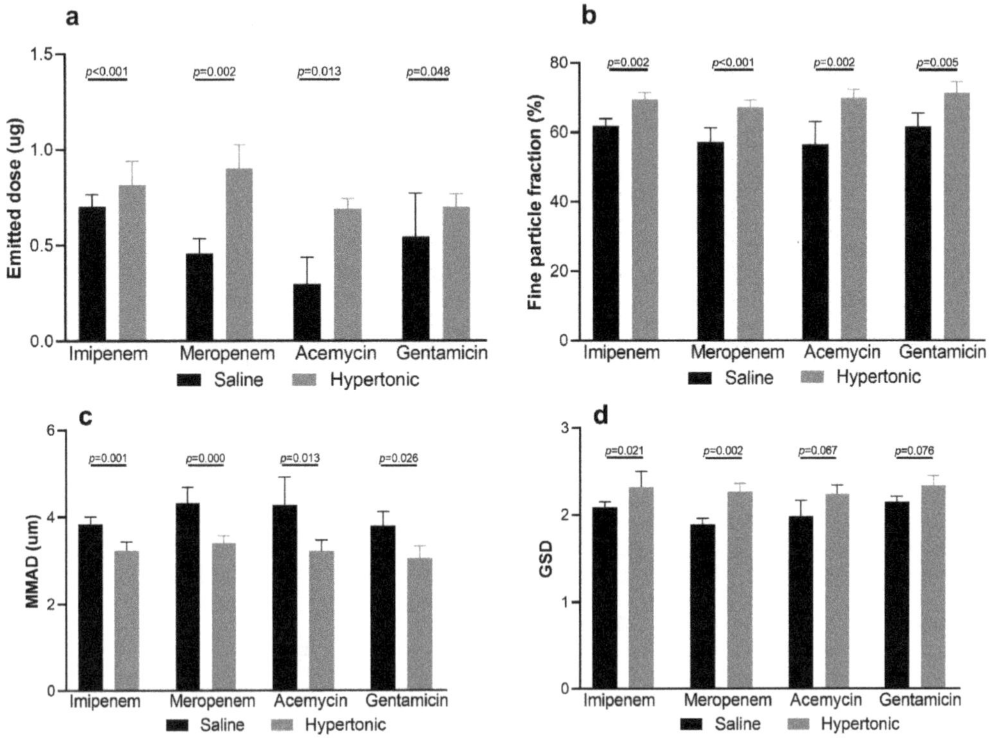

Figure 6. Comparisons of aerosol characteristics: (**a**) emitted doses were higher using hypertonic saline mixtures of all four antibiotics; (**b**,**c**) hypertonic saline generates significantly higher fine particle fraction; (**b**) resulting smaller MMAD; (**d**) the geometric standard deviation of imipenem and meropenem mixed with hypertonic saline was significantly greater.

4. Conclusions

This study demonstrated that aerosolized hypertonic saline hindered biofilm formation by MDR-AB and enhanced the efficacy of gentamicin and acemycin. In our experiments for the MDR-AB-producing biofilm (MDR-087 and MDR-094), the biofilm matrix seemed to contribute to drug resistance. The drug resistance associated with the biofilm matrix can be partially eliminated by aerosolized hypertonic saline. Two potential mechanisms, i.e., the alteration of stable adhesion and biofilm production, have been proposed to interrupt biofilm formation and decrease antibiotic tolerance. In addition, hypertonic saline is known to facilitate the penetration of antibiotic through the mucus layer, which may further enhance its efficacy. On the other hand, we noticed that the impacts of aerosolized hypertonic saline on susceptibility seem to be greater for MDR-ABs with higher biofilm production; one concern is that the high concentration of ions may accelerate the degradation of antibiotics. More detail studies are required to further explore the applications of antibiotic treatment with hypertonic saline aerosol. In summary, we demonstrated that using hypertonic saline aerosol to deliver antibiotics is a promising therapeutic strategy to eliminate MDR-AB infections with currently available antibiotic agents.

Author Contributions: Conceptualization, H.-L.L. and C.-S.C.; Methodology, Y.-T.L.; Software, C.-E.C.; Validation, C.-E.C. and Y.-T.L.; Formal Analysis, M.-C.L.; Investigation, M.-L.K.; Resources, H.-L.L.; Data Curation, Y.-T.L.; Writing—Original Draft Preparation, H.-L.L. and C.-S.C.; Writing—Review and Editing, C.-S.C. and H.-L.L.; Visualization, C.-E.C.; Supervision, C.-S.C.; Project Administration, Y.-T.L.; Funding Acquisition, H.-L.L. All authors have read and agreed to the published version of the manuscript.

Funding: Financial support was provided by the Chang Gung Memorial Foundation (grant number CMRPD1K0181) and Ministry of Science and Technology, Taiwan, R.O.C. (grant numbers MOST-109-2314-B-182-067 and MOST 109-2112-M-007-003).

Data Availability Statement: The datasets used and/or analyzed during the current study are available from the corresponding author on reasonable request.

Conflicts of Interest: The authors declare no conflict of interest. The funders had no role in the design of the study; in the collection, analyses, or interpretation of data; in the writing of the manuscript, or in the decision to publish the results.

References

1. Laessig, K.A. End points in hospital-acquired pneumonia and/or ventilator-associated pneumonia clinical trials: Food and drug administration perspective. *Clin. Infect. Dis.* **2010**, *51* (Suppl. 1), S117–S119. [CrossRef]
2. Moubareck, C.A.; Halat, D.H. Insights into *Acinetobacter baumannii*: A Review of Microbiological, Virulence, and Resistance Traits in a Threatening Nosocomial Pathogen. *Antibiotics* **2020**, *9*, 119. [CrossRef]
3. Cillóniz, C.; Dominedò, C.; Torres, A. Multidrug Resistant Gram-Negative Bacteria in Community-Acquired Pneumonia. *Crit. Care* **2019**, *23*, 79. [CrossRef]
4. Kyriakidis, I.; Vasileiou, E.; Pana, Z.D.; Tragiannidis, A. *Acinetobacter baumannii* Antibiotic Resistance Mechanisms. *Pathogens* **2021**, *10*, 373. [CrossRef]
5. Kurihara, M.N.L.; Sales, R.O.; Silva, K.E.D.; Maciel, W.G.; Simionatto, S. Multidrug-resistant Acinetobacter baumannii outbreaks: A global problem in healthcare settings. *Rev. Soc. Bras. Med. Trop.* **2020**, *53*, e20200248. [CrossRef]
6. Skariyachan, S.; Taskeen, N.; Ganta, M.; Krishna, B.V. Recent perspectives on the virulent factors and treatment options for multidrug-resistant *Acinetobacter baumannii*. *Crit. Rev. Microbiol.* **2019**, *45*, 315–333. [CrossRef] [PubMed]
7. Wood, G.C.; Swanson, J.M. An Update on Aerosolized Antibiotics for Treating Hospital-Acquired and Ventilator-Associated Pneumonia in Adults. *Ann. Pharmacother.* **2017**, *51*, 1112–1121. [CrossRef] [PubMed]
8. Flume, P.A.; VanDevanter, D.R. Clinical applications of pulmonary delivery of antibiotics. *Adv. Drug Deliv. Rev.* **2015**, *85*, 1–6. [CrossRef] [PubMed]
9. Zhou, Q.T.; Leung, S.S.; Tang, P.; Parumasivam, T.; Loh, Z.H.; Chan, H.K. Inhaled formulations and pulmonary drug delivery systems for respiratory infections. *Adv. Drug Deliv. Rev.* **2015**, *85*, 83–99. [CrossRef] [PubMed]
10. Wenzler, E.; Fraidenburg, D.R.; Scardina, T.; Danziger, L.H. Inhaled Antibiotics for Gram-Negative Respiratory Infections. *Clin. Microbiol. Rev.* **2016**, *29*, 581–632. [CrossRef] [PubMed]
11. Gappa, M.; Steinkamp, G.; Tümmler, B.; von der Hardt, H. Long-term tobramycin aerosol therapy of chronic Pseudomonas aeruginosa infection in patients with cystic fibrosis. *Scand. J. Gastroenterol. Suppl.* **1988**, *143*, 74–76. [CrossRef] [PubMed]
12. Chen, Y.M.; Fang, W.F.; Kao, H.C.; Chen, H.-C.; Tsai, Y.-C.; Shen, L.-S.; Li, C.-L.; Chang, H.-C.; Huang, K.-T.; Lin, M.-C.; et al. Influencing factors of successful eradication of multidrug-resistant Acinetobacter baumannii in the respiratory tract with aerosolized colistin. *Biomed. J.* **2014**, *37*, 314–320.
13. Lu, Q.; Luo, R.; Bodin, L.; Yang, J.; Zahr, N.; Aubry, A.; Golmard, J.-L.; Rouby, J.-J.; Nebulized Antibiotics Study Group. Efficacy of high-dose nebulized colistin in ventilator-associated pneumonia caused by multidrug-resistant Pseudomonas aeruginosa and Acinetobacter baumannii. *Anesthesiology* **2012**, *117*, 1335–1347. [CrossRef] [PubMed]
14. Badave, G.K.; Kulkarni, D. Biofilm Producing Multidrug Resistant Acinetobacter baumannii: An Emerging Challenge. *J. Clin. Diagn. Res.* **2015**, *9*, DC08–DC10. [CrossRef] [PubMed]
15. Davies, D. Understanding biofilm resistance to antibacterial agents. *Nat. Rev. Drug Discov.* **2003**, *2*, 114–122. [CrossRef]
16. Flemming, H.C.; Wingender, J.; Szewzyk, U.; Steinberg, P.; Rice, S.A.; Kjelleberg, S. Biofilms: An emergent form of bacterial life. *Nat. Rev. Microbiol.* **2016**, *14*, 563–575. [CrossRef]
17. Lee, H.W.; Koh, Y.M.; Kim, J.; Lee, J.-C.; Lee, Y.-C.; Seol, S.-Y.; Cho, D.-T. Capacity of multidrug-resistant clinical isolates of Acinetobacter baumannii to form biofilm and adhere to epithelial cell surfaces. *Clin. Microbiol. Infect.* **2008**, *14*, 49–54. [CrossRef]
18. Meyer, B. *Approaches to Prevention, Removal and Killing of Biofilms*; International Biodeterioration & Biodegradation: London, UK, 2003; Volume 51, pp. 249–253.
19. Zapotoczna, M.; O'Neill, E.; O'Gara, J.P. Untangling the Diverse and Redundant Mechanisms of Staphylococcus aureus Biofilm Formation. *PLoS Pathog.* **2016**, *12*, e1005671. [CrossRef]
20. Chen, C.S.; Shiu, R.F.; Hsieh, Y.Y.; Xu, C.; Vazquez, C.I.; Cui, Y.; Hsu, I.C.; Quigg, A.; Santschi, P.H.; Chin, W.-C. Stickiness of extracellular polymeric substances on different surfaces via magnetic tweezers. *Sci. Total Environ.* **2021**, *757*, 143766. [CrossRef]
21. Guttenplan, S.B.; Kearns, D.B. Regulation of flagellar motility during biofilm formation. *FEMS Microbiol Rev.* **2013**, *37*, 849–871. [CrossRef]
22. Tsuneda, S.; Aikawa, H.; Hayashi, H.; Yuasa, A.; Hirata, A. Extracellular polymeric substances responsible for bacterial adhesion onto solid surface. *FEMS Microbiol. Lett.* **2003**, *223*, 287–292. [CrossRef]
23. Guo, Y.S.; Furrer, J.M.; Kadilak, A.L.; Hinestroza, H.F.; Gage, D.; Cho, Y.K.; Shor, L.M. Bacterial Extracellular Polymeric Substances Amplify Water Content Variability at the Pore Scale. *Front. Environ. Sci.* **2018**, *6*. [CrossRef]

24. Lin, H.L.; Chiu, L.C.; Wan, G.H.; Huang, C.-C.; Lee, Z.-T.; Lin, Y.-T.; Wu, S.-R.; Chen, C.-S. Hypertonic saline enhances the efficacy of aerosolized gentamicin against Pseudomonas aeruginosa. *Sci. Rep.* **2020**, *10*, 4325. [CrossRef] [PubMed]
25. Harimawan, A.; Rajasekar, A.; Ting, Y.P. Bacteria attachment to surfaces–AFM force spectroscopy and physicochemical analyses. *J. Colloid Interface Sci.* **2011**, *364*, 213–218, Erratum in **2013**, *15*, 392–470. [CrossRef] [PubMed]
26. Klemmer, A.; Krämer, I.; Kamin, W. Physicochemical compatibility of nebulizable drug admixtures containing budesonide and colistimethate or hypertonic saline. *Int. J. Pharm. Compd.* **2013**, *17*, 254–261.
27. Carro, L.M.; Martínez-García, M.A. Use of Hyaluronic Acid (HA) in Chronic Airway Diseases. *Cells* **2020**, *9*, 2210. [CrossRef]
28. Reeves, E.P.; Williamson, M.; O'Neill, S.J.; Greally, P.; McElvaney, N.G. Nebulized hypertonic saline decreases IL-8 in sputum of patients with cystic fibrosis. *Am. J. Respir. Crit. Care Med.* **2011**, *183*, 1517–1523. [CrossRef] [PubMed]

antibiotics

Article

Flavonoid-Coated Gold Nanoparticles as Efficient Antibiotics against Gram-Negative Bacteria—Evidence from In Silico-Supported In Vitro Studies

Hani A. Alhadrami [1,2,3,†], Raha Orfali [4,†], Ahmed A. Hamed [5], Mohammed M Ghoneim [6], Hossam M. Hassan [7,8], Ahmed S. I. Hassane [9,10], Mostafa E. Rateb [9], Ahmed M. Sayed [7,*] and Noha M. Gamaleldin [11,*]

1 Department of Medical Laboratory Technology, Faculty of Applied Medical Sciences, King Abdulaziz University, Jeddah 21589, Saudi Arabia; hanialhadrami@kau.edu.sa
2 Molecular Diagnostic Lab, King Abdulaziz University Hospital, King Abdulaziz University, Jeddah 21589, Saudi Arabia
3 Special Infectious Agent Unit, King Fahd Medical Research Centre, King Abdulaziz University, Jeddah 21589, Saudi Arabia
4 Department of Pharmacognosy, College of Pharmacy, King Saud University, Riyadh 11495, Saudi Arabia; rorfali@ksu.edu.sa
5 National Research Centre, Microbial Chemistry Department, 33 El-Buhouth Street, Dokki, Giza P.O. Box 12622, Egypt; ahmedshalbio@gmail.com
6 Department of Pharmacy Practice, College of Pharmacy, AlMaarefa University, Riyadh 13713, Saudi Arabia; mghoneim@mcst.edu.sa
7 Department of Pharmacognosy, Faculty of Pharmacy, Nahda University, Beni-Suef 62513, Egypt; hossam.mokhtar@nub.edu.eg
8 Department of Pharmacognosy, Faculty of Pharmacy, Beni-Suef University, Beni-Suef 62513, Egypt
9 School of Computing, Engineering & Physical Sciences, University of the West of Scotland, Paisley PA1 2BE, UK; Ahmedsayed.hassane@nhs.scot (A.S.I.H.); mostafa.rateb@uws.ac.uk (M.E.R.)
10 Aberdeen Royal Infirmary, Foresterhill Health Campus, Foresterhill Road, Aberdeen AB25 2NZ, UK
11 Department of Microbiology, Faculty of Pharmacy, The British University in Egypt (BUE), Cairo 11837, Egypt
* Correspondence: Ahmed.mohamed.sayed@nub.edu.eg (A.M.S.); noha.gamaleldin@bue.edu.eg (N.M.G.)
† These authors equally contributed to this work.

Citation: Alhadrami, H.A.; Orfali, R.; Hamed, A.A.; Ghoneim, M.M.; Hassan, H.M.; Hassane, A.S.I.; Rateb, M.E.; Sayed, A.M.; Gamaleldin, N.M. Flavonoid-Coated Gold Nanoparticles as Efficient Antibiotics against Gram-Negative Bacteria— Evidence from In Silico-Supported In Vitro Studies. *Antibiotics* **2021**, *10*, 968. https://doi.org/10.3390/antibiotics10080968

Academic Editors: Anthony William Coleman and Helena Felgueiras

Received: 2 July 2021
Accepted: 9 August 2021
Published: 12 August 2021

Abstract: Flavonoids are a class of bioactive plant-derived natural products that exhibit a broad range of biological activities, including antibacterial ones. Their inhibitory activity toward Gram-positive bacterial was found to be superior to that against Gram-negative ones. In the present study, a number of flavonoid-coated gold nanoparticles (GNPs) were designed to enhance the antibacterial effects of chrysin, kaempferol, and quercetin against a number of Gram-negative bacteria. The prepared GNPs were able to conjugate to these three flavonoids with conjugation efficiency ranging from 41% to 80%. Additionally, they were able to exert an enhanced antibacterial activity in comparison with the free flavonoids and the unconjugated GNPs. Quercetin-coated GNPs were the most active nano-conjugates and were able to penetrate the cell wall of *E. coli*. A number of in silico experiments were carried out to explain the conjugation efficiency and the antibacterial mechanisms of these flavonoids as follows: (i) these flavonoids can efficiently bind to the glutathione linker on the surface of GNPs via H-bonding; (ii) these flavonoids, particularly quercetin, were able to increase the bacterial membrane rigidity, and hence decrease its functionality; (iii) these flavonoids can inhibit *E. coli*'s DNA gyrase (Gyr-B) with IC_{50} values ranging from 0.9 to 3.9 μM. In conclusion, these bioactive flavonoid-based GNPs are considered to be very promising antibiotic candidates for further development and evaluation.

Keywords: gold nanoparticles; flavonoids; Gram-negative bacteria; DNA gyrase; in silico

1. Introduction

One of the major drug delivery challenges is drug selectivity to avoid the potential side effect and reduce the cytotoxic effects of the therapeutic agent [1]. This selectivity plays a significant role in increasing drug efficacy, reducing the drug dosage and frequency, and controlling the release of the therapeutic agent [2]. On the other hand, using large-sized materials for drug delivery faces many challenges, starting from in vivo instability, poor solubility, poor bioavailability, and poor absorption in the body to issues with target-specific delivery [1]. Therefore, searching for a new drug delivery system is crucial for solving these critical issues. In this regard, nanotechnology can provide a variety of solutions. Beside its unlimited applications in construction material, electronics, food production, agriculture, catalysis, and energy production, it can provide unique applications and solutions for many medical and health-based issues [3,4].

Nanobiotechnology is a promising area of nanotechnology that utilizes nano-scale materials in different aspects of biology [5]. Recently, nanomaterials have gained considerable attention from scientists due to their potential applications in medicine and drug formulations [6]. With their nano size, which ranges between 1 and 100 nm, nanomaterials have gained increasing attention in many medical fields such as biosensors, microarray tests, microfluidics, tissue engineering and drug delivery [7]. Furthermore, their chemical and physical properties make them an excellent choice as a drug delivery system when compared with other larger-scale counterparts usually used for drug delivery [8]. Their high surface-area-to-volume ratio increases their affinity for small molecules and facilitates their uptake across the cell membrane [4]. Beside their unique structures, nanoparticles display magnetic, electrical, and biological properties which allow them to be good candidates for a delivery system for encapsulating drugs and deliver them more precisely with a controlled release to target tissues [4,8]. Selection of suitable nanomaterials for drug delivery is based on the drug's physiochemical features [1].

Among all the noble metal nanoparticles, gold has gained great attention due to its unique properties, such as good conductivity, chemical stability, catalytic properties, and biological activity, including antibacterial, antifungal, antiviral and anti-inflammatory activities. It can also be used in a variety of applications, ranging from medical applications (photothermal and radiation therapy, photodynamic therapeutics, biosensors, and X-ray imagery) to food industry, material science, chemistry, and physics [9–11].

As a part of the continuing investigation into safe and effective antibacterial agents from natural products, a number of non-glycosylated flavonoids have been tested for their growth inhibitory activity against some Gram-negative bacteria (*Escherichia coli, Pseudomonas aeruginosa, Proteus vulgaris* and *Klebsiella pneumonia*). This class of compounds has been found to exert antibacterial activity via multiple mechanisms: (i) altering the fluidity of the bacterial membranes (i.e., increasing their rigidity), an effect that was found to be associated with bacterial growth inhibition [12]; (ii) inhibiting DNA gyrase and, in turn, bacterial DNA supercoiling [13]; and (iii) inhibiting the bacterial penicillin-binding proteins (PBPs) and thus inhibiting bacterial cell wall biosynthesis [14].

Combining some of these bioactive flavonoids with biocompatible metallic nanoparticles can improve their pharmacokinetic properties and maximize their antibacterial efficacy. Accordingly, in this investigation, a number of novel flavonoid–gold nano-conjugates were designed and their antibacterial potential against Gram-negative bacteria was explored. Additionally, a number of in silico analyses (e.g., molecular docking and dynamics) were utilized to obtain some insight into the molecular structure of these newly prepared nano-conjugates and the mode of action of their flavonoid components. The results of the present investigation can provide a good starting point to develop flavonoid-based antimicrobial nanomaterials in the future.

2. Results and Discussion

2.1. Screening of Flavonoids against Gram-Negative Bacteria

Firstly, we evaluated the antibacterial potential of a number of flavonoids against some pathogenic Gram-negative bacteria. As shown in Figure 1, some of the tested flavonoids showed weak millimolar activity and some of them were inactive up to 1 mM. However, in our previous report, we found that some of these flavonoids (e.g., chrysin and apigenin) were far more active against Gram-positive bacteria (e.g., *Staphylococcus aureus*), where their minimum inhibitory concentrations (MICs) were in the micromolar range [14]. These significant differences in the antibacterial activity could be attributed to the Gram-negative bacterial outer membrane, which usually acts as a natural protective barrier preventing the passage of unfavourable compounds [15].

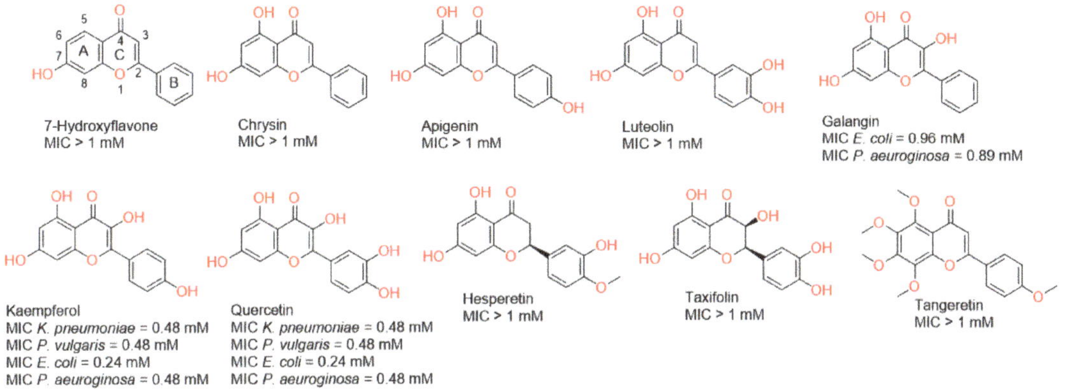

Figure 1. Structures of the tested flavonoids in the present study along with the antibacterial activity of each one against a number of Gram-negative bacteria.

In the present study, all the flavonoids that showed growth inhibitory activity against the tested bacteria (MIC < 1 mM) shared the presence of a hydroxyl group at C-3. Additionally, the hydroxylation at Ring B correlated with enhanced activity (Figure 1). These observations indicated the most important structural elements in the scaffold of this class of compounds may develop more potent antibacterial derivatives in the future.

Our strategy in this investigation was to enhance the antibacterial activity of this class of natural products against Gram-negative bacteria via conjugating them to gold nanoparticles (GNPs). Hence, these bioactive molecules can benefit from the unique properties of the metallic nanoparticles (MNPs): (i) MNPs could act as a very good carrier for these bioactive flavonoids and could easily pass the bacterial outer membrane [16–18]; (ii) MNPs have the ability to concentrate bioactive molecules on their surfaces and hence maximize their activity (i.e., polyvalent effects) [19–23].

Accordingly, we chose the most active flavonoids (i.e., kaempferol and quercetin) against all tested Gram-negative bacteria together with chrysin, which was the most active flavonoid against the Gram-positive bacteria *S. aureus* [14], to be coated on GNPs, and subsequently tested if the new nano-conjugates could exert enhanced growth inhibitory activity towards Gram-negative bacteria. In parallel, we aimed to perform a number of in silico experiments (docking, molecular dynamic simulations, and free energy calculations) to explain the mode of conjugation of these flavonoids and their probable antibacterial mode of actions.

2.2. Gold Nanoparticle Preparation and Conjugation with Flavonoids

Gold nanoparticles (GNPs) were prepared via chemical synthesis using reduced L-glutathione (GSH). The synthesis process was mediated by the formation of a covalent bond between the gold nanoparticles' surfaces in the $HAuCl_4.3H_2O$ compound and the cysteine thiolate of GSH. This binding led to the aggregation of GNPs on GSH molecules and, by the addition of $NaBH_4$ at pH8, the formation of a ruby red colour indicated the formation of GNPs (Figure 2). GSH is a hydrophilic tripeptide, and thus coating GNPs with such molecules makes them more stable and more water-soluble. Additionally, the GSH's carboxylate terminals are a good binder for a variety of molecules, including flavonoids, where they are able to form extensive H-bond networks with such polyhydroxylated molecules, making them a very good carrier of such bioactive chemicals. Being a natural substrate for bacteria, GSH may facilitate the entry of the whole conjugate (i.e., GSH-GNPs) inside bacterial cells [24,25].

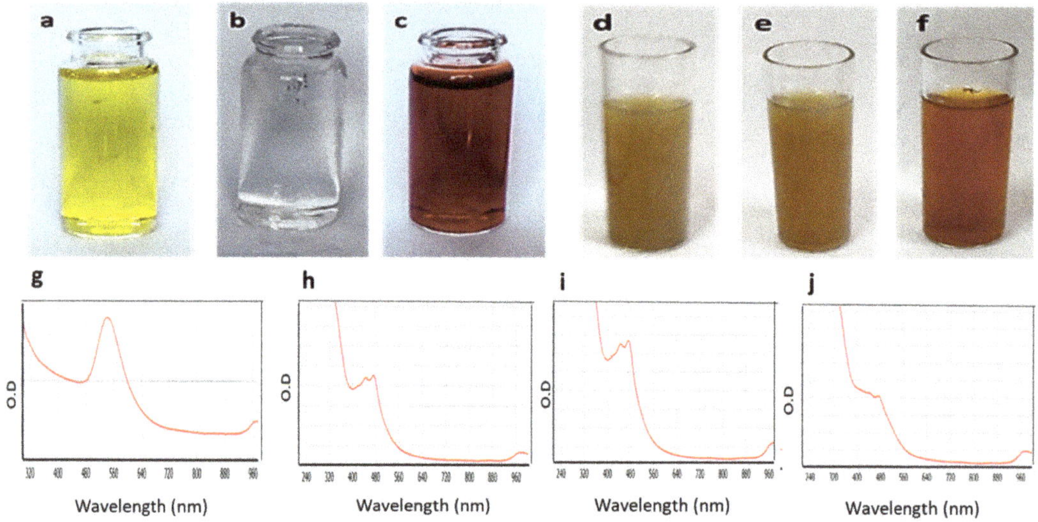

Figure 2. The upper panel shows the gold nanoparticles' preparation steps: (**a**) $HAuCl_4{\cdot}3H_2O$ only, (**b**) $HAuCl_4{\cdot}3H_2O$ + GSH at pH 8, (**c**) formation of gold after the addition of $NaBH_4$, and formation of gold nano-conjugates, (**d**) GNP-kaempferol, (**e**) GNP-chrysin, and (**f**) GNP-quercetin. The lower panels show (**g**) the UV-VIS spectra of the GNPs, (**h**) the UV-VIS spectra of GNP-kaempferol, (**i**) the UV-VIS spectra of GNP-chrysin, and (**j**) the UV-VIS spectra of GNP-quercetin.

Accordingly, the freshly prepared GSH-GNPs were incubated with each selected flavonoid to allow their binding with the GSH's carboxylate groups; in turn, they became coated on the GSH-coated GNPs. The efficiency of conjugation of each flavonoid (in %) was found to be 80%, 71%, and 41% for quercetin, kaempferol, and chrysin, respectively. These results indicated that the degree of a flavonoid's hydroxylation correlates well to its binding efficiency with the prepared GSH-coated GNPs.

2.3. UV-Vis Spectroscopy

To ensure that the GNPs were formed and successfully conjugated to each selected flavonoid, the UV-visible absorbance of the prepared GSH-GNPs and those coated with flavonoids was measured. As shown in Figure 2 (lower panel), the absorption spectrum of the free GNPs showed a λ_{max} at ~540 nm. Such UV absorbance was due to the surface plasmon excitation of the very small GNPs. The flavonoid-coated GNPs showed a considerable shift in their λ_{max} (~480 nm) in comparison with the uncoated ones (~530 nm), indicating successful coating of the flavonoids on the GNPs and, in turn, altering the plasmon resonance absorption band characteristic of GNPs.

2.4. Fourier Transform Infrared Spectroscopy Analysis (FTIR)

Fourier transform infrared spectroscopy (FTIR) is an essential technique to detect different functional groups via measuring the infrared spectra of emission, absorption, and photoconductivity of the materials. The FTIR spectrum is usually between 4000 and 400 cm^{-1}. Supplementary Figure S1a–d presents the FTIR spectra of the GNPs, GNP-kaempferol, GNP-chrysin, and GNP-quercetin. The FTIR spectra of the prepared GNPs display the presence of the OH group at 3367.70 cm^{-1}, which indicates the presence of alcohol. The C=O was measured at 1577.50 cm^{-1}, while the band at 13.8732 cm^{-1} refers to C-C-C stretching. The C-O group appeared at a wavelength of 1279.66 to 1069.89 cm^{-1}. These results were in good agreement with those of Jiang et al. (2007) and Sulaiman et al. (2020) [25,26]. The peaks that appeared after the conjugation of GNPs with kaempferol, chrysin, and quercetin were different in their intensities and shapes, and this might be attributed to the reactions that occurred between each flavonoid and the GNP-GSH. In general, a change in the band absorption intensities means that a physical change has occurred, while an increase in the band intensities means a change in the morphology and chemical composition of that band. The FTIR spectra for flavonoid-coated GNPs showed that the hydroxyl group (O-H) stretching vibration appears at 3399.10, 3402.80, and 3346.14, respectively, while the bands appearing at 2841.57, 2844.74, and 2834.72 cm^{-1} reflected the alkane (C-H) stretching vibration. Additionally, the carbonyl (C=O) stretch vibration was displayed at 1663.90, 1663.77, and 1582.04 cm^{-1}. The aromatic (C=C) stretch bands were observed at 1521.42, 1521.42, and 1416.94 cm^{-1}, respectively. The aromatic C-O stretch was observed at bands 1381.27 to 1131.00 cm^{-1}. All the peaks characterizing flavonoids were observed. These results were in good agreement with those of Kiroula et al. (2016) and Sulaiman et al. (2020) [26,27].

2.5. X-ray Powder Diffraction (XRD)

One of the most important techniques used to study structural properties is X-ray powder diffraction (XRD). The diffraction pattern of the prepared GNPs and GNP-coated flavonoids (i.e., GNP-quercetin, GNP-chrysin, and GNP-quercetin) were analysed. As depicted in Figure 3a–d, the most important characteristic peaks of the Au phase appeared at 38.10°, 44.5°, 64.06° and 77.45°, accredited to the crystallographic planes (111), (200), (220), and (311), respectively. Additionally, the intensity of GSH appeared at 31.53°. Whereas, in flavonoid-coated GNPs (Figure 3), they displayed characteristic peaks for quercetin, kaempferol, and chrysin at 23°, 38°, 44°, 64°, and 77°.

2.6. Electron Microscopy

The particle size and morphology of the prepared GNPs, GNP-kaempferol, GNP-chrysin, and GNP-quercetin were determined via transmission electron microscopy (TEM) (Figure 4a–d) and field emission scanning electron microscopy (FESEM) (Figure 4e–h). The average particle size of the GNPs is about ~4.10 ± 2 to 35 ± 2 nm with monodisperse spherical and hexagonal prism-like shapes (Figure 4a). The TEM and FESEM micrographs of GNP-kaempferol, GNP-chrysin, and GNP-quercetin showed spherical and homogenous structures (Figure 4b–d,f–h).

2.7. Energy Dispersive X-ray Spectroscopy (EDX)

To measure the elemental composition of the prepared GNPs, GNP-kaempferol, GNP-chrysin, and GNP-quercetin, the samples were tested using EDX. The EDX of the GNPs confirmed the presence of Au with different percentages in each sample up to 24.71% in GNP-quercetin (Figure 4i), with the presence of carbon and oxygen in sufficient percentages to confirm the loading of kaempferol, chrysin, and quercetin on GNPs.

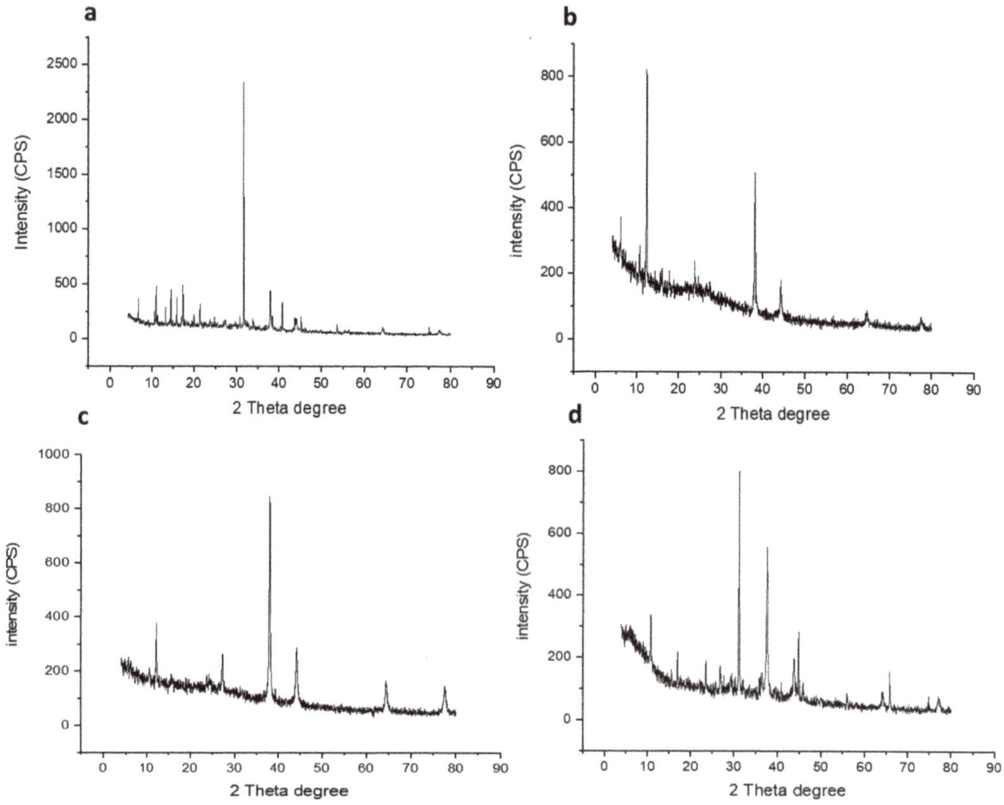

Figure 3. X-ray diffraction analyses for (**a**) prepared GNPs, (**b**) GNP-kaempferol, (**c**) GNP-chrysin, and (**d**) GNP-quercetin.

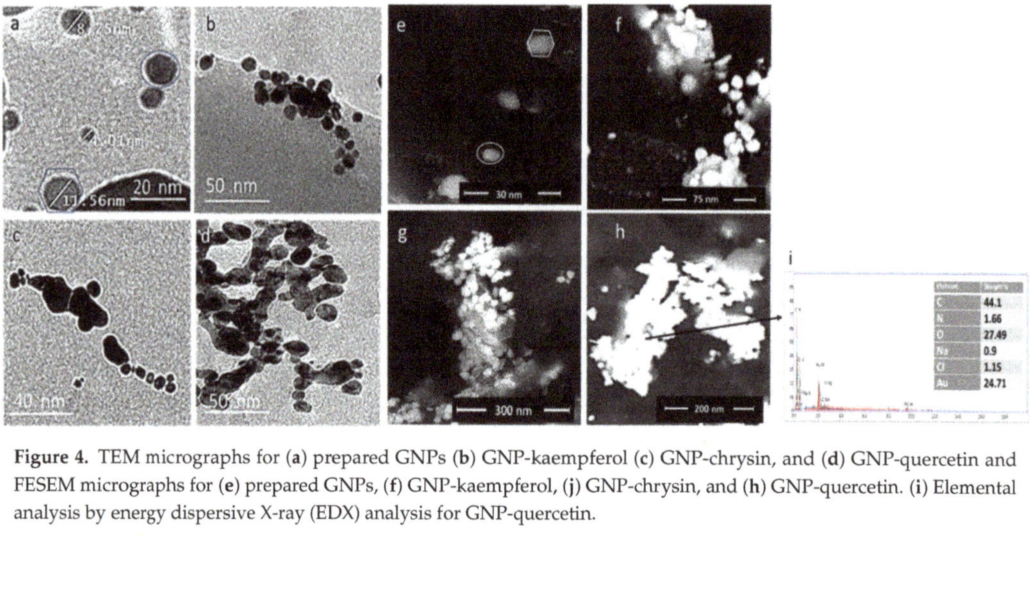

Figure 4. TEM micrographs for (**a**) prepared GNPs (**b**) GNP-kaempferol (**c**) GNP-chrysin, and (**d**) GNP-quercetin and FESEM micrographs for (**e**) prepared GNPs, (**f**) GNP-kaempferol, (**j**) GNP-chrysin, and (**h**) GNP-quercetin. (**i**) Elemental analysis by energy dispersive X-ray (EDX) analysis for GNP-quercetin.

2.8. *In Vitro Investigation*

2.8.1. In Vitro Antibacterial Activity

The antibacterial activity of the GNP conjugates was measured against a panel of clinical isolates comprising Gram-negative bacteria (*E. coli, P. aeruginosa, K. pneumonia* and *P. vulgaris*). The minimum inhibitory concentrations (MIC) were determined by the micro-dilution method using 96-well plates. The MIC results showed that the activity of the tested GNPs (GNP-kaempferol, GNP-chrysin, and GNP-quercetin) was quite diverse. The results showed that GNP-quercetin was generally the most active against all tested Gram-negative bacteria, with pronounced activity against *E. coli, P. aeruginosa* and *P. vulgaris* (MIC = 30 μg/mL) and *K. pneumonia* (MIC = 60 μg/mL). On the other hand, the prepared GNP-kaempferol exhibited good antibacterial properties against *E. coli* and *P. vulgaris* with MICs of 60 and 30 μg/mL, respectively, while it displayed weak activity against *P. aeruginosa* (MIC = 240 μg/mL) and *K. pneumonia* (MIC = 120 μg/mL). The GNP-chrysin showed good inhibitory activity against *E. coli* (MIC = 60 μg/mL) and weak activity against the rest of the tested microbes (MIC > 240 μg/mL). Ciprofloxacin was used as a positive control.

2.8.2. GNP-Induced Disruption of Bacterial Cell Membranes

To explore the antibacterial mechanism of these GNPs, the GNP-quercetin conjugate was selected, since it showed the best antibacterial activities (Table 1). After treating suspensions of *E. coli* or *P. aeruginosa* (5.0 × 105 cfu mL^{-1}) with GNP-quercetin conjugate at a final concentration of 20 μg mL^{-1}, incubated at 37 °C overnight, the antibiotic effect of the GNP-quercetin conjugate on the membrane morphology and nucleic acid leakage of *E. coli* and *P. aeruginosa* was visualized using transmission electron microscopy (TEM). The TEM micrograph clearly displayed the broken membranes of the treated *E. coli* and *P. aeruginosa* (Figure 5a–c) with the clear appearance of GNP-quercetin inside the bacterial cell. Figure 5b,d presents the two bacterial strains without treatment. Free uncoated GSH-GNPs, in contrast, were not able to have similar effects on *E. coli*, in which the membrane integrity remained intact and no particles were seen inside the bacterial cells.

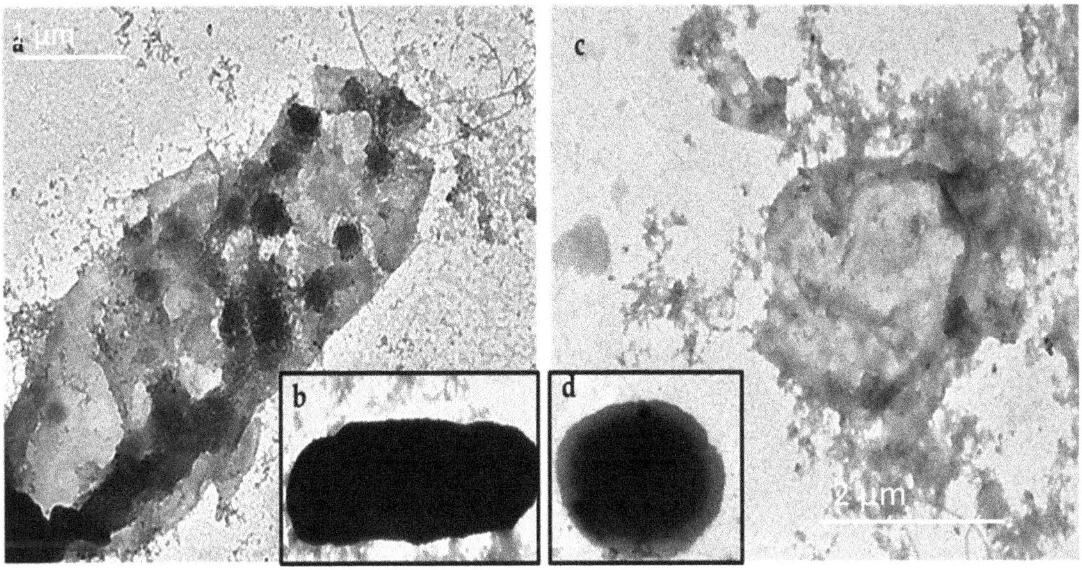

Figure 5. (**a**) *E. coli* + GNP-quercetin, (**b**) *E. coli* without treatment, (**c**) *P. aeruginosa* + GNP-quercetin, and (**d**) *P. aeruginosa* without treatment.

Table 1. Antibacterial activity of the gold nano-conjugates against Gram-negative bacteria.

Tested Compound	MIC (μg/mL)			
	E. coli	*P. aeruginosa*	*K. pneumonia*	*P. vulgaris*
Free GNPs	120	240	120	120
GNP-quercetin	30	30	60	30
GNP-kaempferol	60	240	120	30
GNP-chrysin	60	>240	>240	>240
Cip	1	1	1	2

Cip: ciprofloxacin. MIC values were the same in three independent experiments.

2.8.3. In Vitro DNA Gyrase-B Inhibition

Quercetin, kaempferol, and chrysin have been reported to produce negative supercoiling of the bacterial DNA via the inhibition of DNA gyrase [13]. However, the exact mode of action of these molecules is still elusive. DNA gyrase consists of two subunits: subunit A and B (Gyr-A and -B, respectively). Gyr-A is the subunit that binds to DNA and relaxes its positive supercoils. Additionally, it is targeted by fluoroquinolone antibiotics [28]. On the other hand, Gyr-B is responsible for obtaining the required energy of this process via hydrolysing one molecule of ATP [14].

Upon docking these flavonoids (i.e., quercetin, kaempferol, and chrysin) against the binding site of each subunit (Gyr-A and B), they achieved significantly higher docking scores with Gyr-B (−9.5, −9.5, −9.3 kcal/mol, respectively) than with Gyr-A (−5.1, −4.9, and −5.2, respectively). Accordingly, we tested these flavonoids for their Gyr-B inhibitory activity. As shown in Figure 6, the three flavonoids produced micromolar inhibition of Gyr-B's activity. Quercetin was the most potent inhibitor, with an IC_{50} value of 0.89 ± 0.1 μM, while chrysin was the least potent (IC_{50} = 3.91 ± 0.2 μM), where the flavonoids' degree of hydroxylation apparently correlated to their Gyr-B inhibitory activity.

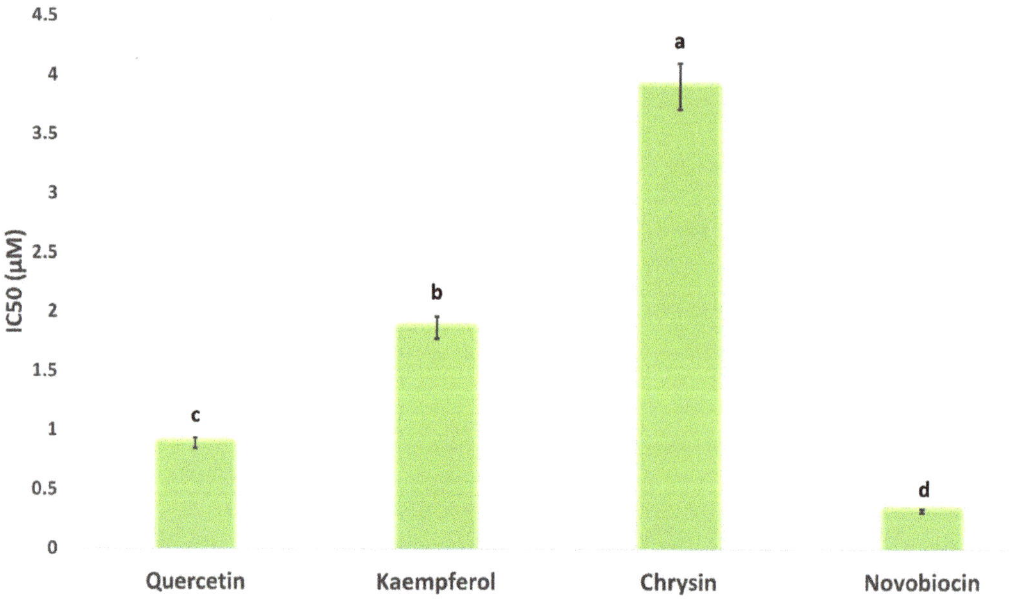

Figure 6. Gyr-B inhibitory activity of quercetin, kaempferol, and chrysin expressed as IC_{50}. Bars represent standard errors. Different letters indicate significant differences from repeated-experiments (n = 3) ANOVA (Hotelling's T^2, $p < 0.05$).

2.9. In Silico Investigation

To gain more insight into the antibacterial mode of action of these flavonoids, we carried out a number of in silico experiments (e.g., docking, molecular dynamic simulations (MDS), and binding free energy calculations).

First, we aimed to study the interaction between each flavonoid and the GSH interface of 5 nm GNP. To do so, we constructed a model consisting of GNP (5 nm) linked to three GSH molecules via covalent bonds between their SH groups and three Au atoms at the surface (Figure 7). Subsequently, we docked each flavonoid against this constructed GSH coating. As shown in Figure 7, the three flavonoids took almost the same orientation between the three GSH molecules, establishing a network of H-bonds between their OH groups and a number of polar moieties in the GSH molecules (e.g., their carboxylate and amide groups) (Figure 7). During the course of MDS (50 ns), these extensive H-bonds kept the binding orientations of both quercetin and kaempferol almost unchanged (RMSD~2.1 Å and 3.8 Å, respectively), while chrysin was far less stable (RMSD~10.3 Å). These binding behaviours appeared to be linked to the Ring B hydroxyl groups that were involved in multiple H-bonds with GSH's carboxylate arms during the course of MDS. Accordingly, the two flavonoids with a hydroxyl group or groups at Ring B were more stable in their interactions with GSH in comparison with chrysin, which had no hydroxyl groups at Ring B. The results of MDS were in good accordance with those of the percent efficiency of conjugation, where the flavonoids with the highest stability with GNP-coated GSH (quercetin and kaempferol) were found to achieve the highest binding efficiency (80% and 71%, respectively), while chrysin, which was significantly less stable, achieved less binding efficiency (41%).

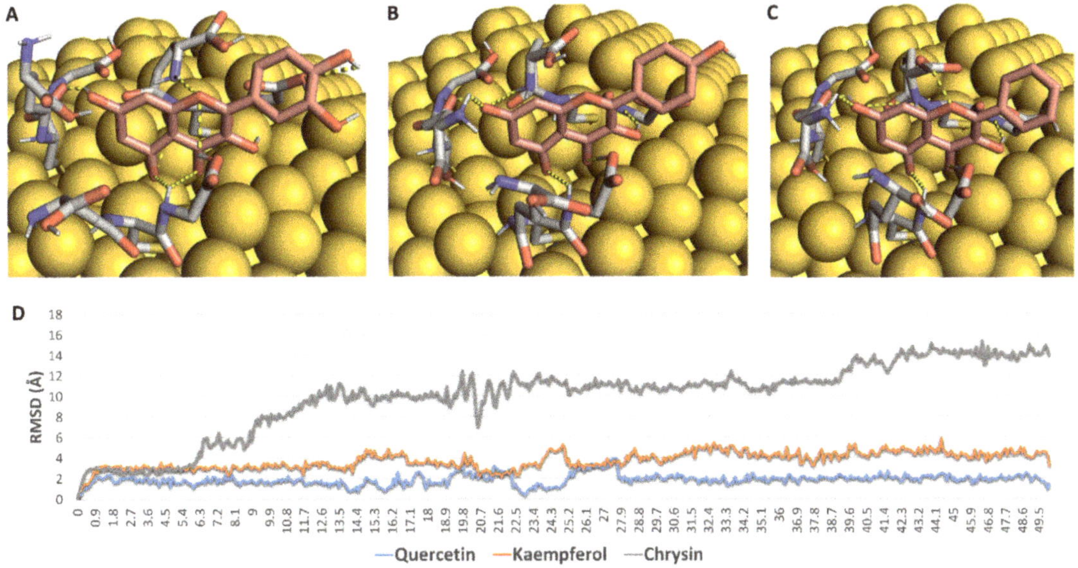

Figure 7. (**A–C**): Binding mode of quercetin, kaempferol, and chrysin with GSH molecules covalently linked to gold molecules on the surface of GNP. (**D**): RMSDs of these flavonoids during the course of 50 ns MDS.

Second, we aimed to study the effect of each flavonoid on the bacterial outer membrane (OM). Previously, it was found that this class of natural products (i.e., flavonoids) exert their antibacterial activity against *E. coli* via increasing the rigidity of its outer membrane (OM) [12,29]. In this study, we found a very good correlation between the growth inhibitory activity of these flavonoids and their effect on the rigidity of a membrane model composed of dipalmitoylphosphatidylcholine (DPPC) and 1,2-dipalmitoyl-sn-glycero-3-

phosphoglycerol (DPPG) (used as a representative of the bacterial membrane), where the increase in this membrane's rigidity was accompanied by increased antibacterial activity.

To study this effect at a molecular level, we performed a number of MDS experiments on lipid bilayer systems consisting of DPPC and DPPG (1:1) with two molecules of each flavonoid inserted inside the core of the lipid bilayer (Figure 8). When each flavonoid was added to the simulations, they spontaneously directed to the head–tail interface, where they partitioned themselves and stayed stable until the end of the simulations. Additionally, each flavonoid molecule attracted a number of water molecules thanks to their hydroxyl groups; hence, the water density at the hydrophilic–hydrophobic interface increased (Figure 8). This increase in water molecules at the head–tail interface was proportional to the degree of hydroxylation, and thus quercetin and kaempferol attracted the highest number of water molecules (~4 molecules), while chrysin attracted the fewest.

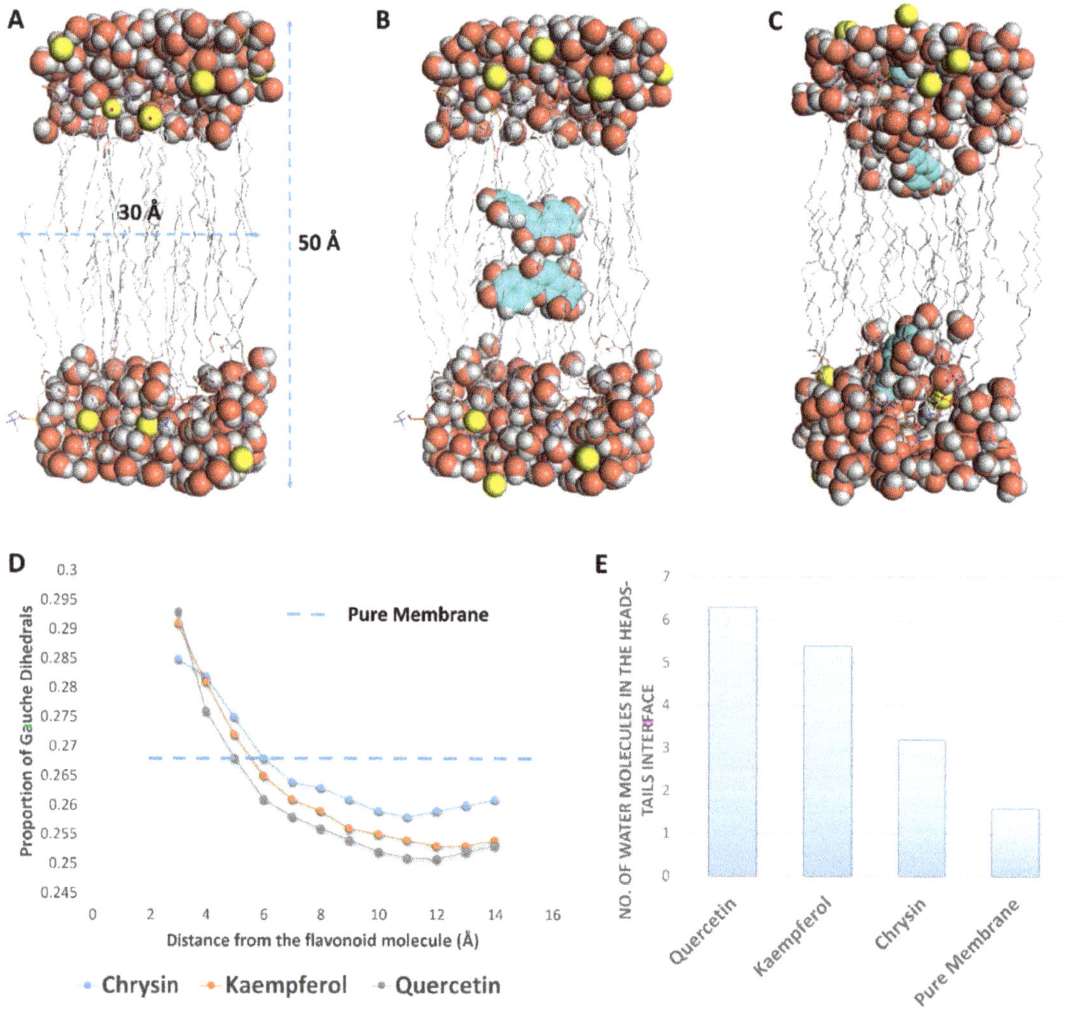

Figure 8. (**A**) The lipid bilayer system used for the MDS. (**B**) The lipid bilayer system with two molecules of quercetin at the beginning of a 100 ns MDS. (**C**) The lipid bilayer system at the end of 100 ns of MDS, where each quercetin molecule was stabilized at the head–tail interface. (**D**) Proportion of gauche dihedrals on lipid tail carbon atoms as a function of the lipid's distance from each flavonoid molecule. (**E**) Number of water molecules per lipid molecule at the head–tail interface.

Hydrated membranes are usually more fluid than less hydrated ones and have higher numbers of gauche defects (distortion in the lipid alkyl chains) [30–32]. Accordingly, polyhydroxylated flavonoids (e.g., quercetin) were able to draw water from the surrounding environment at the hydrophilic–hydrophobic interface, producing a local increase in the water density and, in turn, a local increase in the membrane's fluidity (a high proportion of gauche defects). At the same time, this effect led eventually to a dehydrated membrane with much less fluidity (i.e., increased rigidity) and a low proportion of gauche defects. Quercetin produced the highest proportion of local gauche defects (0.293 at 3 Å from quercetin) but, at the same time, drew the largest number of water molecules (~6 molecules), producing the highest dehydration effect and the lowest proportion of gauche defects (~0.245 at 6 to 10 Å away from quercetin). The proportion of gauche defects in the lipid bilayer without flavonoids was ~0.268, while this proportion, in general, was significantly lower in the presence of each flavonoid (Figure 8). These results were in very good accordance with that reported for caffeine, which was found to increase the rigidity of 1-palmitoyl-2-oleoyl-sn-glycero-3-phosphocholin (POPC) membranes via the same mechanism [32]. Being able to concentrate flavonoids on their surfaces, our prepared GNPs in this study had the ability to significantly increase the effect of each flavonoid on the bacterial OM (i.e., polyvalent effects) and hence maximize their antibacterial potential.

Third, we studied the binding mode of each flavonoid inside the active site of *E. coli*'s Gyr-B to rationalize their inhibitory effects. Quercetin, kaempferol, and chrysin achieved convergent docking scores with Gyr-B's active site (−9.5, −9.5, and −9.3 kcal/mol). Additionally, they took an orientation and exhibited molecular interactions inside the active site that were very close to that of the co-crystalized inhibitor (Figure 9). Being rich in hydroxyl groups, quercetin was able to establish a network of H-bonds with ASP-73, GLY-77, GLY-101, LYS-103, ARG-136, and THR-165. Furthermore, it established a number of hydrophobic interactions with ILE-78, PRO-79, and ILE-94. Both kaempferol and chrysin exhibited the same interactions, except for the H-bond with ARG-136. To further validate these docking results, all of these binding poses were subjected to 50 ns MDS. Both quercetin and kaempferol were able to keep their binding orientation with low deviations (RMSD~1.5 Å), while chrysin deviated more from its docking pose, with an average RMSD of 4.4 Å. The three flavonoids achieved almost identical binding free energies (ΔGs) (i.e., −8.5, −8.5, and −8.2 kcal/mol). All of these in silico analyses explained the low micromolar inhibition of the three flavonoids against *E. coli*'s Gyr-B. The present in vitro and in silico results correlated well with those of Wu and co-workers on flavonoids against DNA gyrase [13].

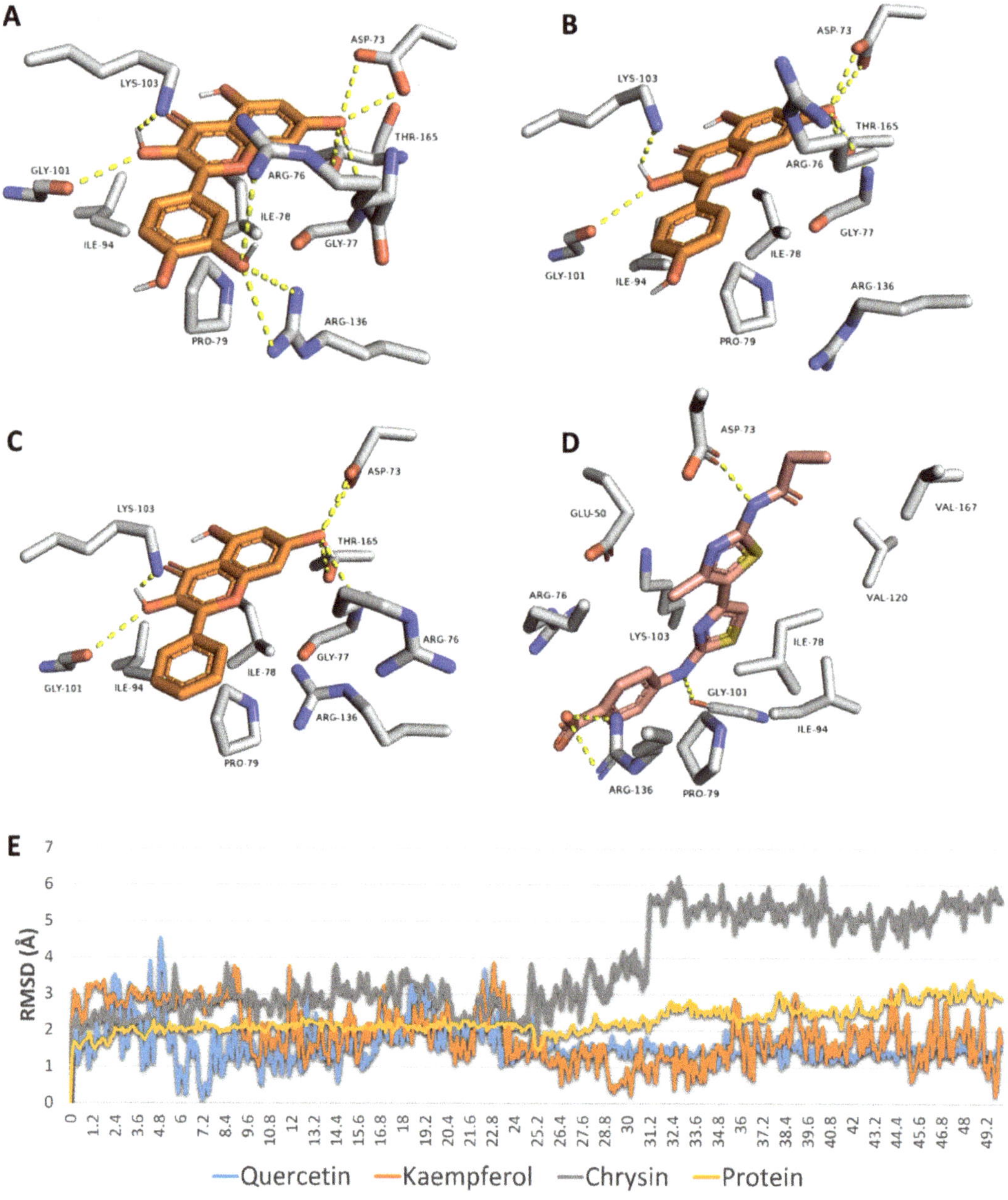

Figure 9. Docking poses of quercetin, kaempferol, and chrysin inside the active site of *E. coli*'s Gyr-B (**A–C**, respectively) alongside the binding pose of the co-crystalized inhibitor (**D**). RMSDs of quercetin, kaempferol, and chrysin inside the active site of *E. coli*'s Gyr-B during 50 ns of MDS (**E**).

3. Materials and Methods

3.1. Chemicals

$HAuCl_4 \cdot 3H_2O$ and reduced L-glutathione (GSH) were purchased from Sigma-Aldrich Chemical Co. (St. Louis, MO, USA), lysogeny broth (LB broth) and (NaOH) were purchased from Merck (Mainz, Germany), while sodium borohydride from Strem Chemicals, Inc. (Newburyport, MA, USA). All other chemicals and reagents were of analytical grade. Regarding the flavonoids used in this study, all of them were isolated from their plant sources [14], except for quercetin, apigenin, and hesperetin, which were purchased from Alfa Aesar, Massachusetts, USA, and Sigma-Aldrich, Saint Louis, USA. All of these flavonoids were of acceptable purity (i.e., >98%).

3.2. Microorganisms

Pseudomonas aeruginosa ATCC10145, *Escherichia coli* ATCC25955, *Proteus vulgaris* ATTC7829, and *Klebsiella pneumonia* ATCCBAA-1705 were obtained from the Faculty of Medicine, Al-Azhar University, Egypt.

3.3. Gold Nanoparticle Preparation

Gold nanoparticles were prepared as described by Wu et al. (2014) and Sulaiman et al. (2020) [26,33], 5 mL of a tetrachloroauric acid aqueous solution (0.025 M) was added to 50 mL of 0.019 M of a reduced L-glutathione (GSH) aqueous solution, and the mixture was vigorously stirred for 30 min. The pH of the mixture was adjusted to 8 using NaOH (0.1 M). To this mixture, freshly prepared aqueous $NaBH_4$ (2 mg·mL^{-1}) was added dropwise under vigorous stirring until the formation of a ruby red colour. To remove the excess GSH and other salts, the GNPs were centrifuged for 3 h at 5000 rpm. After the centrifugation, the supernatant was removed and the gold nanoparticles were dispersed in double-distilled water; the centrifugation was repeated 2 times to obtain clean GNPs that were kept in the dark at 4 °C for 14 days (aggregations were detected after 17 days of storage). Freshly prepared nanoparticles were then conjugated with the flavonoids (i.e., kaempferol, chrysin, and quercetin).

3.4. Conjugation of Kaempferol, Chrysin, and Quercetin with Gold Nanoparticles

Conjugation of kaempferol, chrysin, and quercetin with the prepared GNPs was carried out according to [26]. Here, 1 mL of the prepared GNPs (3.5×10^{13}; GNPs/mL) was mixed with 1 mL of the flavonoid solution (i.e., kaempferol, chrysin, or quercetin) (500 µg mL^{-1}) and stirred overnight at room temperature. After preparation, the conjugates (GNP-kaempferol, GNP-chrysin, and GNP-quercetin) were centrifuged for 1 h at 10,000 rpm to remove any excess of the drug.

The freshly conjugated nanoparticles were used for the antibacterial assay immediately after their preparation. They were also kept in the dark at 0 °C. These conjugated nanoparticles can be used after storage for 10 days (they produced the same results in the antibacterial assay and no aggregation was observed up to 10 days of storage).

3.5. Characterization of Prepared Nanoparticles

3.5.1. UV-Vis Spectroscopy Measurements

The synthesis of GNPs was primarily visualized through the change in colour. The conversion of Au^{3+} to Au^0 was monitored by measuring the UV-vis spectra within wavelengths ranging from 220 nm to 1000 nm in the mixture over time. The UV-vis spectra of the solutions were measured in 96-well flat polystyrene plates by using a SPECTROstar nano absorbance plate reader (BMG LABTECH).

3.5.2. X-ray Diffraction (XRD) Studies

To study the X-ray diffraction pattern of the prepared GNPs and flavonoid–GNPs conjugates, samples were drop-coated onto a glass material. The XRD analysis was performed using a PANalytical X'pert PRO X-ray diffractometer (The Netherlands) with Cu Ka1 radiation under an operating voltage and tubing current of about 40 kV and 30 mA, respectively. The diffracted patterns were recorded at 2θ from 10° to 80° at the scanning speed of 0.02°/min.

3.5.3. Fourier-Transform Infrared Spectroscopy (FTIR)

The ATR-FTIR spectra of GNPs and flavonoid–GNPs conjugates were carried out using a Broker vertex 80 v in the range of 4000–400 cm^{-1} with a resolution of 4 cm^{-1}, according to Brock-Neely (1957).

3.5.4. Transmission Electron Microscopy Analysis (TEM)

Transmission electron microscopy (TEM) was used to measure the size and obtain the morphology of the prepared GNPs and flavonoid–GNPs conjugates. Preparation of the samples was carried out by placing 2–4 μL of the prepared solution on carbon-coated copper grids. The thin film that formed was air-dried at room temperature and observed using a Philips 10 Technai with an accelerating voltage of about 180 keV with a wavelength (λ) of 0.0251 Å. The average size of the prepared nanoparticles was measured using Image J software.

3.5.5. Scanning Electron Microscope (SEM)

Scanning electron microscopy (SEM) was carried out using a field emission scanning electron microscope (FE-SEM) (Quanta FEG-250, Netherlands) with the acceleration voltage at 20 kV, attached to EDX (energy dispersive x-ray analysis) to perform the elemental analysis.

3.6. Determination of the Antimicrobial Activity of Flavonoids, GNPs, and Flavonoid–GNPs Conjugates

The antibacterial activity of the flavonoids (Figure 1), the prepared GNPs and the flavonoid–GNPs conjugates was acquired against four Gram-negative bacteria: *Escherichia coli* ATCC25955, *Pseudomonas aeruginosa* ATCC10145, *Proteus vulgaris* ATTC7829, and *Klebsiella pneumonia* ATCCBAA-1705. The minimal inhibitory concentration was assessed in 96-well flat polystyrene plates by addition of 80 μL of lysogeny broth (LB broth) in each well, followed by the addition of 10 μL of a bacterial culture suspension (log phase), then 10 μL of the test material (the flavonoids, the prepared GNPs, or the flavonoid–GNPs) was added. The final concentrations of the mixture were 960, 480, 240, 120, 60, 30, 15, 7.5, 3.25, 1.62 and 0.81 μg/mL. The plates were incubated at 37 °C for 24 h. After incubation, the positive antibacterial activity of the flavonoids, the prepared GNPs, and the flavonoid–GNPs was observed as clearance in the wells, which was confirmed by measuring the absorbance after about 20 h at OD_{600} in a Spectrostar Nano Microplate Reader (BMG LABTECH GmbH, Allmendgrun, Germany). The MIC experiments were carried out three times and gave the same results each time. Ciprofloxacin was used as a positive control.

3.7. In Vitro Enzyme Assay

Gyrase subunit B (Gyr-B) in vitro inhibitory activity was carried out using the Inspiralis assay kit (Inspiralis, UK) according to previous protocols [34,35]. The procedure of this in vitro assay is described in detail in Supplementary File 1.

3.8. In Silico Investigation

3.8.1. Molecular Docking

Before the docking experiments the gold–GSH model was prepared. First, we used the online nanomaterial modeller software Charm GUI (https://charmm-gui.org/?doc=input/nanomaterial, accessed on 20 June 2021) [36] to construct a 6 nm spherical gold nanoparticle model. Subsequently, we linked three molecules of glutathione (GSH) to three surface gold atoms via covalent bonds (i.e., between the SH group of GSH and the gold atom). We kept a distance of 7 Å between each GSH molecule to avoid steric clashes between them, particularly during molecular dynamic simulations. After that, we enclosed the three GSH molecules in a grid box for docking experiments using the Auto Dock tools 1.5.4 program [37]. Chrysin, kaempferol, and quercetin were docked on this predetermined grid box using AutoDock 4 software [37]. The top scores were then selected and visualized using Pymol software [38].

3.8.2. Molecular Dynamic Simulations

All molecular dynamics experiments were carried out by Desmond v. 2.2 and NAMD software [39,40] using OPLS and Charmm27 force fields, respectively. Further experimental details can be found in the Supplemenatry Table S1.

3.9. Statistical Analysis

Three independent experiments were carried out to provide the results in the present investigation, expressed as the means ± SE (n = 3). Statistical significance was determined by ANOVA ($p < 0.05$).

4. Conclusions

Free uncoated GNPs exhibited moderate antibacterial properties, while flavonoids exhibited weak inhibitory activity against Gram-negative bacteria. The outer membrane may be the shield of Gram-negative bacteria against this type of natural product because several flavonoids have previously shown very good potential against Gram-positive strains. Concentrating flavonoids on the surface of GNPs could maximize their inhibitory potential against Gram-negative bacteria. Accordingly, we formulated novel flavonoid-coated gold nano-conjugates to detect their antibacterial properties. We used GSH as a linker between the surface of GNPs and the flavonoids. To select the best flavonoids to be coated on the surface of GSH-GNPs, we screened a number of flavonoid derivatives against four common pathogenic Gram-negative bacteria. Quercetin, kaempferol, and chrysin were found to be the most active candidates; however, their activity was expressed in the millimolar range. Coating GSH-GNPs with these flavonoids led to the preparation of efficient growth-inhibitory nano-conjugates against Gram-negative bacteria. Quercetin-coated gold nano-conjugate was the most potent one and was able to penetrate the cell wall of *E. coli*. These nano-conjugates were able to fight Gram-negative bacteria via two proposed mechanisms: (i) increasing the bacterial membrane's rigidity, hence decreasing its functionality; and (ii) targeting the bacterial subunit B of DNA gyrase (Gyr-B). By conducting a series of in silico and in vitro experiments, we found that quercetin was the best flavonoid in terms of its binding efficiency to the GSH-GNPs, increasing the membrane rigidity and inhibiting Gyr-B. In conclusion, flavonoid-coated GNPs are considered to be promising antibiotic candidates for further development and evaluation.

Supplementary Materials: The following are available online at https://www.mdpi.com/article/10.3390/antibiotics10080968/s1. Figure S1: Fourier-transform infrared spectroscopy for (a) prepared GNPs, (b) GNP-kaempferol, (c) GNP-chrysin, and (d) GNP-quercetin. Table S1: MIC absorbance data. File 1: In Vitro Enzyme Assay.

Author Contributions: Conceptualization, A.M.S., A.A.H., H.M.H. and M.E.R.; methodology, A.A.H., H.A.A. and A.M.S.; software, A.M.S.; validation, H.A.A., R.O., N.M.G. and M.M.G.; formal analysis, H.A.A. and A.S.I.H.; resources, H.A.A., N.M.G. and M.M.G..; writing—original draft preparation, A.A.H. and A.M.S.; writing—review and editing, all the authors; funding acquisition, H.A.A., N.M.G. and M.M.G. All authors have read and agreed to the published version of the manuscript.

Funding: This research received no external funding.

Data Availability Statement: All relevant data are contained within the article.

Acknowledgments: The authors would like to thank AlMaarefa University for their financial support.

Conflicts of Interest: The authors declare no conflict of interest.

References

1. Patra, J.K.; Das, G.; Fraceto, L.F.; Campos, E.V.R.; del Pilar Rodriguez-Torres, M.; Acosta-Torres, L.S.; Diaz-Torres, L.A.; Grillo, R.; Swamy, M.K.; Sharma, S.; et al. Nano based drug delivery systems: Recent developments and future prospects. *J. Nanobiotechnol.* **2018**, *16*, 71. [CrossRef] [PubMed]
2. Tiwari, G.; Tiwari, R.; Sriwastawa, B.; Bhati, L.; Pandey, S.; Pandey, P.; Bannerjee, S.K. Drug delivery systems: An updated review. *Int. J. Pharm. Investig.* **2012**, *2*, 2–11. [CrossRef]
3. Ditta, A.; Arshad, M. Applications and perspectives of using nanomaterials for sustainable plant nutrition. *Nanotechnol. Rev.* **2016**, *5*, 209–229. [CrossRef]
4. Ditta, A. How helpful is nanotechnology in agriculture? *Adv. Nat. Sci. Nanosci. Nanotechnol.* **2012**, *3*, 033002. [CrossRef]
5. Arayne, M.S.; Sultana, N.; Qureshi, F. Nanoparticles in delivery of cardiovascular drugs. *Pak. J. Pharm. Sci.* **2007**, *20*, 340–348.
6. Patra, J.K.; Baek, K.-H. Green nanobiotechnology: Factors affecting synthesis and characterization techniques. *J. Nanomater.* **2014**, *2014*, 219. [CrossRef]
7. Joseph, R.R.; Venkatraman, S.S. Drug delivery to the eye: What benefits do nanocarriers offer? *Nanomedicine* **2017**, *12*, 683–702. [CrossRef]
8. Lam, P.-L.; Wong, W.-Y.; Bian, Z.; Chui, C.-H.; Gambari, R. Recent advances in green nanoparticulate systems for drug delivery: Efficient delivery and safety concern. *Nanomedicine* **2017**, *12*, 357–385. [CrossRef] [PubMed]
9. Abdelaziz, M.S.; Hamed, A.A.; Radwan, A.A.; Khaled, E.; Hassan, R.Y.A. Biosynthesis and Bio-sensing Applications of Silver and Gold Metal Nanoparticles. *Egypt. J. Chem.* **2021**, *64*, 1057–1063.
10. El-Bendary, M.A.; Abdelraof, M.; Moharam, M.E.; Elmahdy, E.M.; Allam, M.A. Potential of silver nanoparticles synthesized using low active mosquitocidal Lysinibacillus sphaericus as novel antimicrobial agents. *Prep. Biochem. Biotechnol.* **2021**, 1–10. [CrossRef] [PubMed]
11. Hamed, A.A.; Kabary, H.; Khedr, M.; Emam, A.N. Antibiofilm, antimicrobial and cytotoxic activity of extracellular green-synthesized silver nanoparticles by two marine-derived actinomycete. *RSC Adv.* **2020**, *10*, 10361–10367. [CrossRef]
12. Wu, T.; He, M.; Zang, X.; Zhou, Y.; Qiu, T.; Pan, S.; Xu, X. A structure–Activity relationship study of flavonoids as inhibitors of E. coli by membrane interaction effect. *Biochim. Biophys. Acta (BBA)-Biomembr.* **2013**, *1828*, 2751–2756. [CrossRef]
13. Wu, T.; Zang, X.; He, M.; Pan, S.; Xu, X. Structure–activity relationship of flavonoids on their anti-Escherichia coli activity and inhibition of DNA gyrase. *J. Agric. Food Chem.* **2013**, *61*, 8185–8190. [CrossRef]
14. Alhadrami, H.A.; Hamed, A.A.; Hassan, H.M.; Belbahri, L.; Rateb, M.E.; Sayed, A.M. Flavonoids as Potential anti-MRSA Agents through Modulation of PBP2a: A Computational and Experimental Study. *Antibiotics* **2020**, *9*, 562. [CrossRef] [PubMed]
15. Osonga, F.J.; Akgul, A.; Miller, R.M.; Eshun, G.B.; Yazgan, I.; Akgul, A.; Sadik, O.A. Antimicrobial activity of a new class of phosphorylated and modified flavonoids. *ACS Omega* **2019**, *4*, 12865–12871. [CrossRef] [PubMed]
16. Rosi, N.L.; Giljohann, D.A.; Thaxton, C.S.; Lytton-Jean, A.K.; Han, M.S.; Mirkin, C.A. Oligonucleotide-modified gold nanoparticles for intracellular gene regulation. *Science* **2006**, *312*, 1027–1030. [CrossRef] [PubMed]
17. Thomas, M.; Klibanov, A.M. Conjugation to gold nanoparticles enhances polyethylenimine's transfer of plasmid DNA into mammalian cells. *Proc. Natl. Acad. Sci. USA* **2003**, *100*, 9138–9143. [CrossRef]
18. Cho, E.C.; Au, L.; Zhang, Q.; Xia, Y. The effects of size, shape, and surface functional group of gold nanostructures on their adsorption and internalization by cells. *Small* **2010**, *6*, 517–522. [CrossRef]
19. Gu, H.; Ho, P.L.; Tong, E.; Wang, L.; Xu, B. Presenting vancomycin on nanoparticles to enhance antimicrobial activities. *Nano Lett.* **2003**, *3*, 1261–1263. [CrossRef]
20. Kitov, P.I.; Mulvey, G.L.; Griener, T.P.; Lipinski, T.; Solomon, D.; Paszkiewicz, E.; Jacobson, J.M.; Sadowska, J.M.; Suzuki, M.; Yamamura, K.-I.; et al. In vivo supramolecular templating enhances the activity of multivalent ligands: A potential therapeutic against the Escherichia coli O157 AB5 toxins. *Proc. Natl. Acad. Sci. USA* **2008**, *105*, 16837–16842. [CrossRef]
21. Bowman, M.C.; Ballard, T.E.; Ackerson, C.J.; Feldheim, D.L.; Margolis, D.M.; Melander, C. Inhibition of HIV fusion with multivalent gold nanoparticles. *J. Am. Chem. Soc.* **2008**, *130*, 6896–6897. [CrossRef]
22. Yavuz, M.S.; Cheng, Y.; Chen, J.; Cobley, C.M.; Zhang, Q.; Rycenga, M.; Xie, J.; Kim, C.; Song, K.H.; Schwartz, A.G.; et al. Gold nanocages covered by smart polymers for controlled release with near-infrared light. *Nat. Mater.* **2009**, *8*, 935–939. [CrossRef] [PubMed]
23. Zhao, Y.; Tian, Y.; Cui, Y.; Liu, W.; Ma, W.; Jiang, X. Small molecule-capped gold nanoparticles as potent antibacterial agents that target gram-negative bacteria. *J. Am. Chem. Soc.* **2010**, *132*, 12349–12356. [CrossRef]
24. Montoya, M. Bacterial glutathione import. *Nat. Struct. Mol. Biol.* **2013**, *20*, 775. [CrossRef]
25. Jiang, G.; Wang, L.; Chen, W. Studies on the preparation and characterization of gold nanoparticles protected by dendrons. *Mater. Lett.* **2007**, *61*, 278–283. [CrossRef]
26. Sulaiman, G.M.; Waheeb, H.M.; Jabir, M.S.; Khazaal, S.H.; Dewir, Y.H.; Naidoo, Y. Hesperidin Loaded on Gold Nanoparticles as a Drug Delivery System for a Successful Biocompatible, Anti-Cancer, Anti-Inflammatory and Phagocytosis Inducer Model. *Sci. Rep.* **2020**, *10*, 9362. [CrossRef]
27. Kiroula, N.; Negi, J.S.; Singh, K.; Rawat, R.; Singh, B. Preparation and characterization of ganciclovir-loaded glutathione modifed gold nanoparticles. *Indian J. Pharm. Sci.* **2016**, *78*, 313–319. [CrossRef]
28. Zhanel, G.G.; Ennis, K.; Vercaigne, L.; Walkty, A.; Gin, A.S.; Embil, J.; Smith, H.; Hoban, D.J. A critical review of the fluoroquinolones. *Drugs* **2002**, *62*, 13–59. [CrossRef]

29. de Sousa Neto, D.; Tabak, M. Interaction of the meso-tetrakis (4-N-methylpyridyl) porphyrin with gel and liquid state phospholipid vesicles. *J. Colloid Interface Sci.* **2012**, *381*, 73–82. [CrossRef] [PubMed]
30. Dhaliwal, A.; Khondker, A.; Alsop, R.; Rheinstädter, M.C. Glucose can protect membranes against dehydration damage by inducing a glassy membrane state at low hydrations. *Membranes* **2019**, *9*, 15. [CrossRef]
31. Sharma, V.K.; Mamontov, E.; Ohl, M.; Tyagi, M. Incorporation of aspirin modulates the dynamical and phase behavior of the phospholipid membrane. *Phys. Chem. Chem. Phys.* **2017**, *19*, 2514–2524. [CrossRef] [PubMed]
32. Khondker, A.; Dhaliwal, A.; Alsop, R.J.; Tang, J.; Backholm, M.; Shi, A.C.; Rheinstädter, M.C. Partitioning of caffeine in lipid bilayers reduces membrane fluidity and increases membrane thickness. *Phys. Chem. Chem. Phys.* **2017**, *19*, 7101–7111. [CrossRef]
33. Wu, X.; Lu, C.; Zhou, Z.; Yuan, G.; Xiong, R.; Zhang, X. Green synthesis and formation mechanism of cellulose nanocrystal-supported gold nanoparticles with enhanced catalytic performance. *Environ. Sci. Nano* **2014**, *1*, 71–79. [CrossRef]
34. Durcik, M.; Tammela, P.; Barančoková, M.; Tomašič, T.; Ilaš, J.; Kikelj, D.; Zidar, N. Synthesis and Evaluation of N-Phenylpyrrolamides as DNA Gyrase B Inhibitors. *Chem. Med. Chem.* **2018**, *13*, 186–198. [CrossRef] [PubMed]
35. Sayed, A.M.; Alhadrami, H.A.; El-Hawary, S.S.; Mohammed, R.; Hassan, H.M.; Rateb, M.E.; Bakeer, W. Discovery of two brominated oxindole alkaloids as Staphylococcal DNA gyrase and pyruvate kinase inhibitors via inverse virtual screening. *Microorganisms* **2020**, *8*, 293. [CrossRef]
36. Jo, S.; Cheng, X.; Lee, J.; Kim, S.; Park, S.J.; Patel, D.S.; Beaven, A.H.; Lee, K.I.; Rui, H.; Park, S.; et al. CHARMM-GUI 10 years for biomolecular modeling and simulation. *J. Comput. Chem.* **2017**, *38*, 1114–1124. [CrossRef] [PubMed]
37. Morris, G.M.; Huey, R.; Lindstrom, W.; Sanner, M.F.; Belew, R.K.; Goodsell, D.S.; Olson, A.J. AutoDock4 and AutoDockTools4: Automated docking with selective receptor flexibility. *J. Comput. Chem.* **2009**, *30*, 2785–2791. [CrossRef] [PubMed]
38. DeLano, W.L. Pymol: An open-source molecular graphics tool. CCP4 Newsl. *Protein Crystallogr.* **2002**, *40*, 82–92.
39. Bowers, K.J.; Chow, D.E.; Xu, H.; Dror, R.O.; Eastwood, M.P.; Gregersen, B.A.; Klepeis, J.L.; Kolossvary, I.; Moraes, M.A.; Sacerdoti, F.D.; et al. Scalable Algorithms for Molecular Dynamics Simulations on Commodity Clusters. In Proceedings of the 2006 ACM/IEEE Conference on Supercomputing, Tampa, FL, USA, 11–17 November 2006; p. 43.
40. Phillips, J.C.; Braun, R.; Wang, W.; Gumbart, J.; Tajkhorshid, E.; Villa, E.; Chipot, C.; Skeel, R.D.; Kalé, L.; Schulten, K. Scalable molecular dynamics with NAMD. *J. Comput. Chem.* **2005**, *26*, 1781–1802. [CrossRef]

antibiotics

Article

Bioactivity and Control Efficacy of the Novel Antibiotic Tetramycin against Various Kiwifruit Diseases

Qiuping Wang [1], Cheng Zhang [2], Youhua Long [2,*], Xiaomao Wu [2], Yue Su [1], Yang Lei [1] and Qiang Ai [1]

1 Department of Food and Medicine, Guizhou Vocational College of Agriculture, Qingzhen 551400, China; qpwang518@aliyun.com (Q.W.); suyue09136@163.com (Y.S.); gznzyylei@126.com (Y.L.); gznzyaqiang@163.com (Q.A.)
2 Research Center for Engineering Technology of Kiwifruit, Institute of Crop Protection, College of Agriculture, Guizhou University, Guiyang 550025, China; chengz76@aliyun.com (C.Z.); wuxm827@126.com (X.W.)
* Correspondence: gzlyh126@126.com

Abstract: Tetramycin, a novel polyene agriculture antibiotic, has excellent antimicrobial activity against many plant pathogens. In this study, the antimicrobial activities of tetramycin and conventional antibiotics on eight common pathogens and their field control efficacies against four serious diseases in kiwifruit were investigated. The results show that 0.3% tetramycin aqueous solutions (AS) exhibited the superior antibacterial and antifungal activity against *Pseudomonas syringae* pv. *actinidiae*, *Pseudomonas fulva*, *Agrobacterium tumefaciens*, *Botryosphaeria dothidea*, *Phomopsis* sp., *Alternaria tenuissima*, *Armillariella mellea* and *Phytophthora cactorum* of kiwifruit pathogens with EC_{50} values of 1.21, 1.24, 0.72, 0.14, 0.09, 0.16, 0.06 and 0.17 mg kg^{-1}, respectively. These EC_{50} values of tetramycin were much higher than those of conventional kasugamycin, zhongshengmycin or polyoxin. Meanwhile, 0.3% tetramycin AS possessed the good field control efficacies for canker, soft rot, blossom blight and brown spot disease of kiwifruit with 74.45, 83.55, 84.74 and 89.62%. Moreover, 0.3% tetramycin AS application notably increased fruit resistance substances contents, activated fruit superoxide dismutase and polyphenoloxidase activities, as well as remarkably enhanced fruit growth, improved fruit quality and storability. This study highlights that tetramycin can be used as a preferred alternative to conventional antibiotics in kiwifruit production.

Keywords: tetramycin; antimicrobial activity; kiwifruit disease; conventional antibiotics; storage quality

Citation: Wang, Q.; Zhang, C.; Long, Y.; Wu, X.; Su, Y.; Lei, Y.; Ai, Q. Bioactivity and Control Efficacy of the Novel Antibiotic Tetramycin against Various Kiwifruit Diseases. *Antibiotics* **2021**, *10*, 289. https://doi.org/10.3390/antibiotics10030289

Academic Editor: Helena P. Felgueiras

Received: 2 February 2021
Accepted: 7 March 2021
Published: 10 March 2021

1. Introduction

Kiwifruit (*Actinidia*), an emerging, healthy and economical fruit, has been commercially cultivated worldwide on a large scale since the 1970s. The yield and area of kiwifruit cultivation around the world are continuously increasing in the 21st century, and its planting area and annual output reached 381,800 hm^2 and 5,270,000 tons by 2020 [1,2]. However, as commercial cultivation of kiwifruit expanded, many diseases gradually appeared in kiwifruit orchards and have become increasingly prominent and serious problems [3]. These serious diseases include bacterial canker, soft rot, bacterial blossom blight, brown spot and root rot, etc. For instance, *Pseudomonas syringae* pv. *actinidiae* (*Psa*) is the causal agent of destructive canker disease in kiwifruit, whose field symptoms include leaders and trunks often accompanied by oozing exudates, shoot wilting, reddening of the lenticels, twig dieback, blossom necrosis and leaf spotting [4–6]. Soft rot, which mainly caused by *Botryosphaeria dothidea*, *Phomopsis* sp., *Cryptosporiopsis actinidiae*, *Botrytis inereal*, *Cylindrocarpon* sp. and *Phoma exigua*, is a major disease of postharvest kiwifruit [7–12]. The occurrence of these diseases seriously affects the quality and yield of kiwifruit, as well as being a frequent cause of major economic losses worldwide.

Recently, China's kiwifruit industry has developed rapidly, and its planting area has reached over 243,000 hm^2, with an annual output of nearly 2,500,000 tons. In Guizhou

Province of Southwest China, the kiwifruit industry has made great contributions to poverty alleviation and rural revitalization, and its planting area reaches over 40,000 hm^2. Various diseases including canker (*Psa*), soft rot (*B. dothidea* and *Phomopsis* sp.), blossom blight (*Pseudomonas fulva*), brown spot (*Alternaria tenuissima*), crown gall (*Agrobacterium tumefaciens*) and root rot (*Armillariella mellea* and *Phytophthora cactorum*) are common diseases in kiwifruit planted in Guizhou [12–16]. Although some chemical fungicides have good antibacterial activity against these pathogens, there are increasing concerns about the harmful impacts of chemical fungicide residues on human health and the environment. Moreover, the number of effective control fungicides for these diseases is extremely limited, as for example, only streptomycin or copper are effective in controlling bacterial canker [17]. Additionally, chemical fungicides easily induce pathogen resistance [17,18]. Therefore, there is an urgent need to develop safe and effective control technologies for kiwifruit diseases.

Agricultural antibiotics, as a kind of important biological pesticides, have many prominent advantages including high efficiency, easy decomposition, no residue and no environmental pollution, are thus a green, popular and eco-friendly approach to controlling plant diseases [19,20]. Some conventional antibiotics such as streptomycin, kasugamycin, zhongshengmycin and polyoxin (Figure 1), have been widely used to control various plant diseases [17,19–22]. However, we found that these conventional antibiotics exhibited low efficacy in controlling many diseases of kiwifruit, and streptomycin application in agricultural production in China has been already limited. Tetramycin, produced by *Streptomyces hygrospinosus* var. *Beijingensis*, is a novel 26-member tetraene macrolide antibiotic containing two active components (tetramycin A and tetramycin B, Figure 1) [23,24]. It exhibits satisfactory inhibitory bioactivity against numerous plant pathogens, such as *Botrytis cinerea*, *Colletotrichum scovillei*, *Pyricularia oryzae*, *Phytophthora capsici* and *Passalora fulva* [25–30]. Recently, tetramycin was registered for controlling rice and fruit diseases in China [25], and has gradually become a preferred alternative to conventional antibiotics because of its environmental friendliness and low toxicity [31,32]. Up to date, however, there is little attention paid or documentation available about the application of tetramycin for the control of various kiwifruit diseases.

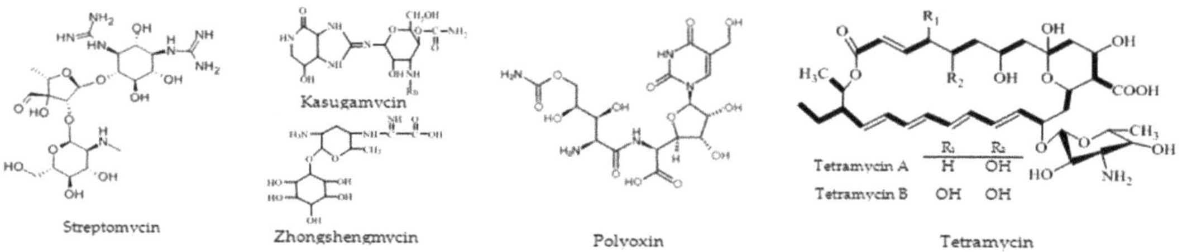

Figure 1. The chemical structures of streptomycin, kasugamycin, zhongshengmycin, polyoxin and tetramycin.

Accordingly, this study was initiated to evaluate the antimicrobial activity of tetramycin and conventional antibiotics against eight common pathogens of kiwifruit, and to assess the control efficacy of tetramycin and the conventional antibiotics against canker, soft rot, blossom blight and brown spot diseases of kiwifruit under field conditions. Moreover, the effects of tetramycin on the disease resistance, growth and quality of kiwifruit were investigated. The findings should provide a technical basis for the registration and application of tetramycin for the control of various kiwifruit diseases.

2. Materials and Methods

2.1. Pathogens and Materials

Psa, *B. dothidea*, *Phomopsis* sp., *P. fulva*, *A. tenuissima*, *A. tumefaciens*, *A. mellea* and *P. cactorum* were provided by the Research Center for Engineering Technology of Kiwifruit, Guizhou University (Guiyang, China), and they had highly pathogenicity. 0.3% tetramycin aqueous solutions (AS) was purchased from Liaoning Microke Biological Engineering Co. Ltd. (Liaoning, China). 5.0% polyoxin AS was obtained from Rushan Hanwei Biotechnology Co., Ltd. (Shandong, China). 4.0% kasugamycin wettable powder (WP) was purchased from Huafeng Chemical Co., Ltd. (Qiqihar, China). 3.0% zhongshengmycin WP was obtained from Noposion Agrochemicals Co., Ltd. (Shenzhen, China). Potato dextrose agar (PDA, potato 200 g, dextrose 20 g, agar 15 g, distilled water 1000 mL) and nutrient agar (NA, beef extract 5.0 g, peptone 10.0 g, NaCl 5 g, distilled water 1000 mL) were purchased from Xiya Reagent Co. Ltd. (Chengdu, China).

2.2. *In Vitro Toxicity Tests*

For bacterial pathogens (*Psa*, *P. fulva* and *A. tumefaciens*), the plate colony counting method was used to determine the in vitro toxicity of bactericides. 1 mL tested solution of bactericide and 9 mL NA were emptied into the glass petri dishes (90 mm in diameter) and mixed, 1 mL sterile water was used as control. After solidification, 200 μL bacterial suspension (1000 cfu mL^{-1}) was evenly coated on the NA plate containing bactericide with three replicates, and then cultured at 28 °C for 48 h. The colony number of each replicate was observed and counted. The formula for calculating the inhibition rate of bacteria was as Equation (1):

$$\text{Inhibition rate (\%)} = 100 \times (\text{Colony counts in control dish} - \text{Colony counts in treatment dish}) / \text{Colony counts in control dish} \tag{1}$$

EC_{50} (effective concentration of 50% inhibition rate) values were estimated statistically using the SPSS 18.0 software.

For fungal pathogens (*B. dothidea*, *Phomopsis* sp., *A. tenuissima*, *A. mellea* and *P. cactorum*), the mycelial growth rate method was used to determine the in vitro toxicity of fungicides. 9 mL PDA was emptied into the glass Petri dishes. After PDA solidification, 1 mL tested solution of fungicides was evenly coated on the PDA plate, sterile water was used as control. Then, a 5 mm diameter disc of pathogen which cut from the actively growing front of a 7 d old colony was placed in the plate center with the inoculum side down and three replicates. Subsequently, the treated plate cultured at 28 °C till the fungal growth was almost complete in the control plates, the diameters of the fungal growth were measured. The formula for calculating the growth inhibition of fungal hyphae was as Equation (2):

$$\text{Inhibition rate (\%)} = 100 \times [(\text{Mycelial growth diameter in control dish} - \text{Mycelial growth diameter in treatment dish}) / (\text{Mycelial growth diameter in control dish} - 5)] \tag{2}$$

The calculation of EC_{50} values was the same as above.

2.3. *Field Experiments*

2.3.1. Study Site

Field experiments were conducted in a kiwifruit garden at Xiuwen Country, Guizhou, China (26°79′80.0″ N, 106°56′58.2″ E), where serious infestations of bacterial canker, soft rot, bacterial blossom blight and brown spot of kiwifruit had occurred in previous years. The cultivar was *A. deliciosa* cv. Guichang, with a tree age of 5 years and spacing of 3.0 m × 3.0 m, cultivated on concrete 'T' type frames. The proportion of male and female kiwifruit plants was 1:8. The annual rainfall, mean temperature and altitude of the kiwifruit garden was about 1293 mm, 15~16 °C and 1267 m, respectively. The loam soils (0~60 cm in deep) had 25.94 g kg^{-1} of organic matter, 1.38 g kg^{-1} of total nitrogen, 1.65 g kg^{-1} of total phosphorus, 1.08 g kg^{-1} of total potassium, 3.96 mg kg^{-1} of available nitrogen, 4.25 mg kg^{-1} of available phosphorus, 3.15 mg kg^{-1} of available potassium, 31.61 mg kg^{-1} of available iron, 19.17 mg kg^{-1} of available manganese, 50.66 mg kg^{-1} of total zinc, 17.63 cmol kg^{-1} of exchangeable calcium, and 5.72 of pH value.

2.3.2. Field Experiment Design of Kiwifruit Canker

The bactericide control experiment of kiwifruit canker was carried out using the smearing disease spot method. The experimental treatments included 0.3% tetramycin AS 50 times dilution liquid, 3.0% zhongshengmycin WP 50 times dilution liquid and clear water (control), and a total of nine plots were arranged randomly with three replicates (the plot distribution figure see Figure S1 in the Supplementary Materials). Each plot had eight kiwifruit trees, and the interior six trees were used for determination. The bactericide was applied in mid-March for three times with an interval of 7 d. The healing rate of the disease spot was observed and recorded after the three months of application, and the healing rate and control effect were calculated according to Equations (3) and (4):

$$\text{Healing rate (\%)} = 100 \times \text{Number of healed disease spots after treatment/Total number of disease spots before treatment} \tag{3}$$

$$\text{Control effect (\%) of canker} = 100 \times (\text{Healing rate of control} - \text{Healing rate of treatment})/(100 - \text{Healing rate of control}) \tag{4}$$

2.3.3. Field Experiment Design of Soft Rot, Blossom Blight and Brown Spot Diseases in Kiwifruit

The fungicide control experiment of soft rot, blossom blight and brown spot diseases in kiwifruit was carried out using the spray method. The experimental treatments included 0.3% tetramycin AS 5000 times dilution liquid, 5.0% polyoxin AS 5000 times dilution liquid and clear water (CK), and a total of nine plots were also arranged randomly with three replicates (the plot distribution figure see Figure S2 in the Supplementary Materials). Similarly, each plot had eight kiwifruit trees, and the interior six trees were used for determination. In our previous report, the pathogens of soft rot have the two infection periods on *A.delicios*. cv. Guichang, one is 20 May to 13 June and other is 2 to 12 August [16]. Moreover, blossom blight often occurs in the flower bud stage (late March to late April), and brown spot often occurs in the fruit growth stage (early June to late August). Thus, about 1.00, 1.50 and 2.00 L of fungicide dilution liquid was sprayed on kiwifruit plants (include bud, leaf and stem) at 19 March, 19 May and 1 August in 2020, respectively. The incidence rate of disease flower bud was observed and recorded at flowering phase (15 April to 15 May), and the incidence rate and control effect of blossom blight in kiwifruit were calculated according to Equations (5) and (6):

$$\text{Incidence rate of disease flower buds (\%)} = 100 \times \text{Number of disease flower buds/Total number of flower buds} \tag{5}$$

$$\text{Control effect (\%) of blossom blight} = 100 \times (\text{Incidence rate of control} - \text{Incidence rate of treatment})/\text{Incidence rate of control} \tag{6}$$

The disease index and control effect of brown spot in kiwifruit were investigated at 15 August according to Equations (7) and (8). The disease grade of 10 leaves of 6 branches in each plot was observed and recorded. The grading standard of the incidence degree: 0 = no incidence; 1 = disease spot area is less than 10% of leaf area; 2 = disease spot area is 10~20% of leaf area; 3 = disease spot area is 20~40% of leaf area; 4 = disease spot area is more than 40% of leaf area; 5 = fallen leaf.

$$\text{Disease index} = 100 \times \sum(\text{Disease grade value} \times \text{Number of leaf within each grade})/(\text{Total number of leaf} \times \text{the highest grade}) \tag{7}$$

$$\text{Control effect of brown spot (\%)} = 100 \times (\text{Disease index of control} - \text{Disease index of treatment})/\text{Disease index of control} \tag{8}$$

Two hundred kiwifruits from each plot were randomly collected and divided into two groups at 1 October in 2020, and stored at 25 ± 1 °C. Fruits of the first group were used to investigate the incidence rate and of control effect soft rot in kiwifruit. Fruits of other group were used for determining the development and quality parameters of fruit.

The incidence rate and control effect of soft rot in kiwifruit were investigated according to Equations (9) and (10).

$$\text{Incidence rate of disease fruits (\%)} = 100 \times \text{Number of disease fruits/Total number of fruits} \quad (9)$$

$$\text{Control effect (\%) of soft rot} = 100 \times (\text{Incidence rate of control} - \text{Incidence rate of treatment})/\text{Incidence rate of control} \quad (10)$$

Because it is difficult to find the continuous occurrence garden of crown gall and root rot diseases in kiwifruit, thus the field control experiments of tetracycline against crown gall and root rot diseases were not carried out.

2.4. Analytical Methods

Total phenolics, total flavonoids, superoxide dismutase (SOD) activity and polyphenoloxidase (PPO) activity of fruits were analyzed according to Zhang et al. [15,16]. The development parameters including longitudinal diameters, transverse diameters, lateral diameters, fruit shape index, single fruit volume and single fruit weight, and the quality parameters including vitamin C, total soluble sugar, soluble solid, dry matter, soluble protein, titratable acidity and fruit firmness were also analyzed as described by Zhang et al. [15,16].

2.5. Statistical Analyses

The mean and standard deviation values of triplicate were presented. All analyses were performed using SPSS statistical software package release 18.0 (SPSS Inc., Chicago, IL, USA). The difference significances between group means were treated statistically by one-way analysis of variance (ANOVA). Charts were plotted with Origin 10.0 (OriginLab Inc., Northampton, MA, USA).

3. Results

3.1. Toxicity Effects of Different Antibiotics against Eight Pathogens of Kiwifruit

The toxicities of tetramycin, polyoxin, kasugamycin or zhongshengmycin against eight pathogens of kiwifruit are shown in Table 1. 0.3% Tetramycin AS exhibited a superior toxicity potential for *Psa*, *P. fulva* and *A. tumefaciens* of bacterial pathogens in kiwifruit with EC_{50} values of 1.21, 1.24 and 0.72 mg kg^{-1}, which were 101.91, 99.12 and 721.17 folds, or 14.01, 209.06 and 3905.39 folds higher than 4.0% kasugamycin WP or 3.0% zhongshengmycin WP, respectively. 0.3% tetramycin AS caused the greatest toxicities of mycelium growth for *B. dothidea* and *Phomopsis* sp. of kiwifruit soft rot with EC_{50} values of 0.14 and 0.09 mg kg^{-1}, which were 603.36 and 438.67 folds, or 5158.64 and 14515.11 folds higher than 5.0% polyoxin AS or 4.0% kasugamycin WP, respectively. Moreover, 0.3% tetramycin AS also possessed superior toxicities for *A. tenuissima*, *A. mellea* and *P. cactorum* of other fungal pathogens in kiwifruit with EC_{50} values of 0.16, 0.06 and 0.17 mg kg^{-1}, which were 91.06, 272.33 and 56.59 folds, or 8513.19, 9306.83 and 4665.71 folds higher than 5.0% polyoxin AS or 4.0% kasugamycin WP, respectively. These results suggest that tetramycin had an extremely superior antimicrobial activity than conventional antibiotics such as kasugamycin, zhongshengmycin and polyoxin.

3.2. Field Control Effects of Tetramycin on Canker Disease of Kiwifruit

Table 2 exhibits the field control effects of tetramycin and zhongshengmycin on canker disease of kiwifruit. Prominently, the healing rate of disease spots in kiwifruit by 0.3% tetramycin AS was 72.68%, which was significantly ($p < 0.01$) higher than that of 3.0% zhongshengmycin WP (50.23%) and control (3.95%). Satisfactorily, the application of 0.3% tetramycin AS exhibited a good control capacity for canker disease of kiwifruit with control effect of 74.45%, which was significantly ($p < 0.01$) higher than 45.24% of 3.0% zhongshengmycin WP.

Table 1. Toxicities of different antibiotics against eight pathogens of kiwifruit.

Diseases	Pathogens	Antibiotic Bactericides	Regression Equation	Determination Coefficient (R^2)	EC_{50} (mg kg^{-1})
Canker	*Psa*	0.3% Tetramycin AS	$y = 4.9514 + 0.5947x$	0.9839	1.21
		4.0% Kasugamycin WP	$y = 1.9636 + 1.4521x$	0.9098	123.31
		3.0% Zhongshengmycin WP	$y = 3.6935 + 1.0628x$	0.9923	16.95
Soft rot	*B. dothidea*	0.3% Tetramycin AS	$y = 6.0759 + 1.2511x$	0.9963	0.14
		5.0% Polyoxin AS	$y = 2.0651 + 1.5223x$	0.9931	84.75
		4.0% Kasugamycin WP	$y = 3.1542 + 0.6457x$	0.9652	722.21
	Phomopsis sp.	0.3% Tetramycin AS	$y = 1.1510 + 9.3601x$	0.9968	0.09
		5.0% Polyoxin AS	$y = 2.3579 + 1.6551x$	0.9684	39.48
		4.0% Kasugamycin WP	$y = 2.6214 + 0.7634x$	0.9857	1306.36
Blossom blight	*P. fulva*	0.3% Tetramycin AS	$y = 4.9404 + 0.6414x$	0.9744	1.24
		4.0% Kasugamycin WP	$y = 3.6968 + 0.6237x$	0.9144	122.91
		3.0% Zhongshengmycin WP	$y = 3.1389 + 0.7711x$	0.9040	259.24
Brown spot	*A. tenuissima*	0.3% Tetramycin AS	$y = 5.7631 + 0.9705x$	0.9928	0.16
		5.0% Polyoxin AS	$y = 2.3767 + 2.2548x$	0.959	14.57
		4.0% Kasugamycin WP	$y = 4.1000 + 0.2867x$	0.9432	1362.11
Crown gall	*A. tumefaciens*	0.3% Tetramycin AS	$y = 7.3724 + 1.0031x$	0.9962	0.72
		4.0% Kasugamycin WP	$y = 3.5950 + 0.6408x$	0.9813	519.24
		3.0% Zhongshengmycin WP	$y = 4.1821 + 0.2371x$	0.9759	2811.88
Root rot	*A. mellea*	0.3% Tetramycin AS	$y = 5.6952 + 0.5530x$	0.9922	0.06
		5.0% Polyoxin AS	$y = 4.3471 + 0.5381x$	0.9866	16.34
		4.0% Kasugamycin WP	$y = 2.8248 + 0.7971x$	0.9801	558.41
	P. cactorum	0.3% Tetramycin AS	$y = 5.2013 + 0.2600x$	0.9942	0.17
		5.0% Polyoxin AS	$y = 4.5736 + 0.4337x$	0.9915	9.62
		4.0% Kasugamycin WP	$y = 0.8490 + 1.4371x$	0.9920	793.17

x and y indicate the concentration of antibiotic bactericide and the inhibition rate of bacteria or fungal, respectively.

Table 2. The control effects of tetramycin and zhongshengmycin on canker disease of kiwifruit.

Treatments	Healing Rate of Disease Spots (%)	Control Effect (%)
0.3% Tetramycin AS	72.68 ± 3.46 ^{aA}	74.45 ± 3.61 ^{aA}
3.0% Zhongshengmycin WP	50.23 ± 2.97 ^{bB}	45.24 ± 3.32 ^{bB}
CK	3.95 ± 0.38 ^{cC}	

Values indicate the mean of three replicates ± standard deviation (SD). Different uppercases and lowercases indicate significant differences between different treatments at 1% level ($p < 0.01$) and 5% level ($p < 0.05$), respectively.

3.3. Field Control Effects of Tetramycin on Soft Rot, Blossom Blight and Brown Spot Diseases of Kiwifruit

The field control effects of tetramycin and polyoxin on soft rot, blossom blight and brown spot diseases of kiwifruit are displayed in Table 3. 0.3% Tetramycin AS and 5.0% polyoxin AS significantly ($p < 0.01$) decreased the incidence rates of disease fruit and flower bud in kiwifruit, and significantly ($p < 0.01$) decreased disease index of brown spot diseases in kiwifruit, as well as 0.3% tetramycin AS was more effective than 5.0% polyoxin AS. The control effects of soft rot, blossom blight and brown spot diseases in kiwifruit by 0.3% tetramycin AS were 83.55, 84.74 and 89.62%, which were significantly ($p < 0.01$) higher than 60.83, 34.73 and 55.51% of 5.0% polyoxin AS, respectively. These results indicate that 0.3% tetramycin AS had a superior prevention and control capacity for various diseases in kiwifruit production.

Table 3. The control effects of tetramycin and polyoxin on soft rot, blossom blight and brown spot diseases of kiwifruit.

Treatments	Soft Rot		Blossom Blight		Brown Spot	
	Incidence Rate of Disease Fruit(%)	Control Effect (%)	Incidence Rate of Disease Flower Bud (%)	Control Effect (%)	Disease Index	Control Effect (%)
0.3% Tetramycin AS	9.00 ± 2.65 cC	83.55 ± 3.47 aA	5.25 ± 0.75 cC	84.74 ± 2.60 aA	3.21 ± 0.99 cC	89.62 ± 2.56 aA
5.0% Polyoxin AS	21.00 ± 1.73 bB	60.83 ± 4.63 bB	22.56 ± 2.28 bB	34.73 ± 5.40 bB	13.67 ± 1.86 bB	55.51 ± 3.31 bB
CK	54.00 ± 6.24 aA		34.56 ± 2.03 aA		30.63 ± 1.96 aA	

Values indicate the mean of three replicates ± standard deviation (SD). Different uppercases and lowercases indicate significant differences between different treatments at 1% level ($p < 0.01$) and 5% level ($p < 0.05$), respectively.

3.4. The Effects of Tetramycin on Defense-Related Substances and Enzyme Activity in Kiwifruit

Figure 2 depicts the effects of tetramycin and polyoxin on the changes of total phenolics and total flavonoids, SOD activity and PPO activity in kiwifruit during storage. Total phenolics content increased gradually during storage, and total phenolics content of 0.3% tetramycin AS-treated fruits was consistently higher than that of 5.0% polyoxin AS-treated and control fruits (Figure 2a). Total flavonoids content in kiwifruit increased gradually over the first 14 d and then decreased on the second 14 d, and total flavonoid content of 0.3% tetramycin AS-treated fruits was also consistently significant ($p < 0.01$) higher than that of 5.0% polyoxin AS-treated and control fruits (Figure 2b). Similarly, SOD and PPO activities of 0.3% tetramycin AS-treated fruits were consistently significant ($p < 0.01$) higher than those of 5.0% polyoxin AS-treated and control fruits (Figure 2c,d). The spray of 0.3% tetramycin AS significantly ($p < 0.01$) inductively enhanced SOD and PPO activities in kiwifruit during storage, the improved effect was significantly ($p < 0.01$) higher than that of 5.0% polyoxin AS. These findings here emphasize that 0.3% tetramycin AS treatment significantly ($p < 0.01$) enhanced total phenolics and total flavonoids contents, as well as SOD and PPO activities of kiwifruit during storage, potentially improving disease resistance.

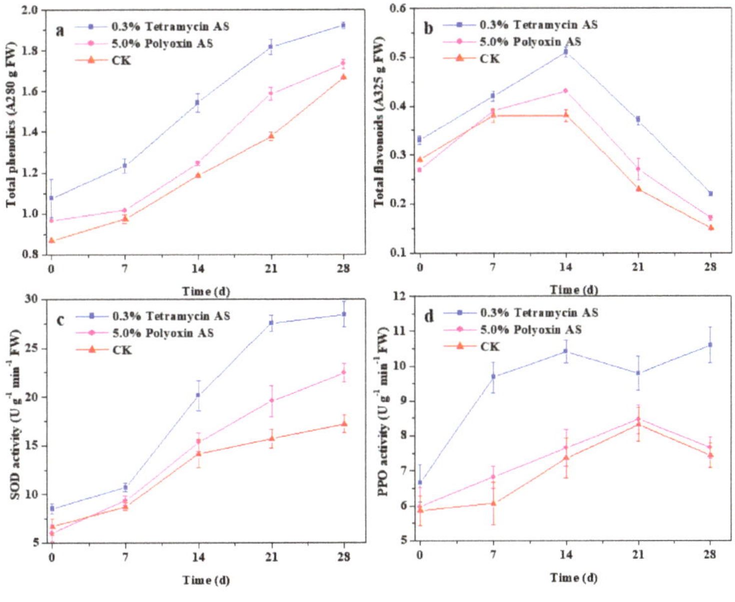

Figure 2. The effects of tetramycin and polyoxin on the changes of total phenolics (**a**) and total flavonoids (**b**), SOD activity (**c**) and PPO activity (**d**) in kiwifruit during storage. Values indicate the mean of three replicates, error bars indicate SD of three replicates.

3.5. The Effects of Tetramycin on Growth and Quality of Kiwifruit

The effect of tetramycin and polyoxin on kiwifruit growth is shown in Table 4. 0.3% tetramycin AS application could significantly ($p < 0.05$) enhance transverse diameter of fruits compared to 5.0% polyoxin AS treatment and control. Longitudinal diameter, lateral diameter and fruit shape index of fruits were no significant ($p < 0.05$) differences in three treatments. Moreover, the single fruit volume and weight of kiwifruit treated by 0.3% tetramycin AS were 71.42 cm^3 and 80.93 g, which was significantly ($p < 0.05$) increased by 2.26 and 4.98%, or 7.34 and 6.22% compared to 5.0% polyoxin AS treatment or control, respectively. Simultaneously, the enhanced effects of fruit growth by 0.3% tetramycin AS was higher than those of 5.0% polyoxin AS. These results indicate that 0.3% tetramycin AS application significantly ($p < 0.05$) enhanced fruit growth and yield formation.

Table 4. The effects of tetramycin and polyoxin on the development of kiwifruit.

Treatments	Longitudinal Diameter (mm)	Transverse Diameter (mm)	Lateral Diameter (mm)	Fruit Shape Index	Single Fruit Volume (cm^3)	Single Fruit Weight (g)
0.3% Tetramycin AS	76.60 ± 1.05 [a]	53.15 ± 0.51 [a]	41.91 ± 0.82 [a]	1.61 ± 0.02 [a]	71.42 ± 1.06 [a]	80.93 ± 0.86 [a]
5.0% Polyoxin AS	76.14 ± 0.74 [a]	51.57 ± 0.50 [b]	42.49 ± 0.70 [a]	1.62 ± 0.03 [a]	69.84 ± 1.69 [b]	77.10 ± 0.14 [b]
CK	75.24 ± 0.17 [ab]	51.05 ± 0.38 [b]	41.35 ± 0.09 [a]	1.63 ± 0.01 [a]	66.50 ± 0.68 [c]	76.19 ± 0.80 [bc]

Values indicate the mean of three replicates ± standard deviation (SD). Different lowercases indicates significant differences between different treatments at 5% level ($p < 0.05$).

Table 5 displays the nutritional parameters of kiwifruits. 0.3% tetramycin AS application significantly ($p < 0.05$) increased vitamin C, total soluble sugar, soluble solid, dry matter and soluble protein of fruits, as well as decreased titratable acidity of fruits compared to 5.0% polyoxin AS treatment and control. While 5.0% polyoxin AS treatment only significant ($p < 0.05$) increased dry matter of fruits compared to control. As shown in Figure 3, firmness decreased more rapidly in 5.0% polyoxin AS treatment and control than in 0.3% tetramycin AS-treated fruit, 0.3% tetramycin AS application effectively maintained higher fruit firmness and delayed its decrease. Meanwhile, the effect of spraying 0.3% tetramycin AS was better than that of 5.0% polyoxin AS. These findings emphasize that 0.3% tetramycin AS application could improve the quality and storability of kiwifruit.

Table 5. The effects of tetramycin and polyoxin on the nutritional quality of kiwifruit.

Treatments	Vitamin C (g kg^{-1})	Total Soluble Sugar (%)	Soluble Solid (%)	Dry Matter (%)	Soluble Protein (%)	Titratable Acidity (%)
0.3% Tetramycin AS	1.89 ± 0.01 [a]	12.44 ± 0.11 [a]	1.89 ± 0.01 [a]	19.50 ± 0.05 [a]	1.76 ± 0.05 [a]	1.01 ± 0.01 [b]
5.0% Polyoxin AS	1.83 ± 0.01 [ab]	12.08 ± 0.02 [b]	1.82 ± 0.01 [b]	19.25 ± 0.10 [a]	1.74 ± 0.01 [a]	1.12 ± 0.06 [a]
CK	1.81 ± 0.01 [b]	12.07 ± 0.02 [b]	1.81 ± 0.01 [b]	18.39 ± 0.08 [b]	1.71 ± 0.01 [ab]	1.13 ± 0.03 [a]

Values indicate the mean of three replicates ± standard deviation (SD). Different lowercases indicates significant differences between different treatments at 5% level ($p < 0.05$).

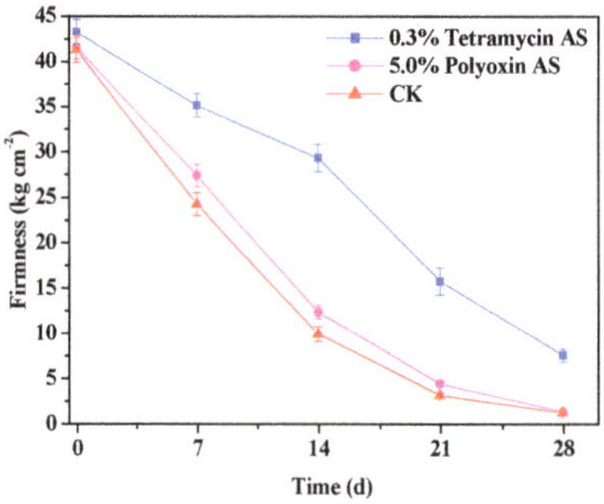

Figure 3. The effects of tetramycin and polyoxin on firmness of kiwifruit during storage. Values indicate the mean of three replicates, error bars indicate SD of three replicates.

4. Discussion

Few reports have discussed the antibacterial activity of tetramycin against the pathogens responsible for plant bacterial diseases. In this study, 0.3% tetramycin AS exhibited significant antibacterial activity against *Psa*, *P. fulva* and *A. tumefaciens*, three bacterial pathogens in kiwifruit, compared to conventional antibiotics such as 4.0% kasugamycin WP and 3.0% zhongshengmycin WP. The results showed that tetramycin also has a superior antibacterial activity against some other pathogens. Previous studies have reported that the mycelial growth of *Botrytis cinerea*, *Colletotrichum scovillei*, *Pyricularia oryzae*, *Phytophthora capsici* and *Passalora fulva* of fungal pathogen were significantly inhibited by tetramycin [25–30]. This study suggests that 0.3% tetramycin AS caused the greatest toxicities of mycelium growth for *B. dothide*, *Phomopsis* sp., *A. tenuissima*, *A. mellea* and *P. cactorum* of fungal pathogens in kiwifruit, and EC_{50} values of tetramycin were much higher than those of conventional antibiotics polyoxin and kasugamycin. These results extend the antimicrobial spectrum of tetramycin and provide a basis for the control of various kiwifruit diseases.

The superior antimicrobial activity of a pesticide is the premise for its good better field control efficacy on plant diseases. In this study, 0.3% tetramycin AS could significantly enhance the healing rate of disease spots caused by canker, decrease the incidence rates of diseased fruit and flower budd caused by soft rot and blossom blight, as well as decrease the disease index caused by brown spot. Satisfactorily, the application of 0.3% tetramycin AS exhibited good field control efficacies for canker, soft rot, blossom blight and brown spot disease of kiwifruit with 74.45, 83.55, 84.74 and 89.62%, which were significantly ($p < 0.01$) higher than those of conventional antibiotics 3.0% zhongshengmycin WP or 5.0% polyoxin AS. Song et al. shown that tetramycin had effective protective and curative activity against *B. cinerea* [26], and the aforementioned results also confirm that tetramycin is an agricultural antibiotic with both protective and curative functions against plant diseases. Moreover, tetramycin, a mixture polyene antibiotic, has excellently antimicrobial activity and unique mode of action, which are unlikely to lead to resistance development [30,32]. The results show that 0.3% tetramycin AS could effectively control various kiwifruit diseases, which successfully achieves the multi-purpose effects of one pesticide and availably reduces the use of various pesticides in kiwifruit production, as well as better implements the "double reduction of chemical fertilizers and pesticides" action in China. In order to evaluate the potential risk of tetracycline application on the imbalance of microbial population in kiwifruit, it is thus essential to study the microbial composition of kiwifruit leaves, stems and fruits after tetracycline application in the future researches.

Phenolics and flavonoids, as two important types of plant secondary metabolites, play extremely important roles in systemic resistance of plants [16]. In this study, 0.3% tetramycin AS significantly ($p < 0.01$) enhanced total phenolics and total flavonoids contents of kiwifruit during storage. The findings emphasize that 0.3% tetramycin AS application promoted the healthy growth of kiwifruit plants and fruits, as well as it possibly induced systemic resistance to inhibit disease development by plant or fruit. SOD and PPO are important defense enzymes associated with plant disease resistance [16]. Zhong et al. [33] reported that tetramycin could induce plant disease resistance by activating PPO, phenylalanine ammonia lyase (PAL) and perox-idase (POD) activities. The results presented here show that 0.3% tetramycin AS significantly enhanced SOD and PPO activities in kiwifruit during storage and increased the disease resistance of fruit, which is consistent with the above report. Moreover, 0.3% tetramycin AS application could significantly ($p < 0.05$) enhance transverse diameter, volume, weight, vitamin C, total soluble sugar, soluble solid, dry matter and soluble protein of fruits and decrease titratable acidity of fruits, as well as maintain high fruit firmness and delay its decrease. These findings imply that 0.3% tetramycin AS application could reliably decrease the occurrence of various kiwifruit diseases, and then promote its favorable growth, yield increase, quality and storability improvement.

Tetramycin is a novel 26-member tetraene macrolide antibiotic with environmental friendliness and low toxicity. Generally, kiwifruit cannot be eaten directly after harvest because of it has a soft ripening period of more than 20 d at room temperature. In this study, the extremely low 0.3% tetramycin AS application concentration (5000 times dilution liquid), long safety interval period (1 August to 1 October, 60 d) and long soft ripening period (more than 20 d) could effectively eliminate tetramycin residues in kiwifruit. The food safety risks caused by tetramycin are extremely low, and the public can rest assured to eat kiwifruit. Therefore, tetramycin can be used as a preferred alternative to conventional antibiotics in kiwifruit production, and 0.3% tetramycin AS 5000 times dilution liquid is a safe, beneficial and suitable concentration.

5. Conclusions

In conclusion, the present study demonstrates that tetramycin has superior antimicrobial activity against eight kiwifruit pathogens, which much higher than that of the conventional antibiotics polyoxin, kasugamycin and zhongshengmycin. 0.3% Tetramycin AS could effectively control the canker, soft rot, blossom blight and brown spot diseases in kiwifruit, and remarkably enhance phenolics and flavonoids contents, as well as SOD and PPO activities of kiwifruit during storage. Moreover, 0.3% tetramycin AS could reliably enhance fruit growth, quality and storability of kiwifruit. This study highlights that the tetramycin is a preferred alternative to conventional antibiotics for controlling kiwifruit diseases.

Supplementary Materials: The following are available online at https://www.mdpi.com/2079-6382/10/3/289/s1. Figure S1. The plot distribution figure of field experiment of kiwifruit canker. Figure S2. The plot distribution figure of field experiment of soft rot, blossom blight and brown spot diseases in kiwifruit.

Author Contributions: Y.L. (Youhua Long) and Q.W. conceived and designed the experiments; Q.W., C.Z., Y.L. (Yang Lei) and Q.A. performed the experiments; Q.W., X.W. and Y.S. analyzed the data; Q.W. and C.Z. wrote the paper. All authors have read and agreed to the published version of the manuscript.

Funding: This work was supported by the Support Plan Projects of Science and Technology Department of Guizhou Province (No. (2020)1Y016, (2019)2703, (2017)2566-1), the Support Plan Projects of Guiyang City (No. (2017)26-1), the scientific and technological achievement transformation project of Guizhou Province (No. (2017)4124), the Science and technology innovation talent project of Guizhou Province [No. (2016)5672].

Data Availability Statement: The data used to support the findings of this study are available from the corresponding author upon request.

Conflicts of Interest: We declare that we do not have any commercial or associative interest that represents a conflict of interest in connection with the work submitted.

References

1. Hu, H.; Zhou, H.; Li, P. Lacquer wax coating improves the sensory and quality attributes of kiwifruit during ambient storage. *Sci. Hortic.* **2019**, *244*, 31–41. [CrossRef]
2. Zhang, M.; Xu, L.; Zhang, L.; Guo, Y.; Qi, X.; He, L. Effects of quercetin on postharvest blue mold control in kiwifruit. *Sci. Hortic.* **2018**, *228*, 18–25. [CrossRef]
3. Huang, H.W. *Kiwifruit: Chapter 7—Cultivation and Management*; Academic Press: Beijing, China, 2016; Volume 7, pp. 265–295.
4. Scortichini, M.; Marcelletti, S.; Ferrante, P.; Petriccione, M.; Firrao, G. *Pseudomonas syringae* pv. *actinidiae*: A re-emerging, multi-faceted, pandemic pathogen. *Mol. Plant Pathol.* **2012**, *13*, 631–640. [CrossRef]
5. Cimmino, A.; Iannaccone, M.; Petriccione, M.; Masi, M.; Evidente, M.; Capparelli, R.; Scortichini, M.; Evidente, A. An ELISA method to identify the phytotoxic *Pseudomonas syringae* pv. *actinidiae* exopolysaccharides: A tool for rapid immunochemical detection of kiwifruit bacterial canker. *Phytochem. Lett.* **2017**, *19*, 136–140. [CrossRef]
6. Prencipe, S.; Nari, L.; Vittone, G.; Gullino, M.L.; Spadaro, D. Effect of bacterial canker caused by *Pseudomonas syringae* pv. *actinidiae* on postharvest quality and rots of kiwifruit 'Hayward'. *Postharvest Biol. Technol.* **2016**, *113*, 119–124. [CrossRef]
7. Hawthorne, B.; Rees-George, J.; Samuels, G.J. Fungi associated with leaf spots and post-harvest fruit rots of kiwifruit (*Actinidia chinensis*) in New Zealand. *N. Z. J. Bot.* **1982**, *20*, 143–150. [CrossRef]
8. Manning, M.A.; Meier, X.; Olsen, T.L.; Johnston, P.R. Fungi associated with fruit rots of Actinidia chinensis 'Hort16A' in New Zealand. *N. Z. J. Crop. Hortic. Sci.* **2003**, *31*, 315–324. [CrossRef]

9. Koh, Y.J.; Hur, J.; Jung, J.S. Postharvest fruit rots of kiwifruit (*Actinidia deliciosa*) in Korea. *N. Z. J. Crop. Hortic. Sci.* **2005**, *33*, 303–310. [CrossRef]
10. Prodi, A.; Sandalo, S.; Tonti, S.; Nipoti, P.; Pisi, A. Phiaphora-like fungi associated with kiwifruit elephantiasis. *Plant Physiol.* **2008**, *90*, 487–494. [CrossRef]
11. Luongo, L.; Santori, A.; Riccioni, L.; Belisario, A. *Phomopsis* sp. associated with post-harvest fruit rot of kiwifruit in Italy. *J. Plant Pathol.* **2011**, *93*, 205–209. [CrossRef]
12. Zhang, C.; Wu, X.M.; Long, Y.H.; Li, M. Control of soft rot in kiwifruit by pre-harvest application of chitosan composite coating and its effect on preserving and improving kiwifruit quality. *Food Sci.* **2016**, *37*, 274–281. [CrossRef]
13. Long, Y.H.; Yin, X.H.; Wang, M.; Wu, X.M.; Li, R.Y.; Tian, X.L.; Li, M. Effects of sulfur on kiwifruit canker caused by *Pseudomonas syringae* pv. *actinidae. Bangladesh J. Bot.* **2017**, *46*, 1183–1192.
14. Li, L.; Pan, H.; Deng, L.; Wang, Z.P.; Li, D.W.; Zhang, Q.; Chen, M.Y.; Zhong, C.H. First Report of *Alternaria tenuissima* Causing Brown Spot Disease of Kiwifruit Foliage in China. *Plant Dis.* **2018**, *103*, 582. [CrossRef]
15. Zhang, C.; Long, Y.-H.; Wang, Q.-P.; Li, J.-H.; An, H.M.; Wu, X.-M.; Li, M. The effect of preharvest 28.6% chitosan composite film sprays for controlling soft rot on kiwifruit and its defense responses. *Hortic. Sci.* **2019**, *46*, 180–194. [CrossRef]
16. Zhang, C.; Long, Y.; Li, J.; Li, M.; Xing, D.; An, H.; Wu, X.; Wu, Y. A Chitosan Composite Film Sprayed before Pathogen Infection Effectively Controls Postharvest Soft Rot in Kiwifruit. *Agronomy* **2020**, *10*, 265. [CrossRef]
17. Cameron, A.; Sarojini, V. *Pseudomonas syringae* pv. *actinidiae*: Chemical control, resistance mechanisms and possible alternatives. *Plant Pathol.* **2013**, *63*, 1–11. [CrossRef]
18. Wicaksono, W.A.; Jones, E.E.; Casonato, S.; Monk, J.; Ridgway, H.J. Biological control of *Pseudomonas syringae* pv. *actinidiae* (*Psa*), the causal agent of bacterial canker of kiwifruit, using endophytic bacteria recovered from a medicinal plant. *Biol. Control.* **2018**, *116*, 103–112. [CrossRef]
19. Ma, X.; Xiang, S.; Xie, H.; He, L.; Sun, X.; Zhang, Y.; Huang, J. Fabrication of pH-Sensitive Tetramycin Releasing Gel and Its Antibacterial Bioactivity against *Ralstonia solanacearum*. *Molecules* **2019**, *24*, 3606. [CrossRef] [PubMed]
20. Fan, C.; Guo, M.; Liang, Y.; Dong, H.; Ding, G.; Zhang, W.; Tang, G.; Yang, J.; Kong, D.; Cao, Y. Pectin-conjugated silica microcapsules as dual-responsive carriers for increasing the stability and antimicrobial efficacy of kasugamycin. *Carbohydr. Polym.* **2017**, *172*, 322–331. [CrossRef]
21. Chen, G.; Qiao, Y.; Liu, F.; Zhang, X.; Liao, H.; Zhang, R.; Dong, J. Dissipation and dietary risk assessment of kasugamycin and saisentong in Chinese cabbage. *Environ. Sci. Pollut. Res.* **2020**, *27*, 35228–35238. [CrossRef]
22. Yi, C.; Chen, J.; Hu, D.; Song, B. First report about the screening, characterization, and fosmid library construction of *Xanthomonas oryzae* pv. *oryzae* strain with resistance to Fubianezuofeng. *Pestic. Biochem. Physiol.* **2020**, *169*, 104645. [CrossRef] [PubMed]
23. Cao, B.; Yao, F.; Zheng, X.; Cui, D.; Shao, Y.; Zhu, C.; Deng, Z.; You, D. Genome Mining of the Biosynthetic Gene Cluster of the Polyene Macrolide Antibiotic Tetramycin and Characterization of a P450 Monooxygenase Involved in the Hydroxylation of the Tetramycin B Polyol Segment. *ChemBioChem* **2012**, *13*, 2234–2242. [CrossRef]
24. Ren, J.; Cui, Y.; Zhang, F.; Cui, H.; Ni, X.; Chen, F.; Li, L.; Xia, H. Enhancement of nystatin production by redirecting precursor fluxes after disruption of the tetramycin gene from *Streptomyces ahygroscopicus*. *Microbiol. Res.* **2014**, *169*, 602–608. [CrossRef]
25. Zhao, X.; Zhong, L.; Zhang, Q.; Xu, C.; Zhu, H.; Lu, Z.; Shen, L.; Wang, G.; Jie, D. Effect of tetramycin on mycelia growth and spore germination of rice blast pathogen. *J. Microbiol.* **2010**, *2*, 43–45.
26. Song, Y.; He, L.; Chen, L.; Ren, Y.; Lu, H.; Geng, S.; Mu, W.; Liu, F. Baseline sensitivity and control efficacy of antibiosis fungicide tetramycin against *Botrytis cinerea*. *Eur. J. Plant Pathol.* **2016**, *146*, 337–347. [CrossRef]
27. Chen, L.L.; Guo, B.B.; Li, B.X.; Mu, W.; Liu, F. Toxicity and control efficacy of tetramycin against *Passalora fulva*. *Chin. J. Pestic. Sci.* **2017**, *19*, 324–330.
28. Ma, D.; Zhu, J.; He, L.; Cui, K.; Mu, W.; Liu, F. Baseline Sensitivity and Control Efficacy of Tetramycin against *Phytophthora capsici* Isolates in China. *Plant Dis.* **2017**, *102*, 863–868. [CrossRef] [PubMed]
29. Gao, Y.; He, L.; Li, X.; Lin, J.; Mu, W.; Liu, F. Toxicity and biochemical action of the antibiotic fungicide tetramycin on *Colletotrichum scovillei*. *Pestic. Biochem. Physiol.* **2018**, *147*, 51–58. [CrossRef]
30. Ma, D.; Zhu, J.; Jiang, J.; Zhao, Y.; Li, B.; Mu, W.; Liu, F. Evaluation of bioactivity and control efficacy of tetramycin against *Corynespora cassiicola*. *Pestic. Biochem. Physiol.* **2018**, *152*, 106–113. [CrossRef]
31. Wang, L.P.; Chang, G.B.; Meng, S.; Sun, C.H. Study on the poplar canker disease controlled using four hygromycin in field. *J. Microbiol.* **2014**, *34*, 68–70.
32. Li, H.; Liu, J.B.; Wang, T.J.; Jiang, H.; Zhang, R.B.; Guan, W.J. Research progress of ATP-binding cassette transporters in Polyene antibiotic biosynthesis Gene Cluster. *Microbiol. China* **2014**, *41*, 950–958.
33. Zhong, L.J. Studies on the rice resistance to rice blast induced by tetramycin. *J. Anhui Agric. Sci.* **2010**, *38*, 6263–6264.

antibiotics

MDPI

Article

Grapefruit Seed Extract as a Natural Derived Antibacterial Substance against Multidrug-Resistant Bacteria

Hee-Won Han [1,2], Jin-Hwan Kwak [3], Tae-Su Jang [4], Jonathan Campbell Knowles [1,5,6], Hae-Won Kim [1,2,7,8,9], Hae-Hyoung Lee [1,2,7,*] and Jung-Hwan Lee [1,2,7,8,9,*]

1 Institute of Tissue Regeneration Engineering (ITREN), Dankook University, Cheonan, Chungcheongnam-do 31116, Korea; 12201075@dankook.ac.kr (H.-W.H.); j.knowles@ucl.ac.uk (J.C.K.); kimhw@dku.edu (H.-W.K.)
2 Department of Biomaterials Science, College of Dentistry, Dankook University, Cheonan, Chungcheongnam-do 31116, Korea
3 Department of Life Science, Handong Global University, 558 Handong-ro, Pohang, Gyeongsangbuk-do 37554, Korea; jhkwak@handong.edu
4 Department of Pre-Medi, College of Medicine, Dankook University, 119 Dandae-ro, Cheonan, Chungcheongnam-do 31116, Korea; jangts@dankook.ac.kr
5 UCL Eastman-Korea Dental Medicine Innovation Centre, Dankook University, 119 Dandae-ro, Cheonan, Chungcheongnam-do 31116, Korea
6 Division of Biomaterials and Tissue Engineering, Eastman Dental Institute, University College London, Rowland Hill Street, London NW3 2PF, UK
7 Department of Nanobiomedical Science and BK21 PLUS NBM Global Research Center for Regenerative Medicine, Dankook University, Cheonan, Chungcheongnam-do 31116, Korea
8 Cell & Matter Institute, Dankook University, Cheonan, Chungcheongnam-do 31116, Korea
9 Department of Regenerative Dental Medicine, College of Dentistry, Dankook University, Cheonan, Chungcheongnam-do 31116, Korea
* Correspondence: haelee@dku.edu (H.-H.L.); ducious@gmail.com (J.-H.L.); Tel.: +82-(0)-41-550-3083 (H.-H.L.); +82-41-550-3081 (J.-H.L.); Fax: +82-(0)-41-559-7839 (H.-H.L.); +82-41-559-7839 (J.-H.L.)

Citation: Han, H.-W.; Kwak, J.-H.; Jang, T.-S.; Knowles, J.C.; Kim, H.-W.; Lee, H.-H.; Lee, J.-H. Grapefruit Seed Extract as a Natural Derived Antibacterial Substance against Multidrug-Resistant Bacteria. *Antibiotics* **2021**, *10*, 85. https://doi.org/10.3390/antibiotics10010085

Received: 24 December 2020
Accepted: 15 January 2021
Published: 18 January 2021

Abstract: Multidrug-resistant (MDR) bacteria are increasing due to the abuse and misuse of antibiotics, and nosocomial infections by MDR bacteria are also increasing. The aim of this study was to identify new substances that can target MDR bacteria among 12 plant extracts that are known to have antibacterial effects. The experiments were performed by the disk diffusion test and microdilution minimum inhibitory concentration (MIC) test, as described by the Clinical and Laboratory Standards Institute (CLSI). By screening against methicillin-sensitive *Staphylococcus aureus* (MSSA), grapefruit seed extract (GSE) was selected from 12 plant extracts for subsequent experiments. GSE showed antibacterial effects against methicillin-resistant *S. aureus* (MRSA) and vancomycin-resistant *S. aureus* (VRSA) in the disk diffusion test. Even at the lowest concentration, GSE showed antibacterial activity in the microdilution MIC test. As a result, we can conclude that GSE is a naturally derived antibacterial substance that exhibits a favorable antibacterial effect even at a very low concentration, so it is a good candidate for a natural substance that can be used to prevent or reduce nosocomial infections as coating for materials used in medical contexts or by mixing a small amount with other materials.

Keywords: multidrug-resistant bacteria; nosocomial infection; plant extract; grapefruit seed extract; antibacterial activity

1. Introduction

The number of bacterial strains that are resistant to antibiotics continues to increase due to the misuse and abuse of antibiotics. Among these, bacteria that are resistant to several antibiotics are called multidrug-resistant (MDR) bacteria. For example, methicillin-resistant *Staphylococcus aureus* (MRSA), which was first identified in the early 1960s [1], is resistant to other beta-lactam antibiotics, including those in the penicillin class and cephalosporin class, in addition to methicillin [2]. MDR bacteria constitute the leading cause of nosocomial infection, and outcomes in patients infected with MDR bacteria tend to be worse than for those infected by more sensitive organisms [3–5]. In addition, the mortality rate from MDR bacteria such as MRSA is significantly higher than for susceptible strains [6]. Therefore, efforts to discover new substances that can target MDR bacteria have become increasingly important.

Antibacterial effects are being studied in various fields, such as tissue engineering [7–9], and many experiments have been conducted to identify new substances that can target antibiotic-resistant bacteria. Recently, antimicrobial activity experiments using nanoparticles (NPs) have been actively conducted. The antibacterial effects of nanoparticles such as silver, gold, and ZnO have already been confirmed for over a decade and are still actively being studied [10–14]. In addition, these nanoparticles have also shown antibacterial effects against MDR bacteria such as vancomycin-resistant *Enterococcus* (VRE) and MRSA [15–19]. In addition to nanoparticles, interest in natural products as substitutes for traditional antibiotics to fight multidrug-resistant pathogens has greatly increased [20]. The antibacterial effect of honeydew honey and the antibacterial effects of plant extracts such as black pepper extract, grapefruit seed extract (GSE), and coral *Hibiscus* extract have been proven in many papers [21–27].

Natural products have long been used as the basis for treatment [28]. Most of the drugs on the market today are natural-based products or their derivatives [29], suggesting that natural-based products may be better accepted by the body and more successful than synthetic chemicals [30]. Therefore, we focused on natural products, especially plant extracts.

In this study, 12 plant extracts known for having antibacterial activity were analyzed by disk diffusion test against MSSA. From this screening test, only GSE showed antibacterial effect. Therefore, the purpose of this study was to evaluate the antibacterial activity of GSE against MDR bacteria such as MRSA and VRSA, which cause serious problems through nosocomial infection, and investigate the cause of the antibacterial effect of GSE.

2. Materials and Methods

2.1. Bacterial Strains and Culture Conditions

S. aureus ATCC6538 (MSSA) and *S. aureus* ATCC33591 (MRSA) were purchased from American Type Culture Collection (ATCC; Manassas, VA, USA). *S. aureus* CCARM3795 (MRSA) was purchased from the Culture Collection of Antimicrobial Resistant Microbes (Nowon-gu, Seoul, Korea). VRSA48, which was clinically isolated, was generously provided by the Korea Research Institute of Bioscience & Biotechnology (KRIBB, Yuseong-gu, Daejeon, Korea) through Prof. Jin-Hwan Kwak of Handong Global University (HGU, Buk-gu, Pohang, Korea). All strains, which had been kept as glycerol stock solutions in a −80 °C deep freezer, were streaked on tryptic soy agar (TSA, Difco Laboratories, Becton Dickinson, Sparks, MD, USA) plates and incubated at 35 °C ± 2 °C for 18 h. A single colony, after incubation, was transferred to tryptic soy broth (TSB, Difco Laboratories, Sparks, MD, USA) and incubated with shaking at 35 °C ± 2 °C for 18 h. To achieve the desired concentration, dilutions were performed with phosphate-buffered saline (PBS; Gibco, Grand Island, NY, USA) for the disk diffusion test and TSB media for the microdilution minimum inhibitory concentration (MIC) test.

2.2. Plant Extracts and Antimicrobial Agents

Among the natural extracts already used in soaps and cosmetics on the market, but not applicable for biomedical settings now, twelve extracts that have antibacterial activity and are considered economical were purchased and used. Bamboo extract was purchased from KoreaSimilac (Pocheon, Gyeonggi-do, Korea). Refined wood vinegar, rosemary, *Pinus densiflora* leaf, *Sophora*, *Cinnamomum cassia* bark, *Hibiscus sabdariffa* flower, *Chamomilla recutita* (*Matricaria*) flower, *Centella asiatica*, *Houttuynia cordata*, and Yucca extracts were purchased from HERBFLORA (Dobong-gu, Seoul, Korea). Grapefruit seed extract (GSE) was purchased from CANDLEIKEA (Jung-gu, Seoul, Korea). Bamboo, rosemary, *Sophora*,

Centella asiatica, *Houttuynia cordata*, and Yucca extracts were extracted by hot water extraction. *Cinnamomum cassia* bark, *Hibiscus sabdariffa* flower, and *Chamomilla recutita* (*Matricaria*) flower extracts were extracted by low temperature extraction. The extraction types for refined wood vinegar, *Pinus densiflora leaf*, and Grapefruit seed extracts are unrevealed due to the company's confidentiality. Vancomycin (VAN), oxacillin (OXA), and linezolid (LZD) were purchased from Sigma-Aldrich (St. Louis, MO, USA).

2.3. *pH Measurements*

The pH of GSE, 76% G (76% glycerol), and pH 76% G (pH-adjusted 76% glycerol) were measured with a pH meter (inoLab pH 7110, WTW, Weilheim, Germany). The 76% glycerol solution was prepared by adding distilled water (DW) to glycerol (≥99.0%, Sigma-Aldrich, St. Louis, MO, USA), and pH 76% G was derived from 76% G using acetic acid. The electrode was soaked in each solution at room temperature (24 °C), and each measurement was repeated three times and averaged.

2.4. *GSE Analysis by LC-MS and LC-MS/MS*

GSE was analyzed by liquid chromatography/mass spectrometry (LC-MS) and liquid chromatography/tandem mass spectrometry (LC-MS/MS) with an Ultimate 3000 RS-Q-Exactive Orbitrap Plus (Thermo Fisher Scientific, Waltham, MA, USA) at the Yonsei Center for Research Facilities (YCRF, Seodaemun-gu, Seoul, Korea). For the negative-mode LC condition, an Acquity UPLC BEH C18 (1.7 µm, 2.1 × 100 mm) was used as an LC column at 40 °C. The injection volume was 3 µL. The run time was 12 min. The mobile phase consisting of solvent A, 6.5 mM ammonium bicarbonate in DW, and solvent B, 6.5 mM ammonium bicarbonate in acetonitrile (ACN) was delivered at a flow rate of 0.4 mL/min. The following linear gradient was used: 0 min, 0% B; 1 min, 10% B; 9 min, 100% B; 12 min; 10% B. The electrospray ionization (ESI) (negative ionization mode) conditions were capillary voltage was 3.0 kV, S-lens RF level was 45, capillary temperature was 370 °C, and aux gas heater temperature was 285 °C. The sheath and aux gas flows were 60 and 20, respectively.

2.5. *In Vitro Studies*

2.5.1. Disk Diffusion Test

All strains that were grown on TSA plates at 35 °C ± 2 °C for 18 h were subcultured separately into 3 mL of TSB media at 35 °C ± 2 °C for 18 h. The cultured bacteria were diluted using PBS to obtain bacterial cell densities of approximately 1~2 × 10^8 CFU (colony forming unit)/mL, and then the diluted bacterial suspensions were spread using sterilized cotton swabs on TSA plates (100 mm × 15 mm). Bacterial concentration was determined by measuring the optical density at 600 nm with a spectrophotometer. The actual number of colonies was confirmed by diluting the bacterial culture solution that was diluted to the desired concentration to 10^3 CFU/mL, dropping 100 µL on an MHA plate, spreading and incubating. After allowing the surface of each medium to dry for 3–5 min, ADVANTEC paper disks (8 mm/0.7 mm) that had been sterilized with ethylene gas were placed on TSA plates and pressed with forceps to ensure complete contact with each agar surface. For the screening test, 20 µL of plant extract and linezolid (1.5 mg/mL) were loaded onto paper disks on agar plates spread with *S. aureus* ATCC6538 (MSSA). To check the antibacterial effect of GSE on MDR bacteria, 20 µL of GSE and linezolid (1.5 mg/mL) were loaded onto paper disks on separate agar plates spread with MSSA and MDR bacteria. To investigate the effects of glycerol and pH on bacterial growth, 20 µL of GSE, 76% G, pH 76% G and linezolid (1.5 mg/mL) were loaded separately onto paper disks on plates spread with MSSA or MDR bacteria, and then agar plates were incubated at 35 °C ± 2 °C for 18 h. After incubation, the diameters of the inhibition zones were measured from edge to edge across the centers of the disks. All experiments were conducted 3 times.

2.5.2. Microdilution MIC Test

The MICs of GSE, 76% G, pH 76% G, pH 76% G with naringin (1.7 mg/mL), and antimicrobial agents were determined using the twofold microdilution broth method. Naringin was dissolved in DMSO first and then diluted with pH 76% G, and all other test compounds were diluted with DW. GSE, 76% G, pH 76% G, and pH 76% G with naringin (1.7 mg/mL) were diluted to yield 10 concentrations from undiluted solution to 1/512, and antimicrobial agents were diluted to yield 10 concentrations from 64 μg to 0.125 μg/mL. All strains that were grown on TSA plates at 35 °C ± 2 °C for 18 h were subcultured into 3 mL of TSB media at 35 °C ± 2 °C for 18 h. The cultured bacterial broth suspensions were diluted using TSB media to obtain bacterial cell densities of approximately 1×10^6 CFU/mL. One-hundred microliters of each diluted bacterial suspension were seeded in 96-well plates containing 100 μL of serially diluted test compounds to achieve a bacterial concentration of 5×10^5 CFU/well, which also resulted in 1/2 dilution of test compounds. The 96-well plates were incubated at 35 °C ± 2 °C for 18 h. MICs were defined as the lowest concentrations that completely inhibited the growth of bacteria when viewed with the unaided eye. As the MIC test was performed by finding the MIC values of the antibiotics for each bacterium several times, each MIC test including GSE was completed in one experiment.

2.6. Statistical Analysis

All data are shown as mean ± SD. In each experiment, n is the number of repeated trials. Statistical significance was determined by unpaired, two-tailed t-tests for differences between two groups and using one-way ANOVA and Dunnett's multiple comparisons tests for differences among more than two groups. GraphPad Prism 8 software (San Diego, CA, USA) was used.

3. Results and Discussion

3.1. Antibacterial Effect of GSE in Disk Diffusion Test

Among the commercially available plant extracts, 12 types of extracts that are known to have antibacterial effects were purchased, and the antibacterial activities of 12 extracts (specified as numbers in Table S1) were analyzed against MSSA ATCC6538 (Figure S1) by the disk diffusion test. The disk diffusion test is a standard method described by the Clinical and Laboratory Standards Institute (CLSI) and is an experimental method that can quickly and easily evaluate the antibacterial activity of many compounds [31]. If an extract exerts an antibacterial effect, an inhibition zone will form around the paper disk where the extract was dropped. A highly effective antibacterial agent produces a wide ring without bacterial growth, whereas an ineffective antibacterial agent shows no change in the concentration of bacteria around it. Except for GSE, the other plant extracts showed no antibacterial effects against MSSA in the disk diffusion test. For subsequent experiments, therefore, only GSE was used. GSE showed inhibition zones against MDR bacteria (MRSA and VRSA) as well as MSSA (Figure 1). The inhibition zones of GSE against MSSA, MRSA 33591, MRSA 3795, and VRSA48 were 18.3 ± 0.6 mm, 16.8 ± 0.6 mm, 18.8 ± 0.3 mm, and 16.4 ± 0.4 mm, respectively (n = 3). In the experiment with VRSA48, there were two circles surrounding the GSE paper disk. One was a small circle (real inhibition zone), and the other was a larger circle (zone of incomplete inhibition of bacterial growth). Therefore, the smaller circle was measured as the inhibition zone. GSE showed antibacterial effects against all tested bacteria. The inhibition zones of LZD, which was used as a control, against MSSA, MRSA 33591, MRSA 3795, and VRSA48, were 28.8 ± 0.3 mm, 29.3 ± 0.6 mm, 24.6 ± 0.5 mm, and 25.7 ± 0.4 mm, respectively (n = 3). These diameter values were illustrated with bar graphs. All tested bacteria were susceptible to LZD, according to the CLSI guidelines (≥21 mm for *Staphylococcus* spp.) [31]. Although the inhibition zone for GSE was smaller than that of LZD, the antibacterial effect of GSE was confirmed through a disk diffusion test. In the next experiment, the pH and percentage of the solvent of the GSE were measured because the antibacterial effect of GSE may occur due to the solvent in which the GSE was dissolved or the acidic properties of the GSE itself.

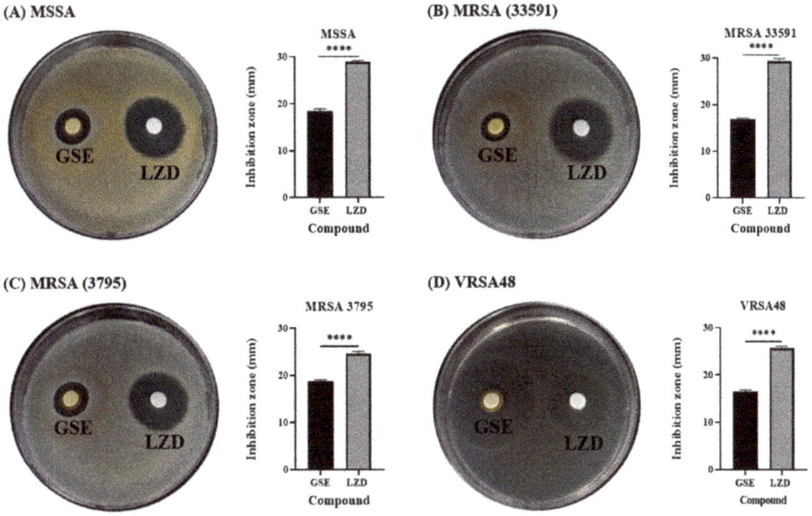

Figure 1. Disk diffusion tests and inhibition zone diameters for Grapefruit seed extract (GSE) and linezolid (LZD) against methicillin-sensitive *Staphylococcus aureus* (MSSA), methicillin-resistant *S. aureus* (MRSA), and VRSA. (**A**) *S. aureus* ATCC 6538 (MSSA), (**B**) *S. aureus* ATCC 33591 (MRSA), (**C**) *S. aureus* CCARM 3795 (MRSA), and (**D**) vancomycin-resistant *S. aureus* (VRSA48). The concentration of LZD was 30 μg/disk, following the CLSI guidelines. The diameters of the inhibition zones for GSE and LZD are illustrated by the bar graphs as the means ± SD ($n = 3$). All tested bacteria were susceptible to LZD, according to the CLSI guidelines (≥21 mm for *Staphylococcus* spp.), and GSE also showed antibacterial effects against all tested bacteria. p values were calculated using two-tailed, unpaired t-tests in this figure. **** $p < 0.0001$.

3.2. GSE Characterization

As the pH or solvent of GSE solutions could affect bacterial growth, the pH of the GSE and the percentage solvent were measured with a pH meter (inoLab pH 7110, Germany) and an LC-MS/MS system (Thermo Fisher Scientific, Waltham, MA, USA), respectively. Glycerol was analyzed quantitatively because we had received information from HERBFLORA (Seoul, Korea) that the GSE extract was dissolved in glycerol that is highly effective for obtaining phenolic compounds [32]. It was confirmed that the pH of GSE was 2.90 ± 0.04 ($n = 3$) and that the GSE extract was dissolved in 76% glycerol (Figure 2). Based on these results, 76% glycerol (76% G throughout the paper) was prepared, and pH-adjusted 76% glycerol (pH 76% G throughout the paper) was prepared from 76% G using acetic acid. The pH of 76% G and pH 76% G were measured using a pH meter (inoLab pH 7110, Germany) and showed pH values of 4.37 ± 0.06 and 2.94 ± 0.01, respectively ($n = 3$). The pH 76% G was prepared carefully without any significant difference from the pH of GSE. The antibacterial effect of GSE is already known, and since it is known that GSE contains flavonoids with antimicrobial effects, flavonoids were also analyzed by LC-MS and LC-MS/MS in addition to glycerol [25,26,33–35]. GSE is known to contain relatively large amounts of the flavonoid naringin, so naringin was quantitatively analyzed. Glycerol and naringin were analyzed by LC-MS/MS, and the other flavonoids hesperidin, eriocitrin, poncirin, and quercetin were analyzed by LC-MS. To measure the concentration of glycerol and naringin in GSE, reference compounds glycerol (≥99.0%, Sigma-Aldrich, St. Louis, MO, USA) and naringin (≥95.0%, Sigma-Aldrich, St. Louis, MO, USA) were purchased. These reagents dissolved in DW were measured by LC-MS/MS, and then compared with GSE analysis results. Glycerol concentration was measured at 762.544 mg/mL (it was considered to be 760 mg/mL, 76%) at 0.63 min, and naringin concentration was determined as 1.726 mg/mL (it was considered to be 1.7 mg/mL) at 3.64 min. From the LC-MS results, quercetin and hesperidin were identified at 0.74 min and 3.70 min, respectively, in GSE (Figure S2). However, because the quercetin and hesperidin concentrations were very low, no peaks were seen in Figure 2B. Eriocitrin and poncirin were not detected in GSE.

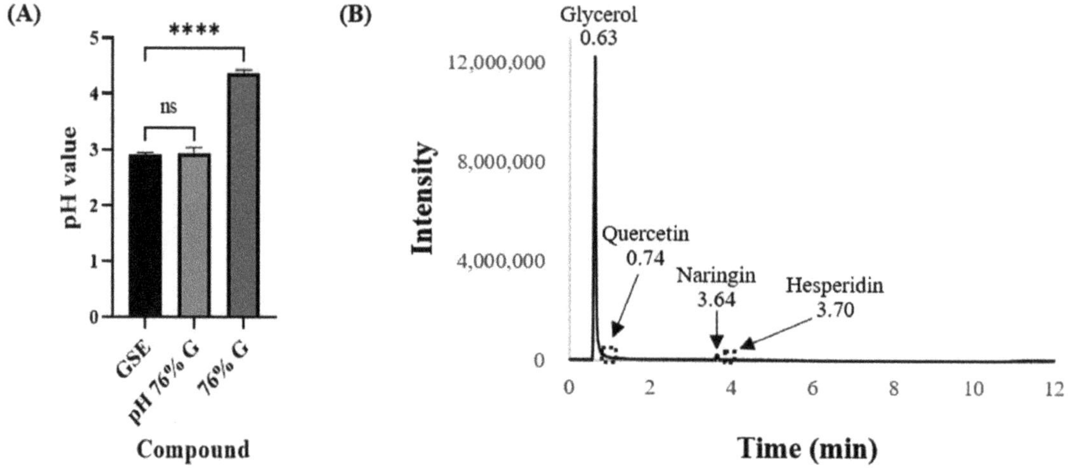

Figure 2. GSE characterization. (**A**) The pH values for GSE, 76% G, and pH 76% G. The pH values of the tested compounds are illustrated by the bar graphs as the means ± SD ($n = 3$). The pH 76% G was prepared from 76% G using acetic acid, and it did not show any significant difference from the pH value of GSE. (**B**) LC-MS/MS results of GSE. Glycerol and naringin were analyzed by LC-MS/MS and LC-MS for quercetin and hesperidin. Because the peaks for quercetin and hesperidin were too small (not visible on the graph), their peaks were replaced by dashed boxes. The numbers above the arrows and peaks represent the retention times. p values were calculated using one-way ANOVA with Dunnett's multiple comparisons test in this figure. ns, not significant; **** $p < 0.0001$.

3.3. *Antibacterial Effects of Solvent and pH of GSE in Disk Diffusion Tests*

GSE dissolved in 76% G was analyzed, and it also had a low pH value. Because high concentrations of glycerol and low pH can affect bacterial growth [36,37], the antimicrobial activity of 76% G and pH 76% G was evaluated along with GSE and LZD. In disk diffusion tests, GSE and LZD showed effects almost identical to those shown in Figure 1, but 76% G and pH 76% G did not show any inhibition zones against any tested bacteria (Figure 3). Therefore, 76% G and pH 76% G were marked as N.D. (not detected) in bar graphs. In the experiment with VRSA48, it appeared that an inhibition zone formed in the glycerol group, but bacterial growth was checked inside the circle which resembled an inhibition zone. From disk diffusion tests, we found that glycerol and the pH of GSE have little effect on the antibacterial effect of GSE.

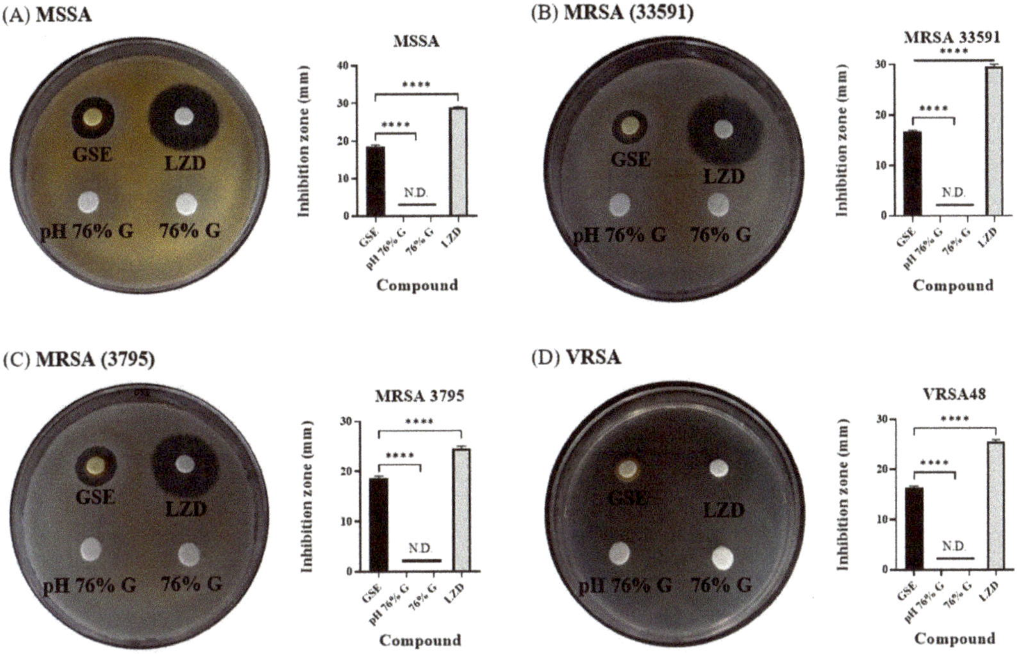

Figure 3. Disk diffusion tests and inhibition zone diameters for the tested compounds and LZD against MSSA, MRSA, and VRSA. (**A**) *S. aureus* ATCC 6538 (MSSA), (**B**) *S. aureus* ATCC 33591 (MRSA), (**C**) *S. aureus* CCARM 3795 (MRSA), and (**D**) VRSA48. The concentration of LZD was 30 μg/disk. N.D. means that an inhibition zone was not detected. The diameters of the inhibition zones for GSE and LZD are illustrated by the bar graphs as means ± SD ($n = 3$). GSE and LZD showed antibacterial effects, as shown in Figure 1, but 76% G and pH 76% G did not show any inhibition zones. This indicates that glycerol and the pH of GSE have little influence on the antibacterial effect of GSE. p values were calculated using one-way ANOVA with Dunnett's multiple comparisons test in this figure. **** $p < 0.0001$.

3.4. Antibacterial Effects of Solvent and pH of GSE in Microdilution MIC Test

To further investigate whether glycerol or the pH of GSE influenced the antimicrobial activity of GSE, microdilution MIC tests were performed. The MIC test is also a standard method described by the CLSI. This method is more detailed than the disk diffusion test because it shows antibacterial effects according to various concentrations. In the 96-well plate figures, the MICs of pH 76% G and 76% G are indicated by red arrows and the MICs of antibiotics by blue arrows. The MIC of GSE and the MIC for >32 μg/mL antibiotic are not indicated. In MIC tests, GSE showed potent antibacterial activity against all tested bacteria. Even at a concentration of 1/1024, the growth of all tested bacteria was suppressed. The red dots that resemble bacterial colonies at the 1/64 and 1/128 concentrations and the turbidity seen in the other concentration groups were the result of the influence of the GSE itself (Figure S3), and it was confirmed that bacteria did not grow in the 1/2 through the 1/1024 concentrations by checking values of CFU (data not shown). The 76% G and pH 76% G treatments showed slight antibacterial effects in MIC tests. pH 76% G showed a MIC value one level lower (1/4 concentration) than that for 76% G (1/2 concentration), except for MRSA. For MRSA, both 76% G and pH 76% G showed a MIC value at 1/2 concentration. Antibiotics were used as controls to check if the experiment was performed properly, and they were also used to check MRSA and VRSA. MSSA and MRSA can be distinguished through the OXA MIC value (≥4 μg/mL, MRSA), and VRSA can be identified through the VAN MIC value

(≥16 μg/mL, VRSA) [31]. VAN, OXA, and LZD showed MIC values of 1 μg/mL, 0.25 μg/mL, and 2 μg/mL against MSSA, respectively. VAN, OXA, and LZD showed MIC values of 1 μg/mL, >32 μg/mL, and 1 μg/mL against MRSA 33591, respectively. VAN, OXA, and LZD showed MIC values of 1 μg/mL, >32 μg/mL, and 1 μg/mL against MRSA 3795, respectively. VAN, OXA, and LZD showed MIC values of >32 μg/mL, >32 μg/mL, and 4 μg/mL against VRSA48, respectively. These results are illustrated as bar graphs. The MICs of GSE, pH 76% G, and 76% G can be read as values of the left *y*-axis (red arrow), and MICs of antibiotics can be read as values of the right *y*-axis (blue arrow). GSE was expressed as <1/1024, as bacteria did not grow even at 1/1024 concentration in any experimental groups. For antibiotics, MIC was expressed as >32 if the growth of bacteria was not inhibited even at a concentration of 32 μg/mL. Based on these antibiotic MIC values, MSSA, MRSA, and VRSA could be identified, and the reliability of the experiment was confirmed. As the MIC test was performed by finding the MIC values of the antibiotics for each bacterial strain several times, each MIC test including that for GSE was completed in one experiment. In disk diffusion tests and MIC tests, it was confirmed that the pH and glycerol did not significantly affect the antimicrobial activity of GSE. This result signifies that there are substances that affect the antibacterial activity of GSE in addition to the pH and solvent of GSE. Several articles related to the antibacterial activity of GSE or other plants have indicated that flavonoids have antibacterial activity [38–40]. GSE contained a large amount of the flavonoid naringin, so the following experiment was conducted by focusing on naringin.

3.5. Antibacterial Effect of Naringin

The antimicrobial activity of naringin against several bacterial species, including *S. aureus*, has already been confirmed in several papers [39,41–43]. The experiment was conducted after preparing a pH 76% G solution containing 1.7 mg/mL naringin. It is indicated as "pH 76% G (naringin)" in figures. In the 96-well plate figures, the MICs of pH 76% G and 76% G are indicated by red arrows, and antibiotic MICs are indicated by blue arrows. The MIC of GSE and the MICs for >32 μg/mL antibiotic are not indicated. In the bar graphs, the MICs of GSE and pH 76% G (naringin) can be read as values of the left *y*-axis (red arrow), and MICs of antibiotics can be read as values of the right *y*-axis (blue arrow). Compared to the results in Figure 4, GSE and antibiotics showed identical MIC values. The pH 76% G (naringin) also showed the same effects as pH 76% G without naringin against MSSA, MRSA 33591, MRSA 3795, and VRSA48. From the results of Figure 5, we knew that naringin did not play an important role in the antibacterial activity of GSE. The antibacterial effect of GSE can be exhibited by benzethonium chloride, a preservative commonly used in commercial GSE [44], but the GSE used in this experiment was confirmed by the manufacturer to be free of benzethonium chloride. Furthermore, the antimicrobial effect of GSE may result from synergistic effects of flavonoids [45]. However, because the concentrations of flavonoids other than naringin are quite small, the probability of a synergistic effect is very low. These our experiments and results can indirectly support the claim that the other phenolic compounds other than flavonoids in GSE contribute to the antimicrobial effects of GSE [46]. However, LC-MS/MS analysis was conducted without removing the solvent (glycerol) to find out the concentration of glycerol and to eliminate the potential risk that the filter to make concentrated GSE could filter out substances with antibacterial activity. Therefore, an experiment to analyze concentrated GSE is required, and then additional experiments to confirm the antibacterial activity of flavonoids and other phenolic compounds are required.

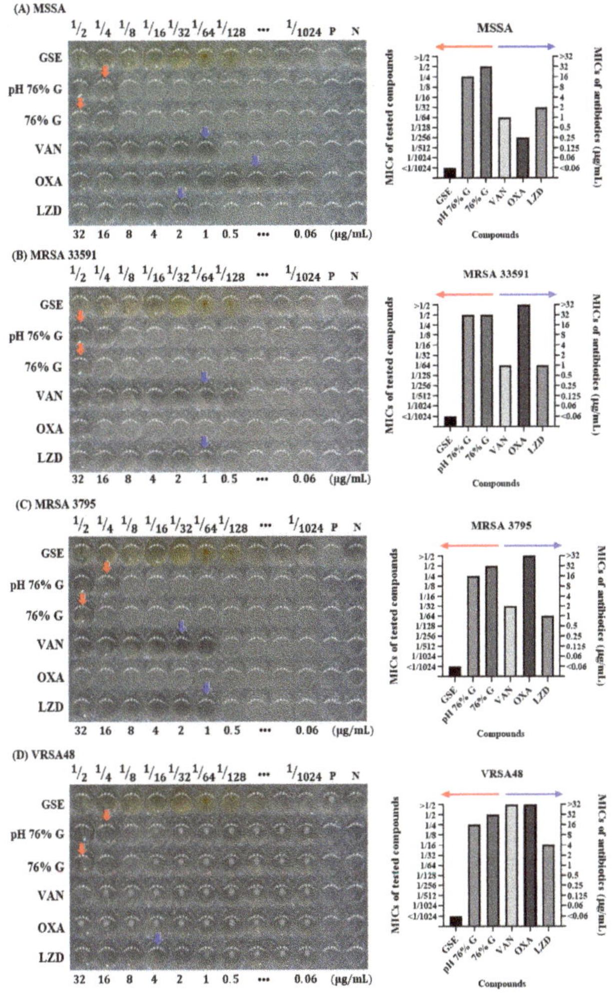

Figure 4. Microdilution minimum inhibitory concentration (MIC) tests for compounds and antibiotics tested against MSSA, MRSA, and VRSA. (**A**) *S. aureus* ATCC 6538 (MSSA), (**B**) *S. aureus* ATCC 33591 (MRSA), (**C**) *S. aureus* CCARM 3795 (MRSA), and (**D**) VRSA48. P is a positive control without any antimicrobial agents, and N is a negative control with only media and DW. In the 96-well plate, from left to right, the tested compound concentrations were 1/2 to 1/1024, and the concentrations of antibiotics were 32 to 0.06 µg/mL. The MICs of pH 76% G and 76% G are indicated by red arrows, and those for antibiotics are indicated by blue arrows. MIC values <1/1024 or >32 µg/mL are not indicated by arrows. The MIC values of the tested compounds and antibiotics for each of the bacterial strains are also illustrated by bar graphs next to the 96-well plate figures. In the bar graph, the MIC values of the tested compounds can be read along the left *y*-axis indicated by the red arrow, and the MIC values of antibiotics along the right *y*-axis are indicated by the blue arrow. MRSA 335591 and 3795 showed OXA MIC values >32 µg/mL, confirmed to be MRSA, and VRSA48 also showed MIC values >32 µg/mL for OXA and VAN, confirming VRSA. The GSE showed MIC values of <1/1024 concentration for all tested bacteria. Excluding MRSA 33591, pH 76% G showed an MIC value (1/4 concentration) lower than 76% G (1/2 concentration), but it was still insufficient to explain the antibacterial effect of GSE.

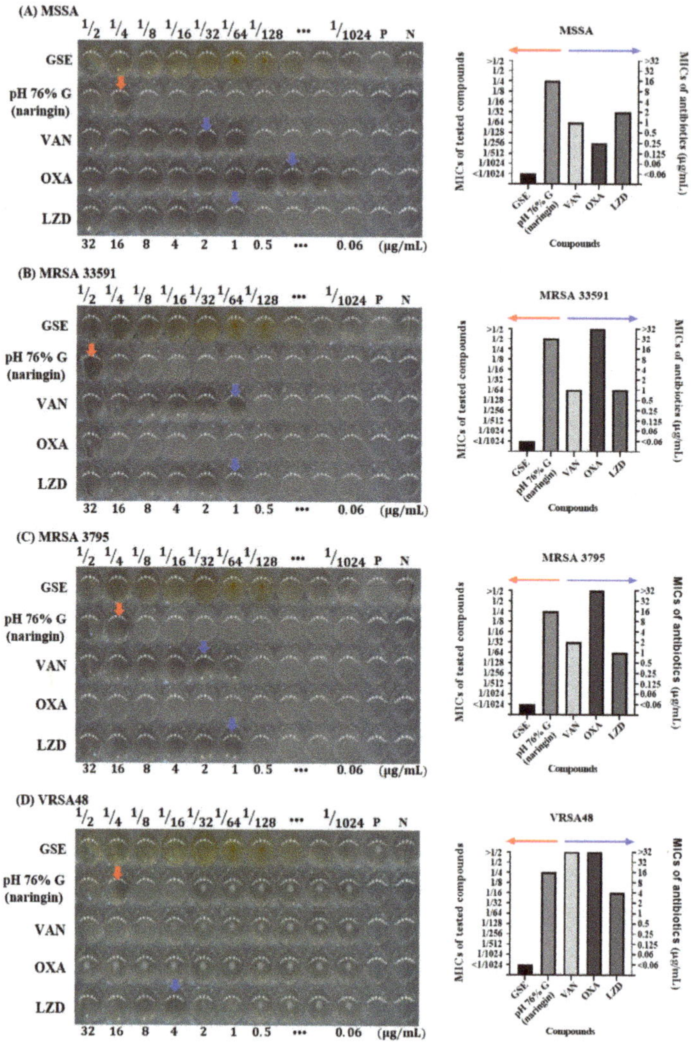

Figure 5. Microdilution MIC test with naringin against MSSA, MRSA, and VRSA. (**A**) *S. aureus* ATCC 6538 (MSSA), (**B**) *S. aureus* ATCC 33591 (MRSA), (**C**) *S. aureus* CCARM 3795 (MRSA), and (**D**) VRSA48. P is a positive control without any antimicrobial agents, and N is a negative control with only media and DW. In the 96-well plate, from left to right, the GSE and pH 76% G (naringin) concentrations were 1/2 to 1/1024, and the concentrations of antibiotics were 32 to 0.06 μg/mL. The MICs of pH 76% G (naringin) are indicated by red arrows, and antibiotic MICs are indicated by blue arrows. MIC values <1/1024 or >32 μg/mL are not indicated by arrows. The MIC values for GSE, pH 76% G (naringin), and antibiotics for each of the bacterial strains are also illustrated by bar graphs next to the 96-well plate figures. In the bar graphs, the MIC values of GSE and pH 76% G (naringin) can be read along the left *y*-axis indicated by the red arrow, and the MIC values of antibiotics can be read along the right *y*-axis indicated by the blue arrow. GSE and the antibiotics showed the same effect, as shown in Figure 4. The pH 76% G (naringin) did not show a better effect than the pH 76% G. This indicates that substances other than naringin in GSE affect the antibacterial activity of GSE.

4. Conclusions

There are many papers on the antibacterial activity of GSE. They have shown antibacterial activity of GSE against MDR bacteria such as MRSA and VRE (vancomycin-resistant enterococci). However, the antibacterial effect of GSE on VRSA was first mentioned in this paper. GSE showed antibacterial activity against MSSA, MRSA, and VRSA in disk diffusion and microdilution MIC tests. The experiments were conducted with glycerol, acidic conditions, and naringin, which were expected to have antimicrobial activity, but the antibacterial effect of GSE was not sufficiently explained. Nevertheless, since GSE exerts favorable antimicrobial activity against not only MSSA but also MDR bacteria, it can be a valuable natural substance for preventing or reducing nosocomial infection, and further analysis is likely to be needed.

Supplementary Materials: The following are available online at https://www.mdpi.com/2079-6382/10/1/85/s1, Figure S1: Antibacterial activity in 12 plant extract screening tests against MSSA; Figure S2. LC-MS Chromatogram of quercetin and hesperidin. LC–MS chromatograms showing; Figure S3. GSE incubation without bacteria and antimicrobial agents Table S1: List of plant extracts used for the antibacterial activity test.

Author Contributions: Conceptualization, H.-W.H., J.-H.K., and J.-H.L.; formal analysis, H.-W.H.; funding acquisition, H.-H.L. and J.-H.L.; investigation, H.-W.H.; project administration, T.-S.J., J.C.K., and J.-H.L.; resources, J.-H.K.; supervision, H.-H.L. and J.-H.L.; writing—original draft, H.-W.H.; writing—review and editing, T.-S.J., H.-W.K., H.-H.L., and J.-H.L. All authors have read and agreed to the published version of the manuscript.

Funding: National Research Foundation of Korea: 2019R1C1C1002490; Ministry of Science and ICT, South Korea: 2020R1A2C1005867; Global Research Development Center: 2018K1A4A3A01064257; Priority Research Center: 2019R1A6A1A11034536; University Innovation Support Program.

Data Availability Statement: Not applicable.

Acknowledgments: This work was supported by a National Research Foundation of Korea (NRF) grant funded by the Ministry of Science and ICT (2019R1C1C1002490 and 2020R1A2C1005867), by the Global Research Development Center Program (2018K1A4A3A01064257) and by the Priority Research Center Program provided by the Ministry of Education (2019R1A6A1A11034536). The present research was also supported by the research fund of Dankook University in 2019 for the University Innovation Support Program.

Conflicts of Interest: The authors declare no conflict of interest. The funders had no role in the design of the study; in the collection, analyses, or interpretation of data; in the writing of the manuscript; or in the decision to publish the results.

References

1. Jevons, M.P. "Celbenin"-resistant staphylococci. *Br. Med. J.* **1961**, *1*, 124. [CrossRef]
2. Magiorakos, A.-P.; Srinivasan, A.; Carey, R.T.; Carmeli, Y.; Falagas, M.T.; Giske, C.T.; Harbarth, S.; Hindler, J.T.; Kahlmeter, G.; Olsson-Liljequist, B. Multidrug-resistant, extensively drug-resistant and pandrug-resistant bacteria: An international expert proposal for interim standard definitions for acquired resistance. *Clin. Microbiol. Infect.* **2012**, *18*, 268–281. [CrossRef] [PubMed]
3. Anudit, C.; Kooltheat, N.; Potup, P.; Sranujit, R.P.; Usuwanthim, K. Nosocomial infection of multidrug-resistant *Acinetobacter baumannii* in Thailand. *Am. J. Infect. Control.* **2016**, *44*, 1161–1163. [CrossRef] [PubMed]
4. Bodi, M.; Ardanuy, C.; Rello, J. Impact of Gram-positive resistance on outcome of nosocomial pneumonia. *Crit. Care Med.* **2001**, *29*, N82–N86. [CrossRef]
5. Vardakas, K.Z.; Rafailidis, P.I.; Konstantelias, A.A.; Falagas, M.E. Predictors of mortality in patients with infections due to multi-drug resistant Gram negative bacteria: The study, the patient, the bug or the drug? *J. Infect.* **2013**, *66*, 401–414. [CrossRef]
6. Gandra, S.; Tseng, K.K.; Arora, A.; Bhowmik, B.; Robinson, M.L.; Panigrahi, B.; Laxminarayan, R.; Klein, E.Y. The mortality burden of multidrug-resistant pathogens in India: A retrospective, observational study. *Clin. Infect. Dis.* **2019**, *69*, 563–570. [CrossRef]
7. Qiao, S.; Wu, D.; Li, Z.; Zhu, Y.; Zhan, F.; Lai, H.; Gu, Y. The combination of multi-functional ingredients-loaded hydrogels and three-dimensional printed porous titanium alloys for infective bone defect treatment. *J. Tissue Eng.* **2020**, *11*. [CrossRef]
8. Singh, R.K.; Knowles, J.C.; Kim, H.-W. Advances in nanoparticle development for improved therapeutics delivery: Nanoscale topographical aspect. *J. Tissue Eng.* **2019**, *10*. [CrossRef]

9. Wang, Z.; Liu, H.; Luo, W.; Cai, T.; Li, Z.; Liu, Y.; Gao, W.; Wan, Q.; Wang, X.; Wang, J. Regeneration of skeletal system with genipin crosslinked biomaterials. *J. Tissue Eng.* **2020**, *11*. [CrossRef]
10. Martínez-Castañon, G.-A.; Nino-Martinez, N.; Martinez-Gutierrez, F.; Martinez-Mendoza, J.; Ruiz, F. Synthesis and antibacterial activity of silver nanoparticles with different sizes. *J. Nanopart. Res.* **2008**, *10*, 1343–1348. [CrossRef]
11. Guzman, M.; Dille, J.; Godet, S. Synthesis and antibacterial activity of silver nanoparticles against gram-positive and gram-negative bacteria. *Nanomed. Nanotechnol. Biol. Med.* **2012**, *8*, 37–45. [CrossRef] [PubMed]
12. Zhou, Y.; Kong, Y.; Kundu, S.; Cirillo, J.D.; Liang, H. Antibacterial activities of gold and silver nanoparticles against *Escherichia coli* and bacillus Calmette-Guérin. *J. Nanobiotechnol.* **2012**, *10*, 19. [CrossRef] [PubMed]
13. Jones, N.; Ray, B.; Ranjit, K.T.; Manna, A.C. Antibacterial activity of ZnO nanoparticle suspensions on a broad spectrum of microorganisms. *FEMS Microbiol. Lett.* **2008**, *279*, 71–76. [CrossRef] [PubMed]
14. Da Silva, B.L.; Caetano, B.L.; Chiari-Andréo, B.G.; Pietro, R.C.L.R.; Chiavacci, L.A. Increased antibacterial activity of ZnO nanoparticles: Influence of size and surface modification. *Colloids Surf. B Biointerfaces* **2019**, *177*, 440–447. [CrossRef]
15. Dasari, T.S.; Zhang, Y.; Yu, H. Antibacterial activity and cytotoxicity of gold (I) and (III) ions and gold nanoparticles. *Biochem. Pharmacol. Open Access* **2015**, *4*, 199. [CrossRef]
16. Lakkim, V.; Reddy, M.C.; Pallavali, R.R.; Reddy, K.R.; Reddy, C.V.; Inamuddin; Bilgrami, A.L.; Lomada, D. Green synthesis of silver nanoparticles and evaluation of their antibacterial activity against multidrug-resistant bacteria and wound healing efficacy using a murine model. *Antibiotics* **2020**, *9*, 902. [CrossRef]
17. Tang, S.; Zheng, J. Antibacterial activity of silver nanoparticles: Structural effects. *Adv. Healthc. Mater.* **2018**, *7*, 1701503. [CrossRef]
18. Tiwari, V.; Mishra, N.; Gadani, K.; Solanki, P.S.; Shah, N.; Tiwari, M. Mechanism of anti-bacterial activity of zinc oxide nanoparticle against carbapenem-resistant Acinetobacter baumannii. *Front. Microbiol.* **2018**, *9*, 1218. [CrossRef]
19. Yang, X.; Yang, J.; Wang, L.; Ran, B.; Jia, Y.; Zhang, L.; Yang, G.; Shao, H.; Jiang, X. Pharmaceutical intermediate-modified gold nanoparticles: Against multidrug-resistant bacteria and wound-healing application via an electrospun scaffold. *ACS Nano* **2017**, *11*, 5737–5745. [CrossRef]
20. Abdallah, E.M.; Koko, W.S. Medicinal plants of antimicrobial and immunomodulating properties. In *Antimicrobial Research: Novelbioknowledge and Educational Programs*; Formatex Research Center: Badajoz, Spain, 2017; pp. 127–139.
21. Ng, W.-J.; Sit, N.-W.; Ooi, P.A.-C.; Ee, K.-Y.; Lim, T.-M. The antibacterial potential of honeydew honey produced by stingless bee (*Heterotrigona itama*) against antibiotic resistant bacteria. *Antibiotics* **2020**, *9*, 871. [CrossRef]
22. Chen, W.; Tang, H.; Jiang, N.; Zhong, Q.; Hu, Y.; Chen, H.; Chen, W. Antibacterial effect of black pepper petroleum ether extract against *Listeria monocytogenes* and *Salmonella typhimurium*. *J. Food Qual.* **2019**, *2019*, 2356161. [CrossRef]
23. Zaki, N.; Al-Oqaili, R.; Tahreer, H. Antibacterial effect of ginger and black pepper extracts (alone and in combination) with sesame oil on some pathogenic bacteria. *World J. Pharm. Pharm. Sci.* **2015**, *4*, 774–784.
24. Zou, L.; Hu, Y.-Y.; Chen, W.-X. Antibacterial mechanism and activities of black pepper chloroform extract. *J. Food Sci. Technol.* **2015**, *52*, 8196–8203. [CrossRef] [PubMed]
25. Heggers, J.P.; Cottingham, J.; Gusman, J.; Reagor, L.; McCoy, L.; Carino, E.; Cox, R.; Zhao, J.-G. The effectiveness of processed grapefruit-seed extract as an antibacterial agent: II. Mechanism of action and in vitro toxicity. *J. Altern. Complement. Med.* **2002**, *8*, 333–340. [CrossRef] [PubMed]
26. Reagor, L.; Gusman, J.; McCoy, L.; Carino, E.; Heggers, J.P. The effectiveness of processed grapefruit-seed extract as an antibacterial agent: I. An in vitro agar assay. *J. Altern. Complement. Med.* **2002**, *8*, 325–332. [CrossRef]
27. El-Shiekh, R.A.; Abdelmohsen, U.R.; Ashour, H.M.; Ashour, R.M. Novel antiviral and antibacterial activities of *Hibiscus schizopetalus*. *Antibiotics* **2020**, *9*, 756. [CrossRef]
28. Cragg, G.M.; Newman, D.J. Medicinals for the millennia: The historical record. *Ann. N. Y. Acad. Sci.* **2001**, *953*, 3–25. [CrossRef]
29. Andrade-Carrera, B.; Clares, B.; Noé, V.; Mallandrich, M.; Calpena, A.C.; García, M.L.; Garduño-Ramírez, M.L. Cytotoxic evaluation of (2S)-5, 7-dihydroxy-6-prenylflavanone derivatives loaded PLGA nanoparticles against MiaPaCa-2 cells. *Molecules* **2017**, *22*, 1553. [CrossRef]
30. Zaid, H.; Raiyn, J.; Nasser, A.; Saad, B.; Rayan, A. Physicochemical properties of natural based products versus synthetic chemicals. *Open Nutraceuticals J.* **2010**, *3*, 194–202. [CrossRef]
31. Wayne, P. Clinical and laboratory standards institute: Performance standards for antimicrobial susceptibility testing: 28th informational supplement. In *CLSI Document M100-S28*; Clinical and Laboratory Standards Institute: Annapolis Junction, MD, USA, 2018.
32. Huamán-Castilla, N.L.; Mariotti-Celis, M.S.; Martínez-Cifuentes, M.; Pérez-Correa, J.R. Glycerol as alternative co-solvent for water extraction of polyphenols from Carménère pomace: Hot pressurized liquid extraction and computational chemistry calculations. *Biomolecules* **2020**, *10*, 474. [CrossRef]
33. Dzoyem, J.; Tchamgoue, J.; Tchouankeu, J.; Kouam, S.; Choudhary, M.; Bakowsky, U. Antibacterial activity and cytotoxicity of flavonoids compounds isolated from Pseudarthria hookeri Wight & Arn. (Fabaceae). *S. Afr. J. Bot.* **2018**, *114*, 100–103.
34. Sahu, N.; Soni, D.; Chandrashekhar, B.; Satpute, D.; Saravanadevi, S.; Sarangi, B.; Pandey, R. Synthesis of silver nanoparticles using flavonoids: Hesperidin, naringin and diosmin, and their antibacterial effects and cytotoxicity. *Int. Nano Lett.* **2016**, *6*, 173–181. [CrossRef]
35. Gutiérrez-Venegas, G.; Gómez-Mora, J.A.; Meraz-Rodríguez, M.A.; Flores-Sánchez, M.A.; Ortiz-Miranda, L.F. Effect of flavonoids on antimicrobial activity of microorganisms present in dental plaque. *Heliyon* **2019**, *5*, e03013. [CrossRef] [PubMed]

36. Nalawade, T.M.; Bhat, K.; Sogi, S.H. Bactericidal activity of propylene glycol, glycerine, polyethylene glycol 400, and polyethylene glycol 1000 against selected microorganisms. *J. Int. Soc. Prev. Community Dent.* **2015**, *5*, 114. [CrossRef] [PubMed]
37. Rousk, J.; Brookes, P.C.; Bååth, E. Contrasting soil pH effects on fungal and bacterial growth suggest functional redundancy in carbon mineralization. *Appl. Environ. Microbiol.* **2009**, *75*, 1589–1596. [CrossRef] [PubMed]
38. Negi, P.; Jayaprakasha, G. Antibacterial activity of grapefruit (*Citrus paradisi*) peel extracts. *Eur. Food Res. Technol.* **2001**, *213*, 484–487.
39. Adamczak, A.; Ożarowski, M.; Karpiński, T.M. Antibacterial activity of some flavonoids and organic acids widely distributed in plants. *J. Clin. Med.* **2020**, *9*, 109. [CrossRef]
40. Rattanachaikunsopon, P.; Phumkhachorn, P. Contents and antibacterial activity of flavonoids extracted from leaves of *Psidium guajava*. *J. Med. Plants Res.* **2010**, *4*, 393–396.
41. Hendra, R.; Ahmad, S.; Sukari, A.; Shukor, M.Y.; Oskoueian, E. Flavonoid analyses and antimicrobial activity of various parts of *Phaleria macrocarpa* (Scheff.) Boerl fruit. *Int. J. Mol. Sci.* **2011**, *12*, 3422–3431. [CrossRef]
42. Tsui, V.; Wong, R.; Rabie, A.B.M. The inhibitory effects of naringin on the growth of periodontal pathogens in vitro. *Phytother. Res. Int. J. Devoted Pharmacol. Toxicol. Eval. Nat. Prod. Deriv.* **2008**, *22*, 401–406.
43. Ab Rahman, S.F.S.; Sijam, K.; Omar, D. Identification and antibacterial activity of phenolic compounds in crude extracts of *Piper sarmentosum* (Kadok). *J. Pure Appl. Microbiol.* **2014**, *8*, 483–490.
44. Takeoka, G.; Dao, L.; Wong, R.Y.; Lundin, R.; Mahoney, N. Identification of benzethonium chloride in commercial grapefruit seed extracts. *J. Agric. Food Chem.* **2001**, *49*, 3316–3320. [CrossRef] [PubMed]
45. Ali, H.; Dixit, S. In vitro antimicrobial activity of flavanoids of Ocimum sanctum with synergistic effect of their combined form. *Asian Pac. J. Trop. Dis.* **2012**, *2*, S396–S398. [CrossRef]
46. Silván, J.M.; Mingo, E.; Hidalgo, M.; de Pascual-Teresa, S.; Carrascosa, A.V.; Martinez-Rodriguez, A.J. Antibacterial activity of a grape seed extract and its fractions against Campylobacter spp. *Food Control* **2013**, *29*, 25–31. [CrossRef]

antibiotics

MDPI

Article

Green Synthesis of Silver Nanoparticles and Evaluation of Their Antibacterial Activity against Multidrug-Resistant Bacteria and Wound Healing Efficacy Using a Murine Model

Vajravathi Lakkim [1], Madhava C. Reddy [2], Roja Rani Pallavali [2], Kakarla Raghava Reddy [3], Ch Venkata Reddy [4,*], Inamuddin [5], Anwar L. Bilgrami [6] and Dakshayani Lomada [1,*]

1 Department of Genetics and Genomics, Yogi Vemana University, Kadapa, AP 516005, India; vajravathi@gmail.com
2 Department of Biotechnology and Bioinformatics, Yogi Vemana University, Kadapa, AP 516005, India; cmreddy@yogivemanauniversity.ac.in (M.C.R.); p.rojarani.virology@gmail.com (R.R.P.)
3 School of Chemical and Biomolecular Engineering, The University of Sydney, Sydney, NSW 2006, Australia; raghava.kakarla@sydney.edu.au
4 School of Mechanical Engineering, Yeungnam University, Gyeongsan 712-749, Korea
5 Advanced Functional Materials Laboratory, Department of Applied Chemistry, Zakir Husain College of Engineering and Technology, Faculty of Engineering and Technology, Aligarh Muslim University, Aligarh, UP 202002, India; inamuddin@zhcet.ac.in
6 Deanship of Scientific Research, King Abdulaziz University, Jeddah 80216, Saudi Arabia; alegman@kau.edu.sa
* Correspondence: cvreddy@ynu.ac.kr (C.V.R.); dlomada@yogivemanauniversity.ac.in (D.L.); Tel.: +91-9652001184 (D.L.)

Received: 2 November 2020; Accepted: 10 December 2020; Published: 13 December 2020

Abstract: Green nanotechnology has significant applications in various biomedical science fields. In this study, green-synthesized silver nanoparticles, prepared by using *Catharanthus roseus* and *Azadirachta indica* extracts, were characterized using UV–Vis spectroscopy, dynamic light scattering, X-ray diffraction, scanning electron microscopy, and transmission electron microscopy. Silver nanoparticles (Ag NPs) synthesized from leaf extracts of *C. roseus* and *A. indica* effectively inhibited the growth of multidrug-resistant (MDR) bacteria isolated from patients with septic wound infections. The maximum bacteriolytic activity of the green-synthesized Ag NPs of *C. roseus* and *A. indica* against the MDR bacterium *K. Pneumoniae* was shown by a zone of inhibition of 19 and 16 mm, respectively. *C. roseus* Ag NPs exhibited more bacteriolytic activity than *A. indica* Ag NPs in terms of the zone of inhibition. Moreover, these particles were effective in healing wounds in BALB/c mice. Ag NPs of *C. roseus* and *A. indica* enhanced wound healing by 94% ± 1% and 87% ± 1%, respectively. Our data suggest that Ag NPs from *C. roseus* and *A. indicia* ameliorate excision wounds, and wound healing could be due to their effective antimicrobial activity against MDR bacteria. Hence, these Ag NPs could be potential therapeutic agents for the treatment of wounds.

Keywords: silver nanoparticles; green synthesis method; *Catharanthus roseus*; *Azadirachta indica*; multidrug-resistant bacteria; wound healing

1. Introduction

Burn injuries, wounds, and diabetic foot ulcers (DFUs) are global public health problems and a leading cause of mortality and amputations. The healing of burns, wounds, and DFUs involves a dynamic and complex network that requires continuous communication between cells in the form of cytokine release, cell-to-cell contacts, and cell-to-matrix interactions. The use of nanomedicines has increased enormously, and nanomaterials have been shown to offer promising strategies to optimize and improve the treatment of numerous disorders, including burns and wounds, owing to their unique small size, large surface area, and large surface-to-volume ratio. Hence, nanoparticles are considered magic bullets that are used in fundamental tasks in science, medicine, and different biotechnological fields, including imaging, biosensors, targeted drug delivery, and disease therapy [1,2]. More importantly, nanoparticles have played a role in delivering drugs, light, heat, and many substances to specific cancer cells in several biological applications. Metal nanoparticles are eminently illustrated as having antioxidant, anticancer, anti-inflammatory, and antimicrobial activities and play a role in wound healing [3–5]. Prior to antibiotic discovery, silver(Ag) was widely used as an antimicrobial agent to treat wound infections [6].However, after the discovery and abundant application of antibiotics, silver usage subsided because of its toxic nature and the easy applicability of antibiotics. Researchers have gained interest in using silver nanoparticles (Ag NPs) coupled with phytochemicals for use as antibacterial, antifungal, and anticancer agents [7].

Green synthesis of nanoparticles has gained attention because of its advantages, including being nontoxic, safe for humans, eco-friendly, and economically viable, compared to chemical and physical synthesis methods [8]. Instead of using silver alone, Ag NPs coupled with phytoextracts have gained more interest because of their action on bacterial and fungal pathogens and promotion of wound healing. Green-synthesized Ag NPs have been extensively used in biomedicine, purification of water, cosmetics, the food industry, numerous household products, and clothing [9,10]. Using plant extracts, Ag NPs synthesis has recently advanced, and it is now safe, allows convenient collection, and can utilize a wide range of metabolites for promoting the bioreduction of Ag^+ (silver ions). Jha et al. demonstrated that plant leaf chemical constituents are precisely implicated in the lessening of silver ions and the formation of silver nanoparticles [11]. It has been shown that Ag NPs and crude phytoextracts successfully inhibit multidrug-resistant (MDR) bacterial growth [12–15]. The antifungal capacity of green-synthesized Ag NPs has gained only marginal attention from researchers in the field of plant pathology [2,16]. Biological methods implicated in Ag NPs synthesis utilize natural plant leaf extracts that act as both reductants and capping agents [17,18].

In folk medicine, *Catharanthus roseus* (*C. roseus*; also known as "Sadabahar" or "Madagascar periwinkle"), which belongs to the "Apocynaceae" family, is widely known as a significant medicinal plant that is used for the treatment of many maladies [19]. *C. roseus* leaves and roots are a source of fundamental anticancer drugs such as vincristine and vinblastine; its phytochemicals, including alkaloids, have been shown to have antihypertensive and anticancer effects [20]. Native to the Indian subcontinent, *Azadirachta indica* (*A. indica*) is another medicinal plant belonging to the "Meliaceae" family; it is typically grown in tropical and subtropical regions. *A. indica* is an abundant source of triterpenoid phytochemicals, like limonoids, that are enriched with powerful medicinal properties, including anti-inflammatory, antioxidant, anticancer, and anti-helminthic activities, as well as natural insecticidal activities [21]. *A. indica* leaves, cork, seeds, and oil are widely used in healthcare products and in Sidda, Unani, and Ayurveda medicine.

To control bacterial infections of septic wounds, many conventional antibiotics have been tested by researchers to maintain sterile conditions on wounds and possibly enhance their healing rate. However, due to the overconsumption of antibiotics, mutations in DNA, transposons, and R-plasmids of bacteria may result in the development of drug resistance [22]. Prolonged antibiotic administration may inhibit the growth of natural flora and also affect the synthesis of various biomolecules such as growth factors and cytokines. Worldwide, even in developed nations, skin infections due to microbes are the cause of approximately 42–65% of total skin-related morbidity, occurring particularly among children [23]. Ansari et al. demonstrated that microbial species such as *Staphylococcus aureus* were frequently colonized on human skin and wounds can cause several types of infections on the skin [24]. *S. aureus* infections on the skin's soft tissue can spread intothe surroundings, causingsevere diseases such as bacteremia [25]. Silver nanoparticles promote the production of free oxygen radicals, which oxidize the bacterial molecular structure through the delivery of silver (Ag^+) ions [26].

Biosynthesized Ag NPs have distinct advantages in medical fields, act as antimicrobials, and are used for drug delivery [27,28]. Because of their size advantage (7–20 nm), Ag NPs act as drug carriers that inhibit the growth of microbes and detoxify most microbial contaminations by disrupting cell membranes and blocking various biological molecules [29]. Biosynthesized Ag NPs are widely utilized as antibacterial components against several MDR bacteria and also reduce the development of antibiotic resistance. Because of their small size, biosynthesized Ag NPs accumulate on the cellular membranes of bacteria and cause an imbalance in microbial membrane integrity, leading to the death of the targeted bacteria, irrespective of their drug-resistant nature [30]. The mechanism of activity of biosynthesized Ag NPs is not completely understood; the significant general approaches of their activity are as follows:

- Biosynthesized Ag NPs release free silver ions that traverse into cells, causing further breakdown of adenosine triphosphate (ATP) generation and promotingthe replication of DNA.
- Ag NPs, along with Ag^+ ions, enhance the production of reactive oxygen species (ROS) in an antioxidant mechanism.
- Ag NPs cause cell membrane damage directly.

Commonly described mechanisms begin with silver ion release [31], followed by ROS generation [13,32] and cell membrane damage, but many ambiguous findings have been reported. Generally, the metal form of silver (Ag) nanocrystallites represents an optical peak at 3KeV because of their surface plasmon resonance [33].

The current study is mainly focused on the green synthesis of Ag NPs from leaf extracts of *C. roseus* and *A. indica* and the characterization of their morphological and structural properties. Antibacterial efficacy of the characterized nanoparticles was evaluated using the isolates of septic wound infections, such as MDR *Escherichia coli*, *Klebsiella pneumoniae*, *Staphylococcus aureus*, and *Pseudomonas aeruginosa*. The wound-healing efficacy of Ag NPs of *C. roseus* and *A. indica* was determined by using in-vivo studies on BALB/c mice through wound excision models. Green-synthesized Ag NPs were produced without using any toxic chemicals or physical approaches and required a low concentration of leaf extract. The method we used to synthesize Ag NPs is easy, inexpensive, and simple to implement. Currently, there is an improved awareness of green synthesis as eco-friendly, stable, safe, and economical, and successful antimicrobial agents have a wide range of applications in healthcare products [34]. Phyto-derived Ag NPs are an especially important resource in the medical research field [35]. We synthesized Ag NPs from aqueous leaf extracts of *C. roseus* and *A. indica*; then, we characterized them via X-ray diffraction (XRD), Fourier-transform infrared spectroscopy (FT-IR), dynamic light scattering (DLS), scanning electron microscopy (SEM) with energy dispersive X-ray analysis (SEM-EDX), and transmission electron microscopy (TEM) analyses; finally, we showed their antibacterial efficacy against MDR bacteria and wound healing capacity using an animal model.

2. Results and Discussion

2.1. Bioreduction and Synthesis of Ag NPs

Ag NPs were synthesized from *C. roseus* (C Ag NPs) and *A. indica* (A Ag NPs) leaf extracts; the development of a brownish color was observed immediately after adding phytoextracts to 1 mM silver nitrate ($AgNO_3$) due to the bioreduction of silver (Ag^+) ions into silver nanoparticles (Ag NPs). Different concentrations (1to 5 mM) of $AgNO_3$ with phytoextracts exhibited the appearance of a dark brown color, confirming the formation of Ag NPs, as shown in Figure 1A. The development of color was enhanced with time because of Ag^+ reduction. During the synthesis of Ag NPs, due to the presence of biomass in the reaction mixture, the color changed from yellow-brown to darkish-brown. Here, biomass plays an essential role in the biosynthesis of Ag NPs. According to Mulvaney, the color change in the suspensions is due to the Ag NPs excitation of surface plasmonresonance vibrations [35].

Phytochemicals such as alkaloids, phenolic compounds, terpenoids, enzyme proteins, coenzymes, and sugars reduce metal (Ag) salts from a positive-oxidation state to a zero-oxidation state. The size and size distribution of metallic silver nanoparticles significantly depend on the biocompounds present in the extract. The presence of a strong reductantin the leaf extract enhances the bioreduction rate and favors the formation of smaller nanoparticles.

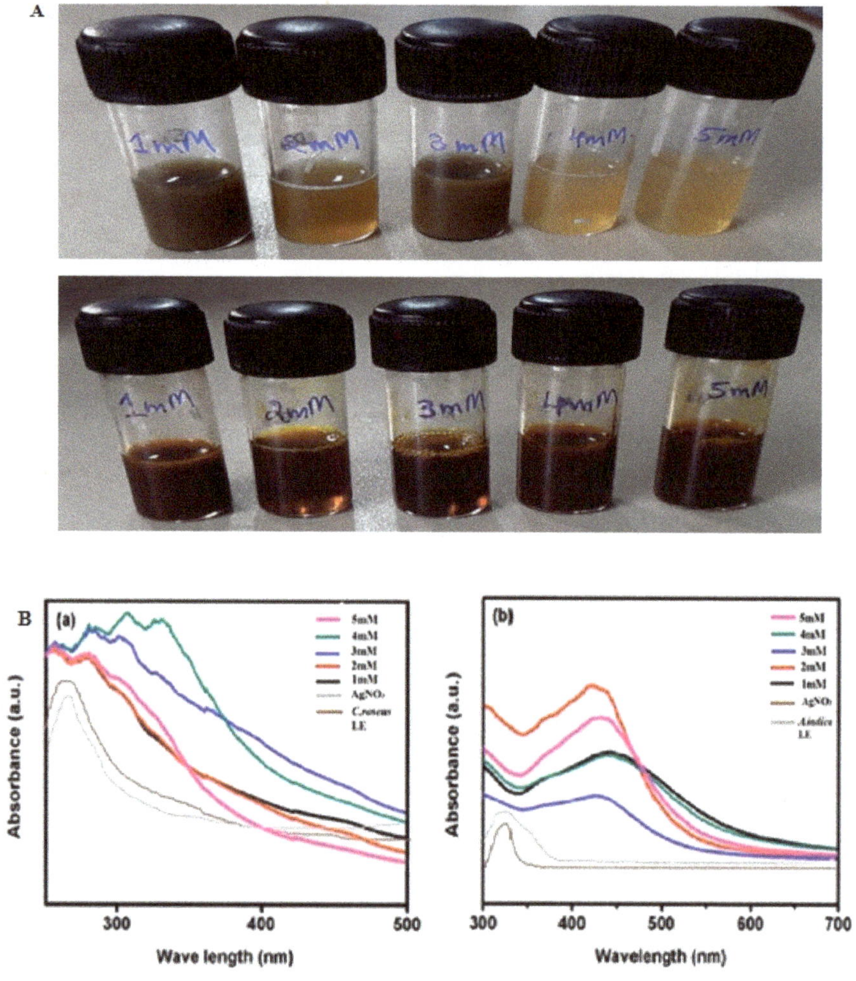

Figure 1. (**A**) Bioreduction of silver nanoparticles from *Catharanthus roseus* (top panel) and *Azadirachta indica* (bottom panel) leaf extracts. (**B**) UV–Vis spectroscopy analysis of biosynthesized silver nanoparticles of *Catharanthus roseus* (**a**) and *Azadirachta indica* (**b**) plant leaf extracts.

2.2. UV–Vis Spectra Analysis of Ag NPs

The structural characterization of green-synthesized nanoparticles was performed by UV–Vis spectral analysis. Mixing *C. roseus* and *A. indica* leaf extract suspensions with 1 to 5mM $AgNO_3$ changed the color from light yellow-brown to dark brown, as mentioned above Figure 1A. As the reaction progressed, the color transformation revealed a reduction of Ag^+ from silver nitrate to nanosilver, which was detected by the absorption maxima peak in the range of 300to 500 nm. The samples were observed periodically in the UV–Vis spectrometer at various concentrations of $AgNO_3$ (1 to

5 mM), along with $AgNO_3$ alone and phytoextracts without the addition of $AgNO_3$. At the same time, the samples were monitored by UV–Vis spectroscopy, which revealed a sharp peak at 315–360 nm in *C. roseus* and at 410–440 nm in *A. indica*, as shown in Figure 1B. These data confirmed the formation of Ag NPs from the phytoextracts. We did not observe an increase in absorbance with increasing concentrations of $AgNO_3$ with C Ag NPs. The lack of dependence on increasing concentration in C Ag NPs may be due to their particle size formation during the synthesis of Ag NPs from *C. roseus* phytoextract with $AgNO_3$. This may be because an increase in concentration increases the density of nanoparticles. Furthermore, the surface plasmonresonance (SPR) peak gradually shifted towards red with respect to the concentration. The shift towards red indicates that the particle size gradually increases with concentration. Curve sharpness also increased with concentration, which may be due to the formation of spherical and cubical nanoparticles. This is illustrated in the UV–Vis spectra through the rise in absorbance and shift of the SPR peaks [36–38]. In biologically synthesized nanoparticles, there was a considerable shift in the absorption maxima. Narayan et al. showed that the free electrons in metal nanoparticles allowed the SPR absorption band in the UV–Vis spectrum [7]. Such a characteristic change in color was due to the excitation of SPR in the metal nanoparticles of the plant leaf extracts that reacted with the 1 mM silver nitrate ($AgNO_3$) suspension. The UV–Vis spectra of the reaction mixture, at a range of wavelengths varying within 300–600 nm, showed a sharp peak at 320–335 and 420–440 nm in *C. roseus* and *A. indica*, respectively [36,37]. According to Udayasoorian et al., a sharp absorption band illustrates a spherical shape, and two other SPR bands are related to anisotropic particles [38]. According to Wiley et al., this method was used to investigate the shape and size of nanoparticles in liquid solutions [39].Hence, the UV–Vis spectroscopic findings verified that *C. roseus* and *A. indica* phytoextracts reduce silver-to-silver nanoparticles (Ag NPs). Bhakya and coworkers observed that peaks exploit the cubic structure and crystalline properties of biosynthesized silver nanoparticles in nanoscale units [40].

2.3. X-ray Diffraction Studies

The crystalline nature of the green-synthesized Ag NPs from plant leaf extracts demonstrated that specific peaks were observed in the spectra analysis using the X-ray diffraction (XRD) method (Rigaku, Miniflex). The Ag NPs X-ray diffraction spectrum demonstrated sharp scattering peaks at 2θ = 27.9°, 32.2°, 34.6°, 38.4°, 44.2°, 57.8°, 64.7°, and 77.4°, corresponding to the (210), (113), (200), (111), (124), (240), (226), and (300) planes of the face-centered cubic crystal structure for silver (Ag), as depicted in Figure 2A. Four Bragg's reflection patterns at 2θ = 32.2°, 38.4°, 44.2°, and 64.7° and in the spectrum varying in the range of 10–90 are represented by the conventional XRD method. The XRD spectrum patterns were considerably associated with (113), (111), (124), and (240). The lattice planes in the XRD spectrum were confirmed and crosschecked with the standard referral peak values (JCPDS Files no. 84-0173 and 04-0783), demonstrating that the synthesized Ag NPs were crystalline. The XRD spectra showed that the *C. roseus* and *A. indica* leaf extracts produced Ag NPs, and their crystalline nature was confirmed through the XRD method. The XRD peaks of the green-synthesized Ag NPs, with reference values, showed that Ag NPs were produced. The formed nanoparticles were confirmed via sharp peaks, and their 2θ values were 27.9°, 32.2°, 34.6°, 38.4°, 44.2°, 57.8°, 64.7°, and 77.4°, corresponding to (210), (113), (200), (111), (124), (240), (226), and (300), respectively, for Ag. Our XRD results demonstrated that the Ag NPs produced through the reduction of silver (Ag^+) ions with *C. roseus* and *A. indica* extracts were crystalline in nature. Our data are consistent with earlier reports [41,42]. Unidentified peaks (peaks 27.9°, 34.6°, and 57.9°) were observed, and it was recognized that the phytochemicals acted as capping agents for Ag NPs production [43]. In addition, Ag NPs (around 20 nm) with a face-centered crystalline cubic structure were confirmed. Shameli et al. demonstrated that the XRD pattern of Ag NPs showed a crystalline property in cubic form [44]. Bhakya and coworkers observed that peaks indicate a cubic structure and the crystalline properties of biosynthesized Ag NPs in nanoscale units [40].

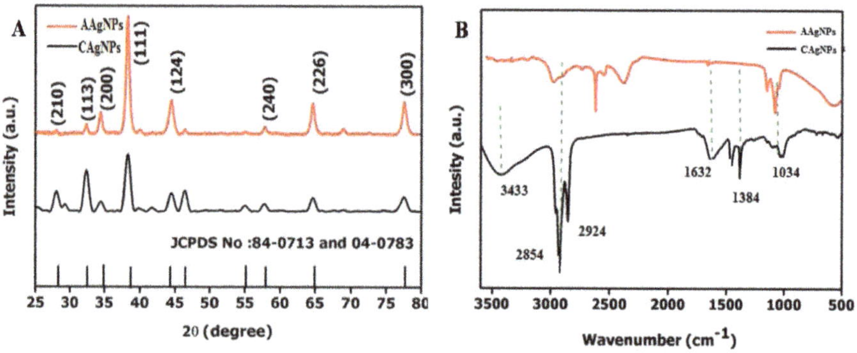

Figure 2. (**A**) X-ray diffraction (XRD) analysis of *Catharanthus roseus* silver nanoparticles (C Ag NPs) and *Azadirachta indica* silver nanoparticles (A Ag NPs).(**B**) FTIR spectra of *Catharanthus roseus* silver nanoparticles (C Ag NPs) and *Azadirachta indica* silver nanoparticles (A Ag NPs).

2.4. FTIR Analysis

A conventional Fourier transform infrared (FTIR) approach was used to identify secondary metabolites involved in reducing and capping for the synthesis of Ag NPs. FTIR spectra were recorded by employing potassium bromide (KBr) disks using an FTIR spectrometer (Perkin Elmer, Spectrum 2) with a wavenumber of 4000 to 400 cm^{-1}. The characteristic FTIR spectrum of green-synthesized Ag NPs, as depicted in Figure 2B, showed peaks at 3433, 2854, 2924, 1632, 1384, and 1034 cm^{-1}. In this spectrum, a sharp absorption signal peak at 3433 cm^{-1} is related to the N–H bond of amine groups of green-synthesized Ag NPs and provides stabilization of Ag NPs. Hence, the occurrence of N–H group-specific proteins and enzymes correspond to the reduction of $AgNO_3$ to Ag [32]. A comparative study of the FTIR spectrum ofthe control shows the most important signal peaks of ~3433, 1632, and 1384 cm^{-1}, illustrating the N–H group's presence on the surface of Ag NPs. According to Mishra et al., the cell-free extract might contain biomolecules such as peptides and proteins that affect the formation of Ag NPs through reduction [45].

The wide peak at 3433 cm^{-1} demonstratesan amide (N–H) stretching vibration of the NH_2 group, and OH with overlapping stretching vibration for water is recognized in *A. indica*. FTIR visible peaks with N–H and OH bond stretching at 3433 cm^{-1} clearly illustratesthe functional groups present in the green-synthesized *C. roseus* and *A. indica* Ag NPs, as shown individually in Appendix A and Figure A1. Another peak at 1632 cm^{-1} belongs to the stretching of C=O and a sharp signal peak at 2854 cm^{-1} could berelatedto the alkyne group in the leaf extracts of *C. roseus* and *A. indica*. The visible sharp signals at 1384 cm^{-1} represent C–O–C and C–O bonds. These visible signals are mainly related to flavonoids and terpenoids specifically present in plant extracts of *C. roseus* and *A. indica* [46,47]. These findings are in agreement with existing literature and confirmed that many bioorganic constituents from *C. roseus* and *A. indica* extracts produced persistent capping agents on green-synthesized Ag NPs [48].

2.5. Dynamic Light Scattering

We measured the distribution, typical particle size, and polydispersity index (PDI) of green-synthesized Ag NPs using dynamic light scattering (DLS).DLS data illustrated that the Ag NPs produced by the green route had a 31.4 diameter with Z, as reported by the distributions of size in number percentage. Briefly, 20.5 nm is related to q^O (number density distribution) and is based on the number percentage correlated with a polydispersity index of 0.65, demonstrating that the green-synthesized Ag NPs were greatly diffusive in suspensions (Figure 3). Using this approach, it was found that the nanoparticles hydrodynamic diameter was greater than the original diameter obtained from SEM and TEM images. Hence, due to electrostatic repulsions of the green-synthesized Ag NPs, the zeta potential value −15.2 represents great stability in water. The bioorganic constituents in the suspension serve as spacers to avoid agglomeration between Ag NPs. The TEM images assist the steric stabilization process, and the DLS study showed that Ag NPs biosynthesized through the green route resulted in a 35.69 nm average diameter. A polydispersity index (PDI) of 0.56 demonstrated that the green-synthesized Ag NPs were widely dispersed in a liquid medium. In DLS, the average particle size of C Ag NPs was 110 nm, with a range of 80–250 nm, and the average particle size of A Ag NPs was 60 nm, with various ranges of 40–80 nm, as indicated in Figure A2.

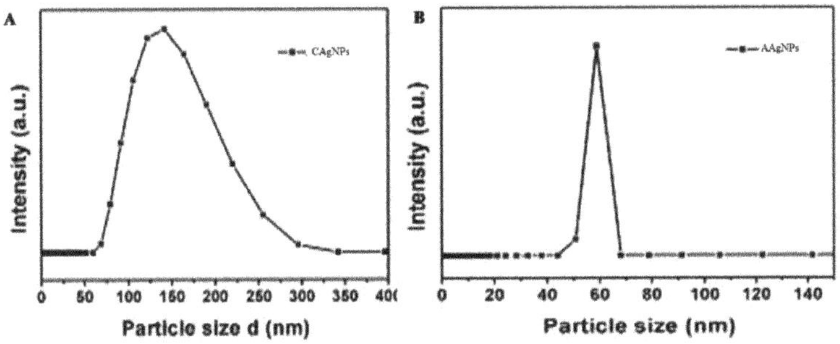

Figure 3. The hydrodynamic size determination of green-synthesized Ag NPs of *Catharanthus roseus* (**A**) and *Azadirachta indica* (**B**) by dynamic light scattering (DLS).

2.6. Scanning Electron Microscopy

The morphology of the green-synthesized Ag NPs was analyzed by scanning electron microscopy [49], and the pictures showthe cubic structure and unique shape of the nanoparticles produced with a 48–67 nm diameter range.

Analysis by the energy-dispersive X-ray (EDX) spectrum revealed that the incidence of silver elemental signals confirmed that the formed particles were Ag NPs through the bioreduction mechanism of leaf extracts with $AgNO_3$. The *y*-axis represents the number of X-ray counts, and the *x*-axis represents energy in keV. The sharp elemental signal peaks showed the most significant emission energies for Ag, and these lines in the EDX spectrum confirmed that Ag had been properly recognized.

The silver peak was from Ag NPs, and its atomic percentage was 13.1% in *C. roseus* and 19.9% in *A. indica*, as shown in Figures 4 and 5, respectively. In *C. roseus*, except for Ag, the atomic percentages of carbon (C), chlorine (Cl), oxygen (O), and aluminum (Al) were 48.5%, 30%, 6.7%, and 0.9%, respectively. In *A. indica*, except for Ag, the atomic percentages of carbon (C), chlorine (Cl), oxygen (O), and aluminum (Al) were 38.5%, 38.5%, 1.7%, and 1.2%, respectively.The peak of carbon in the spectrum represents the adsorbed constituents of the leaf extracts, and the other peaks of oxygen and chlorine are formed because of plant element adsorption over Ag NPs. Carbon is a fundamental chemical constituent in both the *C. roseus* and *A. indica* leaf chemical structures. In *C. roseus* and *A. indica*, carbon sources are abundant in leaf extracts. The synthesized Ag NPs were washed several times with double-distilled water after synthesis to minimize contamination. Because ofthe agglomeration of phytochemicals present on the Ag NPs, there was a high amount of carbon on the green-synthesized Ag NPs. The presence of a high content of aluminum (Al) was probably due to the inclusion of the microscope stage in the analysis. Apart from carbon, the remaining elements showed a drastically decreased atomic percentage compared with silver; the EDX spectrum gives evidence of formed particles through bioreduction of plant leaf extracts, with $AgNO_3$ confirmed as Ag NPs.

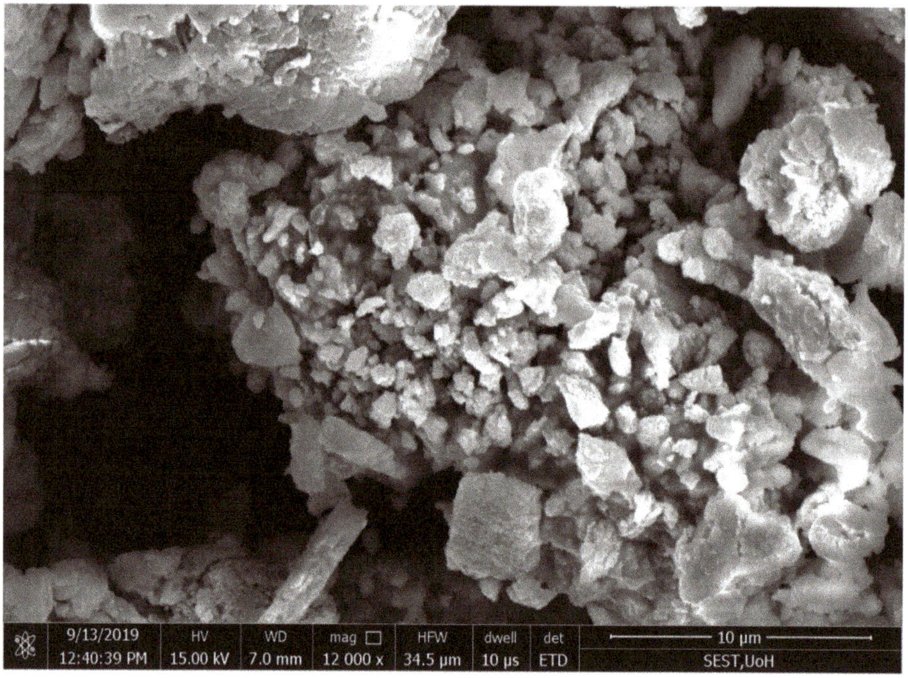

(a)

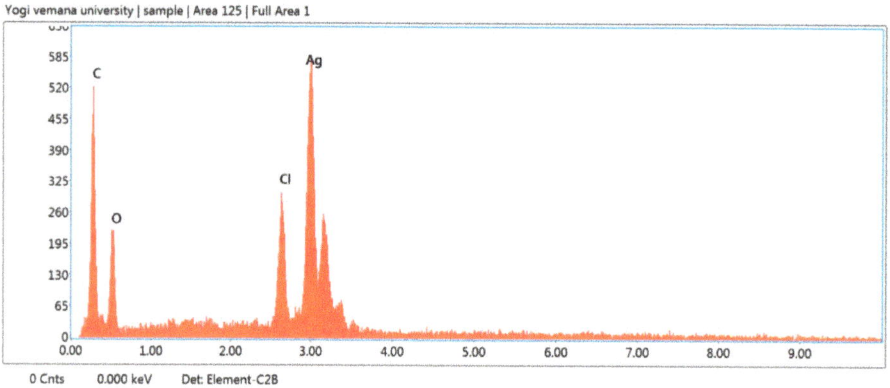

(b)

Figure 4. (**a**) Scanning electron microscopy(SEM) images of synthesized Ag NPs from *Catharanthus roseus*; (**b**) energy dispersive X-ray (EDX) spectrum of C Ag NPs showing the presence of different phytoelements as capping agents.

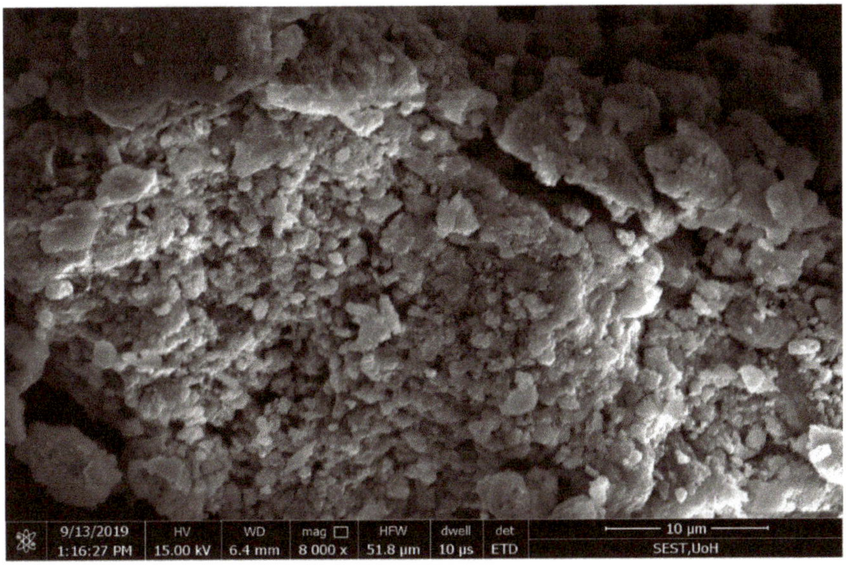

(**a**)

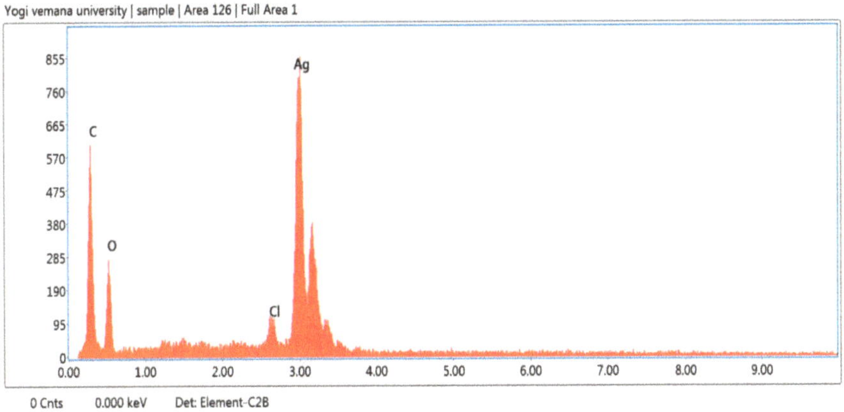

(**b**)

Figure 5. (**a**) Scanning electron microscopy (SEM) images of synthesized Ag NPs from *Azadirachta indica*; (**b**) energy dispersive X-ray (EDX) spectrum of A Ag NPs showing the presence of different phytoelements as capping agents.

2.7. Transmission Electron Microscopy

The morphology (size and shape) of C Ag NPs and A Ag NPs were analyzed using TEM (JEOL, Japan) at an operating voltage of 200 kV. The synthesized C Ag NPs and A Ag NPs were transferred into a new vial. The sample was prepared by mixing with 95% alcohol and then 15 min of ultra-sonication in an ultrasonic water bath. A nanoparticlesaqueous solution (5 µL) was placed on coated carbon grids and air-dried immediately before screening. TEM grids were prepared by placing a drop of particle solution on a carbon-coated Cu grid and drying under a lamp. The characteristics of the Ag NPs synthesized using *C. roseus* and *A. indica* leaf aqueous extracts were examined using TEM. Ag NPs acquired through the green route with 10% (*w*/*v*) of *C. roseus* and *A. indica* leaf extracts in 1 mM $AgNO_3$ showed particle sizes ranging 10–200 nm (average diameter 30 nm), as shown in Figure 6.

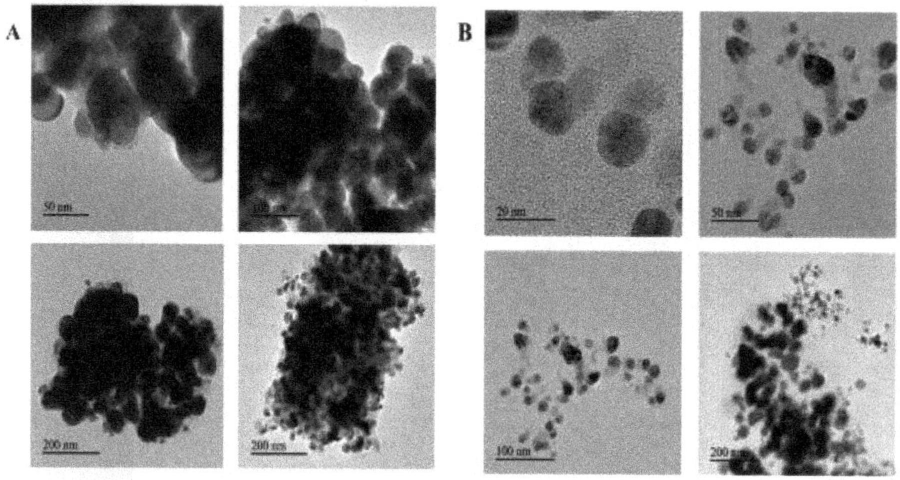

Figure 6. Transmission electron microscopy (TEM) images of biosynthesized silver nanoparticles from (**A**) *Catharanthus roseus* and (**B**) *Azadirachta indica* plant extracts.

TEM images of the green-synthesized Ag NPs revealed that silver nanoparticles were predominantly spherical in shape; a few agglomerated Ag NPs were also observed, which indicates possible sedimentation at a later time. *C. roseus* TEM images revealed that there was variation in particle sizes, with a range from 20 to 50 nm, and the average particle size was found to be 30 nm [50]. The TEM images showed that the Ag NPs were agglomerated and embedded in a dense, thick pattern, possibly acting as stabilizing chemical constituents in the leaf extracts of *C. roseus* and *A. indica*.

2.8. Antibacterial Activity of Silver Nanoparticles

2.8.1. Antibiotic Susceptibility Test

The green-synthesized C Ag NPs and A Ag NPs showed effective bacteriolytic activity against MDR bacteria (*E. coli*, *K. pneumoniae*, *S. aureus*, and *P. aeruginosa*) isolated from wound infections. The green-synthesized C Ag NPs showed high antibacterial activity against both gram-negative (*E. coli*, *K. pneumonia*, *P. aeruginosa*) and gram-positive (*S. aureus)* bacteriaby showing a wider range of inhibitory zones compared to A Ag NPs at various concentrations (10, 30, 60, 90, and 120 μg/μL), as shown in Figure 7 and Table 1. The maximum bacteriolytic activity of green-synthesized C Ag NPs and A Ag NPs was shown as 19and 16-mm zones of inhibition at the highest concentration against *K. pneumoniae*, respectively. C Ag NPs showed more bacteriolytic activity at all tested concentrations compared to A Ag NPs, as described in Table 1.The saturation dose of Ag NPs for that specific tested species was optimized at lower concentrations, so the inhibition zone did not increase even when the doses of Ag NPs were increased. The exact mechanism of green-synthesized Ag NPs dose-exclusion in MDR bacteria is still unknown.

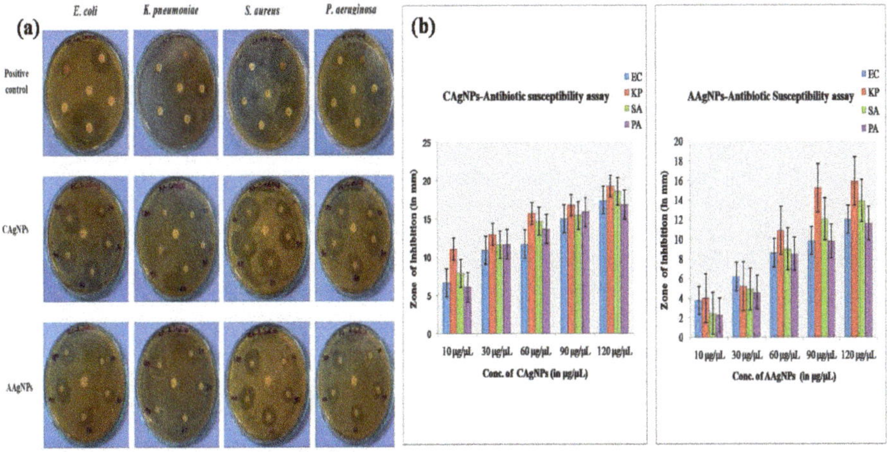

Figure 7. (**a**)Antibiotic susceptibility activity of biosynthesized silver nanoparticles (C Ag NPs and A Ag NPs) demonstrated by the disc diffusion method in multidrug-resistant (MDR) bacteria. (**b**) Graphical representation of antibiotic susceptibility activity of green-synthesized Ag NPs. EC—*Escherichia coli*, KP—*Klebsiella pneumoniae*, SA—*Staphylococcus aureus*, and PA—*Pseudomonas aeruginosa*.

Table 1. Antibiotic susceptibility test of MDR bacteria and the zone of inhibition for different concentrations of green-synthesized silver nanoparticles.

Ag NPs Conc.	*C. roseus* Silver Nanoparticles (Mean Zone of Inhibition in mm)				*A. indica* Silver Nanoparticles (Mean Zone of Inhibition in mm)			
	EC	KP	SA	PA	EC	KP	SA	PA
10 µg/µL	7	11	8	6	4	4	2	2
30 µg/µL	11	13	12	12	6	5	5	5
60 µg/µL	12	16	15	14	9	11	9	8
90 µg/µL	15	17	15	16	10	15	12	10
120 µg/µL	17	19	19	17	12	16	14	12

EC—*Escherichia coli*, KP—*Klebsiella pneumoniae*, SA—*Staphylococcus aureus*, and PA—*Pseudomonas aeruginosa*.

2.8.2. Bacterial Reduction Assay

The bacterial growth inhibitory activity of C Ag NPs and A Ag NPs against MDR bacteria (*E. coli*, *K. pneumoniae*, *S. aureus*,and *P. aeruginosa*) at various time points (1, 3, 5, and 7 h of incubation) and concentrations (ranging from 10 to 100 µg/µL) were measured using a bacterial reduction assay. Interestingly, *P. aeruginosa* (80 µg/µL) required a higher amount of green-synthesized nanoparticles of *C. roseus* and *A. indica* to inhibit growth than the gram-positive bacteria *S. aureus* (10 µg/µL). For *K. pneumoniae* and *E. coli*, 10 µg/µL of synthesized nanoparticles was required for the inhibition of growth of MDR bacteria. The nanoparticles that were green-synthesized with different concentrations of *A. indica* and *C. roseus* were proven effective antibacterial agents against MDR bacteria. The results for C Ag NPs and A Ag NPs are represented in Figure 8A,B, respectively. The bacterial growth on MH-Agar (Mueller-Hinton agar) of *E. coli* and *K. pneumoniae* showed that lower concentrations of C Ag NPs (40–50 µg/µL) are optimum for inhibition. There is no significant inhibitory action obtained by increasing the concentration of C Ag NPs on MH-Agar for *E. coli* and *K. pneumoniae*. Therefore, 50 µL is the optimum/saturated concentration required for inhibitory action on *S. aureus* and *P. Aeruginosa* by C Ag NPs. No significant inhibitory action on bacterial growth was observedby increasing the dose volume of C Ag NPs. The tested species, especially *S. aureus* and *P. aeruginosa*, probably follow the dose-exclusion mechanism.However, at the highest concentration (100 µL), we found bacteriolytic activity in almost all strains. The exact mechanism of the inhibitory action of green-synthesized Ag NPs on bacterial growth is not known. The green-synthesized C Ag NPs and A Ag NPs showed significant bacteriolytic activity compared with several other plant extracts alone or silver nitrate alone. Yliniemi et al. demonstrated that the biosynthesized Ag NPs effectively cause cell death of MDR bacteria through various mechanisms of action on bacterial respiration and cell membrane permeability [51]. Rai et al. and other groups revealed that the smaller size of biosynthesized Ag NPs provides a large surface area, which ensures a more significant outcome compared with commercial silver (Ag) on bacteria [52–54]. Gurunathan et al. demonstrated the dose-dependent bactericidal activity of Ag NPs at concentrations ranging from 0.1 to 1.0 µg mL^{-1} against two gram-negative and two gram-positive bacterial strains. They showed that the antibacterial activity of Ag NPs at low concentrations was more effective against gram-negative bacteria than gram-positive bacteria. They found that cell viability was reduced, and no growth at MIC values was observed for both strains. Thus, the bactericidal effect depends on the concentration, and it is specific for each bacterial strain. Positively charged Ag NPs show bactericidal and bacteriostatic activity, as reviewed by Roy et al. (2019). They found that the antibacterial activity of Ag NPs at a 100 µg mL^{-1} concentration was slightly higher than that at 450 µg mL^{-1} compared to the control [55,56]. Our data demonstrated that although there was no dependence on concentration, at a higher concentration (100 µL), we observed bactericidal activity using a bacterial reduction assay.

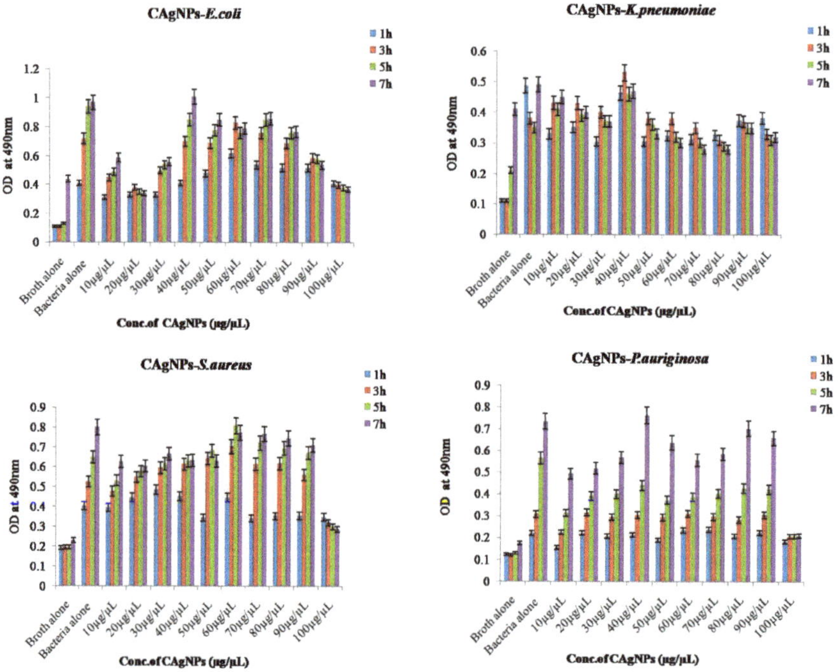

(A)

Figure 8. *Cont.*

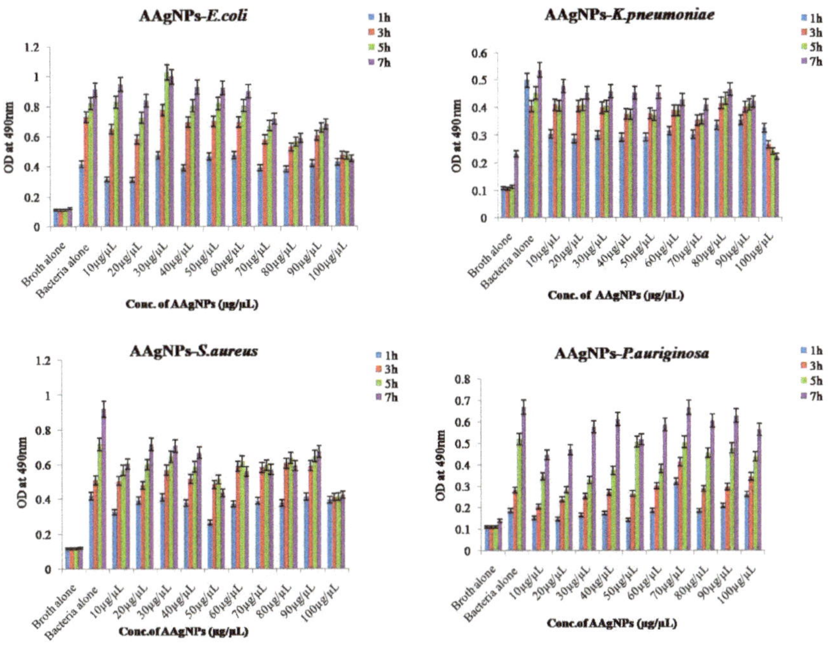

(B)

Figure 8. (**A**) Turbidity test for *C. roseus* Ag NPs (C Ag NPs) in MDR bacteria. (**B**) Turbidity test for *A. indica* Ag NPs (A Ag NPs) in MDR bacteria.

According to Sahayaraj et al., biosynthesized Ag NPs further attached to the cell surface of bacteria and entered the bacteria, leading to DNA replication, interruption of adenosine triphosphate (ATP) production, and ROS generation, directly affecting the cell framework [57]. Moreover, the silver bactericidal effect was possibly related to the inactivation of phosphomannose isomerase catalysis and is involved in the transition of mannose-6-phosphate to fructose -6-phosphate, a key arbitrate in glycolysis and a common sugar catabolism mechanism in microorganisms [58].

2.9. *Wound-Healing Efficacy of Silver Nanoparticles In Vivo*

The wound-healing efficacy of C Ag NPs and A Ag NPs was evaluated using female BALB/c mice using an excision wound-healing model with 5 mm biopsy punches. The wounds were generated on the skin surface dorsally, nano-formulations were applied on alternate days (on days 1, 3, 5, 7, 9, 11), and pictures were taken. Povidone–iodine ointment that is available on the market was used as a positive control for treated mice. As depicted in Figure 9A, green-synthesized silver nanoparticles (C Ag NPs and A Ag NPs)-treated mice showed enhanced wound constriction efficacy when compared to control and positive-control groups. The wound beds where the green-synthesized Ag NPs were topically applied showed no microbial growth, hemorrhage, or formation of pus throughout treatment, while the control group wounds showed remarkable irritation. The green-synthesized silver-nanoparticles-treated animals showed better wound-healing capacity from day 1 onwards and decreased wound size throughout the remaining days of treatment when compared to control group animals. At the end of the study, the wounds exhibited approximately 94% ± 1% ($p < 0.01$) constriction after treatment with C Ag NPs and 87% ± 1% ($p < 0.01$) closure in the A Ag NPs group, whereas the control wound exhibited approximately 74% ± 1% closure and the positive control (povidone–iodine) and vehicle control (Vaseline) wounds showed 79% ± 1% and 76% ± 1% wound constriction, respectively (Figure 9B and Table 2).The decreased size of wounds and increased healing efficacy could possibly be explained by the green-synthesized Ag NPs microbial efficacy towards microbial infection surrounding the region of the wound. Mondal et al. demonstrated that tissue regeneration of damaged sites is well-recognized in wound healing experiments, and the outcomes were satisfactory in earlier studies of wound constriction [59].The C Ag NPs-treated group showed an improvement in whole wound appearance following decreased irritation, as shown by alleviated inflammation and negligible bruising on day 11 of the experiment. The experimental results revealed that the healing capacity of wounds treated with *C. roseus* silver nanoparticles was greater than that of *A. indica* silver nanoparticles.

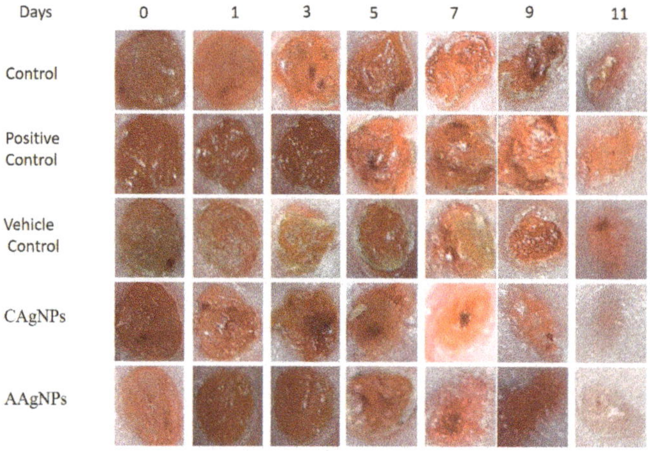

(A)

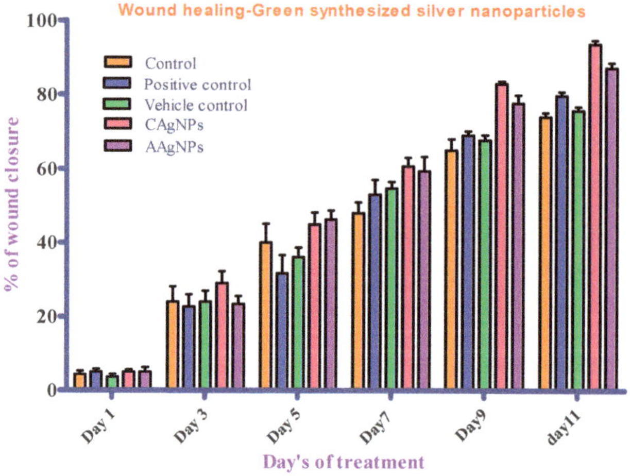

(B)

Figure 9. (**A**) Representative photographs showing wound closure after treatment with green-synthesized silver nanoparticles of *C. roseus* and *A. indica* (1% *w*/*w*) and control groups on days 0, 1, 3, 5, 7, 9, and 11. (**B**) Effect of topical application of green-synthesized silver nanoparticles of *C. roseus* and *A. indica* (1% *w*/*w*) on percent wound closure on different days in BALB/c mice.

Table 2. Percentage of wound contraction in BALB/c mice excision wound model. Note: mean± SE.

Group	Treatment Groups	% of Wound Contraction in Days					
		1	3	5	7	9	11
Group-I	Control	4 ± 1	24 ± 4	40 ± 5	48 ± 3	65 ± 3	74 ± 1
Group-II	Betadine (Povidone–Iodine)	5 ± 1	23 ± 3	32 ± 5	53 ± 4	69 ± 1	79 ± 1
Group-III	Vaseline	4 ± 1	24 ± 3	36 ± 3	55 ± 2	68 ± 1	76 ± 1
Group-IV	1% *C. roseus* Ag NPs	5 ± 1	29 ± 3	45 ± 3	60 ± 2	83 ± 1	94 ± 1
Group-V	1% *A. indica* Ag NPs	5 ± 1	23 ± 2	46 ± 2	59 ± 4	78 ± 2	87 ± 1

According to Tian et al., the significant action of green-synthesized Ag NPs in the healing of wounds in mice is attributed to faster regeneration, which is preferred for improved appearanceand occurs in a dose-dependent manner. In addition, green-synthesized Ag NPs showed positive results throughout the experiment due to their antibacterial efficacy and ability to decrease inflammation of wounds by diminishing the infiltration of mast cells and lymphocytes and the modification of cytokines with a fibrogenic nature [60]. Correspondingly, Liu et al. showed the efficacy of green-synthesized Ag NPs in epidermal re-epithelialization and dermal contraction, demonstrating that green-synthesized Ag NPs might enhance the percentage of wound constriction. Their characteristic wound-healing nature was explained by enhanced keratinocytes production and their movement in damaged wound sites [61]. Additionally, green-synthesized Ag NPs may possibly improve the differentiation of fibroblasts to myofibroblasts, thus increasing the healing capacity of wounds [62].

In the current study, the biosynthesized Ag NPs demonstrated significant potency in wound healing by enhancing the proliferation and migration of fibroblasts. The Ag NPs synthesized from *C. roseus* and *A. indica* enhanced the differentiation of fibroblasts into myofibroblasts and eventually improved wound contraction [63]. Nowadays, Ag NPs coated with biomedical products are commonly used to avoid microbial ailments by enhancing the healing capacity of wounds [64]. Current in vitro and in vivo studies have proven that the synthesized Ag NPs show effective antimicrobial activity against MDR bacteria that causes infections on the skin.

3. Materials and Methods

3.1. Leaf Extracts Preparation from C. roseus and A. indica

Leaf extracts from *C. roseus* and *A. indica* plants were prepared and used to synthesize silver nanoparticles. Young leaves of *C. roseus* and *A. indica* were obtained from Yogi Vemana University (14.473786° N, 78.711482° E; premises in Kadapa, Andhra Pradesh, India). Leaves were cleaned thoroughly to remove the debris and other organic constituents and dried at 37 °C. Powder was made from dried leaves, and 10 g of this powder was mixed with 100 mL distilled water (10% *w*/*v*) in a conical flask and then boiled for 1 h at 80 °C. The brown leaf extract was filtered through Whatmann No. 1 paper and preserved at 4 °C.

3.2. Preparation of Silver Nanoparticlesfrom Leaf Extract

Green synthesis of silver nanoparticles (AgNPs) was performed following the method of Sulaiman et al. [65]. Phytoextracts (1 mL) were mixed with different concentrations of silver nitrate ($AgNO_3$) (GR Merck, India), ranging from 1–5 mM. This step was carried out at 37 °C in the dark to reduce $AgNO_3$. The reduction of silver ions to silver nanoparticles was determined by the change in color to dark brown. The prepared Ag NPs were also validated using spectroscopy.

3.3. *Microbial Strains*

Prevalent MDR bacterial strains were generously gifted to us by the Microbiology Department of Yogi Vemana University. The potent drug-resistant bacterial strains of *E. coli*, *K. pneumoniae*, *S. aureus*, and *P. aeruginosa* were utilized to evaluate the antibacterial and wound healing properties of silver nanoparticles of *C. roseus* and *A. indica*.

3.4. *Silver Nanoparticles Characterization*

Ag NPs were characterized by X-ray diffraction (XRD) using Rigaku Miniflex with Cu Kα radians at 2θ angles varying from 20° to 80°. Optical properties were investigated using DRS UV Visible spectra, with a frequency varying from 500 to 4000 cm^{-1} and 4 cm^{-1} resolution.FTIR spectra were recorded by employing KBr disks using an FTIR spectrometer (Perkin Elmer, Spectrum 2) with a wave number of 4000–400 cm^{-1} [66]. Dynamic light scattering was performed using a Zetasizer-Nano ZS based on a conventional approach with several variations. Silver nanoparticles (100 µg/mol) were sonicated for 2 min, and dynamic particle sizes were assessed by adding two drops of nanoparticles into 10 mL of Millipore water. Once the nanoparticles were widely dispersed in water, the nanoparticles size was measured with a DLS analyzer. The analyses were repeated many times to attain a standard size of nanoparticles. Ag NPs (1 mg/mL) were prepared in Milli-Q water and used for further analysis. The morphology, particle size, and microstructure of Ag NPs were examined by high-resolution scanning electron microscopy [46] (Nikon, Japan). Briefly, 1 mg/mL of Ag NPs was sonicated to obtain a homogenous suspension. A sonicated stock solution was used for the size measurement of silver, which was diluted many times. Images were captured using one drop of dried gold-coated sample. Particle size, shape morphology, and fine pattern were evaluated with higher resolution TEM in a JEOL3010 (Japan) operated at 200 kV, following the protocol reported by Chattopadhyay et al. [67]. The solution was developed by adding 95% alcohol and performing 15 min of ultra-sonication. One drop of Ag NPs was placed on a carbon-coated grid and allowed to dehydrate prior to examination. TEM grids were made by adding a drop of Ag NPs onto carbon-coated Cu grids and allowing them to dry. Images were then taken.

3.5. *Antibacterial Activity of Silver Nanoparticles*

The antibacterial activities of Ag NPs were evaluated using previously isolated MDR bacterial isolates such as *E. coli*, *K. pneumoniae*, *S. aureus*, and *P. aeruginosa* from wound infection patients [12]. Different concentrations, ranging from 10 to 120 µg/µL of Ag NPs obtained from *C. roseus* and *A. indica*, were tested for antibacterial activity against MDR bacteria using the agar well diffusion method and the micro titer plate method. The positive controls used were tetracycline (30 µg), ampicillin (30 µg), and erythromycin (20 µg), and the negative control was deionized water. Antibacterial activity was measured by the zone of inhibition, and the experiment was performed in triplicate.

3.6. *Wound Healing Activity of Silver Nanoparticles*

Female BALB/c mice were procured from Mahaveera Enterprises (Reg.no:1656/PO/Bt/S/12/CPCSEA, Hyderabad, India). BALB/c mice (20–25 g) aged 8–10 weeks were housed at the YVU animal house following the laboratory animal procedures approved by the Institute Animal Ethics Committee (IAEC; CPCSEA no: 1841/GO/Re/S/51/CPCSEA). All procedures were conducted in accordance with the Guide for the Care and Use of Laboratory Animals. The anesthesia dose was 5 mL, with 2 mL ketamine (50 mg/mL), 0.5 mL xylazine (2%), and 2.5 mL saline (9%). The hair on the dorsal skin of the animalwas removed with an artificial hair removal cream [68] and wiped with 70% ethanol. Mice were anesthetized with 40–50 µL of a ketamine and xylazine mixture, depending on the weight of the animal, and a full-thickness open excision wound was made with a 5-mm biopsy punch. Following recovery from anesthesia, micewere housed separately in appropriately sanitized cages. The laboratory mice were distributed evenly and randomly separated into five groups as follows: Group I as the PBS- negative control, Group II as the betadine-positive control (povidone–iodine ointment-treated), Group III as the vehicle control (Vaseline-treated), GroupIV as 1% *w/w* nano-formulation-1 (*C. roseus* Ag NPs-treated), and Group V as the 1% *w/w* nano-formulation-2 (*A. indica* Ag NPs-treated). We pre-formulated 1 mg of green-synthesized silver nanoparticles (C Ag NPs and A Ag NPs), ground in 1 g of Vaseline (1 mg Ag NPs per 1 g Vaseline), and prepared a fine paste using a motor and pestle (~50 μL) for topical application towound surfaceson alternative days for 14 days. Wound constriction was observed by monitoring the wounds at days 0, 1, 3, 5, 7, 9, and 11, and wound closure (in mm) was measured alternatively using a digital Vernier caliper. Wound recovery efficacy is represented as the percentage of wound contraction rate (WCR).

The percentage of wound contraction rate = original wound area - actual wound area/original wound area ×100.

4. Conclusions

The current study demonstrates the biological production of Ag NPs via phytosynthesis using bioreductant, eco-friendly, and renewable *C. Roseus* and *A. indica* leaf extracts. Silver nanoparticleswere quickly and inexpensively synthesizedusing this method. Ag NPs were prepared from aqueous leaf extracts of *C. roseus* and *A. indica* and characterized by XRD, FT-IR, DLS, SEM-EDX, and TEM analyses and their antibacterial efficacy against MDR bacteria and ability to promote wound healing in BALB/c mice. Physical characterization methods revealed that the produced Ag NPs were extremely small and had a highly pure form in nature. Phytoderivatives such as leaf constituents and proteins of plants act as masking agents on nanoparticles. Green-synthesized Ag NPs exhibited *in-vivo* wound healing efficacy and antibacterial activity against MDR *E. coli*, *K. pneumoniae*, *S. aureus*, and *P. aeruginosa* strains. Green-synthesized Ag NPs are one alternative for the management of MDR microbial inflammation; thus, green-synthesized Ag NPs may be used for the management of wounds. Using emerging applicable nanotechnology, we synthesized metallic Ag NPs through a green route and evaluated the antibacterial and wound healing properties. Based on our current results, green-synthesized Ag NPs may have potential applications as pharmaceutical agents for antibacterial activity against MDR bacteria and wound healing.

Author Contributions: V.L., M.C.R., and R.R.P. conceived the experiment; V.L., M.C.R., and R.R.P. performed the experiments; M.C.R., K.R.R., I., A.L.B. and D.L. interpreted the results; V.L., M.C.R., K.R.R., I., C.V.R., and D.L. wrote the first version, and all authors contributed to improving the paper. All authors have read and agreed to the published version of the manuscript.

Funding: The Deanship of Scientific Research (DSR) at King Abdulaziz University, Jeddah, Saudi Arabia has funded this project under grant no. FP-77-42.

Conflicts of Interest: The authors of this manuscript declare no conflict of interest.

Appendix A

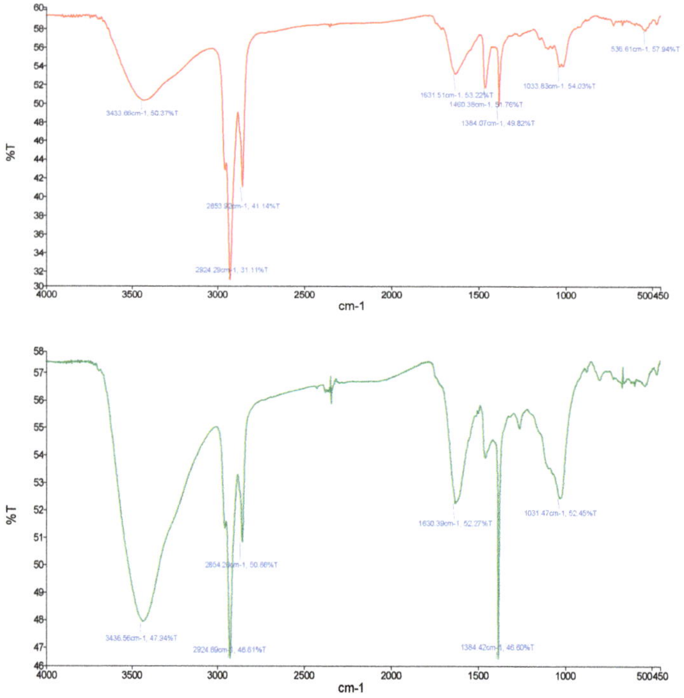

Figure A1. FTIR spectra of *C. roseus* (upper panel) and *A. indica* (lower panel) silver nanoparticles.

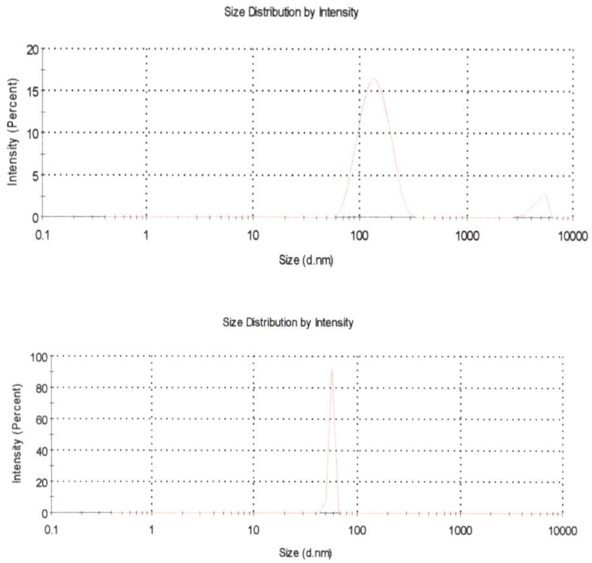

Figure A2. Hydrodynamic size determination of green-synthesized Ag NPs of *C. roseus* (upper panel) and *A. indica* (lower panel), as determined by dynamic light scattering (DLS).

References

1. Latha, T.S.; Lomada, D.; Dharani, P.K.; Muthukonda, S.V.; Reddy, M.C. Ti–O based nanomaterials ameliorate experimental autoimmune encephalomyelitis and collagen-induced arthritis. *RSC Adv.* **2016**, *6*, 8870–8880. [CrossRef]
2. Gao, W.; Wang, J. Synthetic micro/nanomotors in drug delivery. *Nanoscale* **2014**, *6*, 10486–10494. [CrossRef] [PubMed]
3. Latha, T.S.; Reddy, M.C.; Muthukonda, S.V.; Srikanth, V.V.; Lomada, D. In vitro and in vivo evaluation of anti-cancer activity: Shape-dependent properties of TiO2 nanostructures. *Mater. Sci. Eng. C* **2017**, *78*, 969–977. [CrossRef] [PubMed]
4. Palaniselvam, T.; Valappil, M.O.; Illathvalappil, R.; Kurungot, S. Nanoporous graphene by quantum dots removal from graphene and its conversion to a potential oxygen reduction electrocatalyst via nitrogen doping. *Energy Environ. Sci.* **2014**, *7*, 1059–1067. [CrossRef]
5. Schröfel, A.; Kratošová, G.; Šafařík, I.; Šafaříková, M.; Raška, I.; Shor, L.M. Applications of biosynthesized metallic nanoparticles—A review. *Acta Biomater.* **2014**, *10*, 4023–4042. [CrossRef]
6. Singh, M.; Singh, S.; Prasad, S.; Gambhir, I. Nanotechnology in medicine and antibacterial effect of silver nanoparticles. *Dig. J. Nanomater. Biostructures* **2008**, *3*, 115–122.
7. Narayanan, K.B.; Sakthivel, N. Green synthesis of biogenic metal nanoparticles by terrestrial and aquatic phototrophic and heterotrophic eukaryotes and biocompatible agents. *Adv. Colloid Interface Sci.* **2011**, *169*, 59–79. [CrossRef]
8. Mohanpuria, P.; Rana, N.; Yadav, S. Biosynthesis of nanoparticles: Technological concepts and future applications. *J. Nanopart. Res.* **2008**, *10*, 507–517. [CrossRef]
9. Kuppusamy, P.; Yusoff, M.M.; Maniam, G.P.; Govindan, N. Biosynthesis of metallic nanoparticles using plant derivatives and their new avenues in pharmacological applications—An updated report. *Saudi Pharm. J.* **2016**, *24*, 473–484. [CrossRef]
10. Mukunthan, K.; Elumalai, E.; Patel, T.N.; Murty, V.R. Catharanthusroseus: A natural source for the synthesis of silver nanoparticles. *Asian Pac. J. Trop. Biomed.* **2011**, *1*, 270–274. [CrossRef]
11. Jha, A.K.; Prasad, K.; Kumar, V.; Prasad, K. Biosynthesis of silver nanoparticles using Eclipta leaf. *Biotechnol. Prog.* **2009**, *25*, 1476–1479. [CrossRef] [PubMed]
12. Pallavali, R.R.; Avula, S.; Degati, V.L.; Penubala, M.; Damu, A.; Durbaka, V.R.P. Data of antibacterial activity of plant leaves crude extract on bacterial isolates of wound infections. *Data Brief* **2019**, *24*, 103896. [CrossRef] [PubMed]
13. Kim, J.S.; Kuk, E.; Yu, K.N.; Kim, J.-H.; Park, S.J.; Lee, H.J.; Hwang, C.-Y. Antimicrobial effects of silver nanoparticles. *Nanomedicine* **2007**, *3*, 95–101. [CrossRef] [PubMed]
14. Raffi, M.; Hussain, F.; Bhatti, T.; Akhter, J.; Hameed, A.; Hasan, M. Antibacterial characterization of silver nanoparticles against *E. coli* ATCC-15224. *J. Mater. Sci. Technol.* **2008**, *24*, 192–196.
15. Sondi, I.; Salopek-Sondi, B. Silver nanoparticles as antimicrobial agent: A case study on *E. coli* as a model for Gram-negative bacteria. *J. Colloid Interface Sci.* **2004**, *275*, 177–182. [CrossRef]
16. Carisse, O.; Van Der Heyden, H. Relationship of airborne *Botrytis cinerea* conidium concentration to tomato flower and stem infections: A threshold for de-leafing operations. *Plant. Dis.* **2015**, *99*, 137–142. [CrossRef]
17. Li, S.; Shen, Y.; Xie, A.; Yu, X.; Qiu, L.; Zhang, L.; Zhang, Q. Green synthesis of silver nanoparticles using *Capsicum annuum* L. extract. *Green Chem.* **2007**, *9*, 852–858. [CrossRef]
18. Sanghi, R.; Verma, P. Biomimetic synthesis and characterisation of protein capped silver nanoparticles. *Bioresour. Technol.* **2009**, *100*, 501–504. [CrossRef]
19. Singh, S.N.; Vats, P.; Suri, S.; Shyam, R.; Kumria, M.; Ranganathan, S.; Sridharan, K. Effect of an antidiabetic extract of *Catharanthusroseus* on enzymic activities in streptozotocin induced diabetic rats. *J. Ethnopharmacol.* **2001**, *76*, 269–277. [CrossRef]
20. El-Sayed, M.; Verpoorte, R. Methyljasmonate accelerates catabolism of monoterpenoid indole alkaloids in *Catharanthusroseus* during leaf processing. *Fitoterapia* **2005**, *76*, 83–90. [CrossRef]
21. Sidhu, O.P.; Kumar, V.; Behl, H.M. Variability in triterpenoids (nimbin and salanin) composition of neem among different provenances of India. *Ind. Crops Prod.* **2004**, *19*, 69–75. [CrossRef]
22. Melaiye, A.; Youngs, W.J. Silver and its application as an antimicrobial agent. *Expert Opin. Ther. Pat.* **2005**, *15*, 125–130. [CrossRef]

23. Tong, S.Y.C.; Davis, J.S.; Eichenberger, E.; Holland, T.L.; Fowler, V.G. Staphylococcus aureus Infections: Epidemiology, Pathophysiology, Clinical Manifestations, and Management. *Clin. Microbiol. Rev.* **2015**, *28*, 603–661. [CrossRef] [PubMed]
24. Ansari, S.; Jha, R.K.; Mishra, S.K.; Tiwari, B.R.; Asaad, A.M. Recent advances in *Staphylococcus aureus* infection: Focus on vaccine development. *Infect. Drug Resist.* **2019**, *12*, 1243–1255. [CrossRef]
25. Ki, V.; Rotstein, C. Bacterial Skin and Soft Tissue Infections in Adults: A Review of Their Epidemiology, Pathogenesis, Diagnosis, Treatment and Site of Care. *Can. J. Infect. Dis. Med. Microbiol.* **2008**, *19*, 173–184. [CrossRef]
26. Dakal, T.C.; Kumar, A.; Majumdar, R.S.; Yadav, V. Mechanistic Basis of Antimicrobial Actions of Silver Nanoparticles. *Front. Microbiol.* **2016**, *7*, 1831. [CrossRef]
27. Shaikh, R.; Zainuddin Syed, I.; Bhende, P. Green synthesis of silver nanoparticles using root extracts of *Cassia toral* L. and its antimicrobial activities. *Asian J. Green Chem.* **2019**, *3*, 70–81.
28. Bhowmick, S.; Koul, V. Assessment of PVA/silver nanocomposite hydrogel patch as antimicrobial dressing scaffold: Synthesis, characterization and biological evaluation. *Mater. Sci. Eng. C* **2016**, *59*, 109–119. [CrossRef]
29. Pérez-Díaz, M.; Alvarado-Gomez, E.; Magaña-Aquino, M.; Sánchez-Sánchez, R.; Velasquillo, C.; Gonzalez, C.; Martinez-Gutierrez, F. Anti-biofilm activity of chitosan gels formulated with silver nanoparticles and their cytotoxic effect on human fibroblasts. *Mater. Sci. Eng. C* **2016**, *60*, 317–323. [CrossRef]
30. Hwang, E.T.; Lee, J.H.; Chae, Y.J.; Kim, Y.S.; Kim, B.C.; Sang, B.I.; Gu, M.B. Analysis of the toxic mode of action of silver nanoparticles using stress-specific bioluminescent bacteria. *Small* **2008**, *4*, 746–750. [CrossRef]
31. Sedki, M.; Mohamed, M.B.; Fawzy, M.; Abdelrehim, D.A.; Abdel-Mottaleb, M.M. Phytosynthesis of silver–reduced graphene oxide (Ag–RGO) nanocomposite with an enhanced antibacterial effect using Potamogetonpectinatus extract. *RSC Adv.* **2015**, *5*, 17358–17365. [CrossRef]
32. Femi-Adepoju, A.G.; Dada, A.O.; Otun, K.O.; Adepoju, A.O.; Fatoba, O.P. Green synthesis of silver nanoparticles using terrestrial fern (Gleichenia Pectinata (Willd.) C. Presl.): Characterization and antimicrobial studies. *Heliyon* **2019**, *5*, e01543. [CrossRef] [PubMed]
33. Srour, J.; Berg, E.; Mahltig, B.; Smolik, T.; Wollenberg, A. Evaluation of antimicrobial textiles for atopic dermatitis. *J. Eur. Acad. Dermatol. Venereol.* **2019**, *33*, 384–390. [CrossRef] [PubMed]
34. Kanchi, S.; Inamuddin; Khan, A. Biogenic synthesis of selenium nanoparticles with edible mushroom extract: Evaluation of cytotoxicity on prostate cancer cell lines and their antioxidant, and antibacterial activity. *Biointerface Res. Appl. Chem.* **2020**, *10*, 6629–6639.
35. Mulvaney, P. Surface plasmon spectroscopy of nanosized metal particles. *Langmuir* **1996**, *12*, 788–800. [CrossRef]
36. Sundarrajan, M.; Jeelani, A.; Santhanam, V.; Durgadevi, S.; Abirami, S. Effect of Concentration, pH and Time on the Morphology of Silver Nanoparticles Synthesized by Green Method using *Phyllanthus niruri* and *Solanum nigrum* Leaf Extracts. *Int. J. Curr. Res. Rev.* **2018**, *10*, 25–29. [CrossRef]
37. Al-Shmgani, H.S.A.; Mohammed, W.H.; Sulaiman, G.M.; Saadoon, A.H. Biosynthesis of silver nanoparticles from *Catharanthus roseus* leaf extract and assessing their antioxidant, antimicrobial, and wound-healing activities. *Artif. Cells Nanomed. Biotechnol.* **2017**, *45*, 1234–1240. [CrossRef]
38. Udayasoorian, C.; Kumar, R.; Jayabalakrishnan, M. Extracellular synthesis of silver nanoparticles using leaf extract of *Cassia auriculata*. *Dig. J. Nanomater. Biostruct.* **2011**, *6*, 279–283.
39. Wiley, B.J.; Im, S.H.; Li, Z.-Y.; McLellan, J.; Siekkinen, A.; Xia, Y. Maneuvering the surface plasmon resonance of silver nanostructures through shape-controlled synthesis. *J. Phys. Chem. B* **2006**, *110*, 15666–15675. [CrossRef]
40. Bhakya, S.; Muthukrishnan, S.; Sukumaran, M.; Muthukumar, M. Biogenic synthesis of silver nanoparticles and their antioxidant and antibacterial activity. *Appl. Nanosci.* **2016**, *5*, 755–766. [CrossRef]
41. Muthukrishnan, S.; Bhakya, S.; Kumar, T.S.; Rao, M. Biosynthesis, characterization and antibacterial effect of plant-mediated silver nanoparticles using *Ceropegia thwaitesii*—An endemic species. *Ind. Crops Prod.* **2015**, *63*, 119–124. [CrossRef]
42. Vanaja, M.; Annadurai, G. *Coleus aromaticus* leaf extract mediated synthesis of silver nanoparticles and its bactericidal activity. *Appl. Nanosci.* **2013**, *3*, 217–223. [CrossRef]

43. Shankar, S.S.; Ahmad, A.; Pasricha, R.; Sastry, M. Bioreduction of chloroaurate ions by geranium leaves and its endophytic fungus yields gold nanoparticles of different shapes. *J. Mater. Chem.* **2003**, *13*, 1822–1826. [CrossRef]
44. Shameli, K.; Ahmad, M.B.; Zargar, M.; Yunus, W.M.Z.W.; Ibrahim, N.A.; Shabanzadeh, P.; Moghaddam, M.G. Synthesis and characterization of silver/montmorillonite/chitosan bionanocomposites by chemical reduction method and their antibacterial activity. *Int. J. Nanomed.* **2011**, *6*, 271–284. [CrossRef]
45. Mishra, A.; Kumari, M.; Pandey, S.; Chaudhry, V.; Gupta, K.; Nautiyal, C. Biocatalytic and antimicrobial activities of gold nanoparticles synthesized by *Trichoderma* sp. *Bioresour. Technol.* **2014**, *166*, 235–242. [CrossRef]
46. Banerjee, P.; Satapathy, M.; Mukhopahayay, A.; Das, P. Leaf extract mediated green synthesis of silver nanoparticles from widely available Indian plants: Synthesis, characterization, antimicrobial property and toxicity analysis. *Bioresour. Bioprocess.* **2014**, *1*, 3. [CrossRef]
47. Prathna, T.; Chandrasekaran, N.; Mukherjee, A. Studies on aggregation behaviour of silver nanoparticles in aqueous matrices: Effect of surface functionalization and matrix composition. *Colloids Surf. A Physicochem. Eng. Asp.* **2011**, *390*, 216–224. [CrossRef]
48. Pourmortazavi, S.M.; Taghdiri, M.; Makari, V.; Rahimi-Nasrabadi, M. Procedure optimization for green synthesis of silver nanoparticles by aqueous extract of *Eucalyptus oleosa*. *Spectrochim. Acta Part A Mol. Biomol. Spectrosc.* **2015**, *136*, 1249–1254. [CrossRef]
49. Amanzadeh, E.; Esmaeili, A.; Abadi, R.E.N.; Kazemipour, N.; Pahlevanneshan, Z.; Beheshti, S. Quercetin conjugated with superparamagnetic iron oxide nanoparticles improves learning and memory better than free quercetin via interacting with proteins involved in LTP. *Sci. Rep.* **2019**, *9*, 1–19. [CrossRef]
50. Gopinath, K.; Gowri, S.; Arumugam, A. Phytosynthesis of silver nanoparticles using *Pterocarpus santalinus* leaf extract and their antibacterial properties. *J. Nanostructure Chem.* **2013**, 3, 68. [CrossRef]
51. Yliniemi, K.; Vahvaselka, M. Antimicrobial activity of colloidal silver nanoparticles prepared by sol-gel method. *Chem* **2008**, *18*, 199.
52. Rai, M.; Yadav, A.; Gade, A. Silver nanoparticles as a new generation of antimicrobials. *Biotechnol. Adv.* **2009**, *27*, 76–83. [CrossRef] [PubMed]
53. Dosoky, N.S.; Setzer, W.N. Chemical composition and biological activities of essential oils of *Curcuma* species. *Nutrients* **2018**, *10*, 1196. [CrossRef] [PubMed]
54. Akarchariya, N.; Sirilun, S.; Julsrigival, J.; Chansakaowa, S. Chemical profiling and antimicrobial activity of essential oil from *Curcuma aeruginosa* Roxb., *Curcuma glans* K. Larsen & J. Mood and *Curcuma* cf. xanthorrhizaRoxb. collected in Thailand. *Asian Pac. J. Trop. Biomed.* **2017**, *7*, 881–885.
55. Roy, A.; Bulut, O.; Some, S.; Mandal, A.K.; Yilmaz, M.D. Green synthesis of silver nanoparticles: Biomolecule-nanoparticle organizations targeting antimicrobial activity. *RSC Adv.* **2019**, *9*, 2673–2702. [CrossRef]
56. Gurunathan, S.; Han, J.W.; Kwon, D.-N.; Kim, J.-H. Enhanced antibacterial and anti-biofilm activities of silver nanoparticles against Gram-negative and Gram-positive bacteria. *Nanoscale Res. Lett.* **2014**, *9*, 373. [CrossRef]
57. Sahayaraj, K.; Rajesh, S. Bionanoparticles: Synthesis and antimicrobial applications. *Sci. Microb. Pathog. Commun. Curr. Res. Technol. Adv.* **2011**, *23*, 228–244.
58. Beddy, D.; Watson, R.; Fitzpatrick, J.; O'connell, P. Increased vascular endothelial growth factor production in fibroblasts isolated from strictures in patients with Crohn's disease. *Br. J. Surg.* **2004**, *91*, 72–77. [CrossRef]
59. Mondal, N.K.; Chowdhury, A.; Dey, U.; Mukhopadhya, P.; Chatterjee, S.; Das, K.; Datta, J.K. Green synthesis of silver nanoparticles and its application for mosquito control. *Asian Pac. J. Trop. Dis.* **2014**, *4*, S204–S210. [CrossRef]
60. Tian, J.; Wong, K.K.; Ho, C.M.; Lok, C.N.; Yu, W.Y.; Che, C.M.; Tam, P.K. Topical delivery of silver nanoparticles promotes wound healing. *ChemMedChem* **2007**, *2*, 129–136. [CrossRef]
61. Liu, X.; Lee, P.Y.; Ho, C.M.; Lui, V.C.; Chen, Y.; Che, C.M.; Wong, K.K. Silver nanoparticles mediate differential responses in keratinocytes and fibroblasts during skin wound healing. *ChemMedChem* **2010**, *5*, 468–475. [CrossRef] [PubMed]
62. Vivek, R.; Thangam, R.; Muthuchelian, K.; Gunasekaran, P.; Kaveri, K.; Kannan, S. Green biosynthesis of silver nanoparticles from *Annona squamosa* leaf extract and its in vitro cytotoxic effect on MCF-7 cells. *Process.Biochem.* **2012**, *47*, 2405–2410. [CrossRef]

63. Paladini, F.; Pollini, M. Antimicrobial Silver Nanoparticles for Wound Healing Application: Progress and Future Trends. *Materials* **2019**, *12*, 2540. [CrossRef] [PubMed]
64. Keat, C.L.; Aziz, A.; Eid, A.M.; Elmarzugi, N.A. Biosynthesis of nanoparticles and silver nanoparticles. *Bioresour. Bioprocess.* **2015**, *2*, 1–11. [CrossRef]
65. Sulaiman, G.M.; Mohammed, W.H.; Marzoog, T.R.; Al-Amiery, A.A.A.; Kadhum, A.A.H.; Mohamad, A.B. Green synthesis, antimicrobial and cytotoxic effects of silver nanoparticles using *Eucalyptus chapmaniana* leaves extract. *Asian Pac. J. Trop. Biomed.* **2013**, *3*, 58–63. [CrossRef]
66. Das, B.; Dash, S.K.; Mandal, D.; Ghosh, T.; Chattopadhyay, S.; Tripathy, S.; Roy, S. Green synthesized silver nanoparticles destroy multidrug-resistant bacteria via reactive oxygen species mediated membrane damage. *Arab. J. Chem.* **2017**, *10*, 862–876. [CrossRef]
67. Chattopadhyay, S.; Chakraborty, S.; Laha, D.; Baral, R.; Pramanik, P.; Roy, S. Surface-modified cobalt oxide nanoparticles: New opportunities for anti-cancer drug development. *Cancer Nanotechnol.* **2012**, *3*, 13. [CrossRef]
68. Srivastava, S.; Somasagara, R.R.; Hegde, M.; Nishana, M.; Tadi, S.K.; Srivastava, M.; Raghavan, S.C. Quercetin, a Natural Flavonoid Interacts with DNA, Arrests Cell Cycle and Causes Tumor Regression by Activating Mitochondrial Pathway of Apoptosis. *Sci. Rep.* **2016**, *6*, 24049. [CrossRef]

antibiotics MDPI

Article

Poly-ε-caprolactone Nanoparticles Loaded with 4-Nerolidylcatechol (4-NC) for Growth Inhibition of *Microsporum canis*

Vanessa Raquel Greatti [1], Fernando Oda [1], Rodrigo Sorrechia [1], Bárbara Regina Kapp [1], Carolina Manzato Seraphim [1], Ana Carolina Villas Bôas Weckwerth [2], Marlus Chorilli [1], Patrícia Bento Da Silva [1], Josimar O. Eloy [3], Marcelo J. Kogan [4,5], Javier O. Morales [4] and Rosemeire Cristina Linhari Rodrigues Pietro [1,*]

1 Department of Drugs and Medicines, School of Pharmaceutical Sciences, School of Pharmaceutical Sciences of São Paulo State University (UNESP), Rodovia Araraquara-Jaú, Km 1, Araraquara, SP 14800-903, Brazil; vanessagreatti@hotmail.com (V.R.G.); Fernando.oda@unesp.br (F.O.); rodrigo.sorrechia@unesp.br (R.S.); barbara.kapp@unesp.br (B.R.K.); camanzato@hotmail.com (C.M.S.); marlus.chorilli@unesp.br (M.C.); patrbent@yahoo.com.br (P.B.D.S.)

2 Department of Mycology, Lauro de Souza Lima Institute, Bauru, SP 17034-971, Brazil; anaweck@terra.com.br

3 Department of Pharmacy, School of Pharmacy, Dentistry and Nursing, Federal University of Ceará, University Avenue, 2853 Rodolfo Teófilo, Fortaleza, CE 60430160, Brazil; josimar.eloy@ufc.br

4 School of Chemical and Pharmaceutical Sciences, University of Chile, Santos Dumont 964, Independencia, Santiago 8380492, Chile; mkogan@ciq.uchile.cl (M.J.K.); jomorales@ciq.uchile.cl (J.O.M.)

5 Advanced Center for Chronic Diseases, Sergio Livingstone 1007, Santiago 8380492, Chile

* Correspondence: rosemeire.pietro@unesp.br; Tel.: +55-16-3301-6965

Received: 1 November 2020; Accepted: 6 December 2020; Published: 11 December 2020

Abstract: Dermatophyte fungal infections are difficult to treat because they need long-term treatments. 4-Nerolidylcatechol (4-NC) is a compound found in *Piper umbellatum* that has been reported to demonstrate significant antifungal activity, but is easily oxidizable. Due to this characteristic, the incorporation in nanostructured systems represents a strategy to guarantee the compound's stability compared to the isolated form and the possibility of improving antifungal activity. The objective of this study was to incorporate 4-NC into polymeric nanoparticles to evaluate, in vitro and in vivo, the growth inhibition of *Microsporum canis*. 4-NC was isolated from fresh leaves of *P. umbellatum,* and polymer nanoparticles of polycaprolactone were developed by nanoprecipitation using a 1:5 weight ratio (drug:polymer). Nanoparticles exhibited excellent encapsulation efficiency, and the antifungal activity was observed in nanoparticles with 4-NC incorporated. Polymeric nanoparticles can be a strategy employed for decreased cytotoxicity, increasing the stability and solubility of substances, as well as improving the efficacy of 4-NC.

Keywords: nanoparticles; 4-Nerolidylcatechol; antifungals; *Microsporum canis*; polycaprolactone; nanoprecipitation

1. Introduction

Dermatophyte fungal infections affect keratinized tissues and are difficult to combat. The long period of treatment, in addition to the adverse effects caused by systemic antifungal drugs, frequently leads to poor adherence to medication, favoring refractory disease [1,2]. The mycoses caused by *Microsporum canis* are more frequent in dogs and cats, but can extend the contamination to humans due to the contact between them since the pets are present inside the houses and inserted into the family.

4-Nerolidylcatechol (4-NC) is the major compound of the plant *Piper umbellatum*, popularly known in Brazil as pariparoba or caapeba. The molecule is an unstable natural product [3], and the extracts of this plant have demonstrated important biological properties, photoprotective action, leishmanicide, anti-inflammatory, anti-ulcer, anticancer, and antimicrobial activities [4–8]. Studies have demonstrated the high antifungal potential of 4-NC against dermatophyte fungi [9], which has motivated interest to develop this study.

4-NC belongs to the sesquiterpenes class and it is considered practically insoluble in water (solubility of −4303 (log mol/L)) [10]. The mechanism for antimicrobial action is not yet well defined, but a study with derivatives of this compound evaluating antimalarial activity showed mechanisms such as inhibition of isoprenoid biosynthesis and inhibition of hemozoin formation [11]. In human cells, it has a proteasome inhibition mechanism, with the accumulation of ubiquitinated proteins, damage to DNA, and changes in the mitochondrial membrane's potential. These mechanisms may possibly be related to antifungal activity since the cells are eukaryotic [12].

The drug's high antioxidant activity requires attention regarding its stability, and the lipophilic characteristic causes certain difficulties in its incorporation into formulations. To overcome these problems, the development of nanostructured delivery systems can be a viable strategy. Nanoparticles are colloidal systems, have nanometric size, and because of this, have the ability to permeate barriers in the body and protect molecules of interest, giving the incorporated molecule a higher solubility. They are acceptable for loading of both lipophilic and hydrophilic drugs [13,14].

Several polymers, either natural or synthetic, can be used for drug encapsulation. Regarding synthetic polymers, there are biodegradable aliphatic polyesters such as polylactides (PLA), poly (lactide/glycoside) copolymers (PLGA), and poly (ε-caprolactone), as well as non-degradable polymers such as poly (methyl methacrylate) and polyacrylates. Naturally occurring polymers have been widely used as carriers for dermatological disorders; however, polymers of synthetic origin such as poly-ε-caprolactone (PCL) have the advantage of higher encapsulation efficiency, purity, and high reproducibility, being more suitable for molecules with non-polar characteristics [15]. Studies using PCL showed low toxicity and compatibility with many drugs, as well as excellent solubility in organic solvents, heat stability, and good permeability, in addition to allowing slow release [16,17]. However, to the best of our knowledge, PCL has not been previously employed for 4-NC encapsulation.

Polymeric nanoparticles exhibit versatility in their structures, which can be modulated to protect/carry molecules to the action site or respond to physiological or external stimuli. Hydroxypropyl-ß-cyclodextrin (HP-ß-CD), which is a well-known membrane protector, has been shown to increase liposome solubility with 4-Nerolidylcatechol [18].

The mode of incorporation can modulate the response of the nanoparticles in biological environments under different pH conditions, as well as enzymatic, oxidative, reducing, temperature variation, and irradiation [19]. The properties and characteristics of nanostructured systems allow its use for several objectives, such as for mycoses.

Nanotechnology is an interesting strategy to improve the efficacy of traditional antifungals, reduce toxicity, improve biodistribution and drug targeting, and bring promising results in in-vitro and in vivo studies. In view of this, plant extracts can benefit from the association of this technology [20]. Liposomes containing 4-Nerolidylcatechol showed a controlled release, and modulation of hemocompatibility, in addition to a higher biocompatibility in the formulation providing stability and solubility [21].

The polymer PCL (polycaprolactone) has been successfully used for drug delivery, evaluated both in vitro and in vivo. After demonstrating in vivo biocompatibility and efficacy, PCL-based formulations have been approved by the FDA [22]. Furthermore, the reproducible production of biocompatible medical devices, including in the nanoscale, can employ the electrospinning process. For instance, Tammaro et al. (2015) [23] prepared linesolid loaded in electrospun PCL fibers for topically controlled drug delivery to inhibit *Staphylococcus aureus*. Wang et al. (2020) prepared PCL-based nanofibers for delivery of O-D-glucopyranosyl-L-ascorbic acid and heparin to treat inflammation and thrombosis [24].

This study aimed to develop polymeric nanoparticles containing 4-NC for growth inhibition of *M. canis*, evaluating the activity in vitro and in vivo.

2. Materials and Methods

2.1. 4-NC Isolation

The plant material was collected in the Horticultural Medicinal and Toxic Plants "Profa. Dra. Célia Cebrian Araujo Reis", School of Pharmaceutical Sciences, UNESP-Araraquara, and identified and authenticated in the Laboratory of Botany of the School of Pharmaceutical Sciences—UNESP, Araraquara, Brazil. Isolation of 4-NC was performed as described by Iwamoto et al. (2015) [7], with adaptations. The fresh leaves were extracted by maceration with dichloromethane (used proportion of plant material and solvent was 0.25 Kg/L) at room temperature. The extract was filtered and evaporated to remove the solvent completely. After evaporation of the solvent, liquid/liquid was partitioned with acetonitrile/hexane (1:1). Then the acetonitrile phase was subjected to solvent evaporation for column separation. The column separation was made using a 2 cm/2 cm glass column, with C18 (octadecylsilane) as the stationary phase, and ACN:H_2O (50:50) as the mobile phase.The isolation was confirmed by high-performance liquid chromatography and infrared spectroscopy. The analysis of 4-NC by NMR was performed with a Fourier 300 spectrometer, capable of obtaining ^{1}H and ^{13}C nuclei. For the infrared analysis, a Bruker® Spectrophotometer (Billerica, MA, USA) model IV-FT—Alpha Platinum ATR was used, and the data were treated with OriginPro 9 SR2. The application was made directly, without dilution.

2.2. Development of Nanoparticles

The nanoparticles were developed by the classical nanoprecipitation methodology, using a 1:5 weight ratio (drug:polymer). The polycaprolactone polymer and 4-NC were both dissolved in 50 mL of acetone, and the Poloxamer 407 surfactant was dissolved in 100 mL of deionized water (0.5%), the aqueous phase. The organic phase was dipped into the aqueous phase with stirring in a laminar flow hood for approximately 16 h for total evaporation of the organic solvent. The final volume was 50 mL [25].

2.3. Encapsulation Efficiency

The experiment was performed in the laboratory of Drug Delivery at the University of Chile (UCHILE). The high-performance liquid chromatography was performed using a Perkin–Elmer Flexar apparatus, analytical mode with quaternary pumping system, equipped with a Rheodyne 6-way automatic injector with 20uL loop, PDA detector (photodiode array), and degasser. A C-18 ($250 \times 4.6 \times 5$) GL Sciences column was used, and mobile phase composed of a gradient of acetonitrile: water with 0.1% trifluroacetic acid (30:70) for 10 min, (5:95) for 15 min, flow 1 mL/min, 20 µL of injection was used. Data acquisition and processing were performed using Chromera® CD N5188000-T, version 4.1.0 (Perkin–Elmer, Waltham, MA, USA) software.

To evaluate the encapsulation efficiency (EE%), an indirect method based on ultrafiltration, was employed. For this purpose, the free 4-NC was separated from 4-NC-loaded nanoparticles after centrifugation (Centrifuge 5804 R, Eppendof, Hamburg, Germany) performed in Amicon® tubes for 20 min at 3800× *g* at the temperature of 26 ± 1 °C. Then the filtrate was directly chromatographed and the nanoparticles retained in the filter were suspended in 5 mL of acetonitrile to dissolve the particles, sonicated for 5 min, filtered (0.45 μm, PTFE). The efficiency was calculated based on the calibration curve performed, and followed the equation [25].

$$\text{EE\%} = \frac{\text{ultracentrifuged pellet}(\mu\text{g}) - \text{supernatant}(\mu\text{g})\text{drug}}{\text{theoretical mass of the ''drug''}} \times 100 \quad (1)$$

2.4. *Dynamic Light Scattering (DLS) and Zeta Potential (Zeta)*

The mean size and zeta potential of nanoparticles were measured by dynamic light scattering (DLS) using a Zetasizer Nano ZS (Malvern Instruments Ltd., Malvern, Worcestershire, UK). The samples were applied without dilution. Measurements were made at 25 °C with a fixed scattering angle of 173°, the refractive index (RI) at 1.330, and absorbance at 0.01. All analyses were performed in triplicate (n = 3), and the data were expressed as the mean values and standard deviations.

2.5. *Nano Tracking Analysis (NTA)*

The nanoparticles were also analyzed by nano tracking analysis (NTA), a complementary technique to DLS. The samples were applied directly on the NanoSight NS300 (Malvern Instruments Ltd., Malvern, UK). The software traces several particles individually under Brownian motion and relates the velocity of particle movement, and calculates their hydrodynamic diameters using the Stokes-Einstein equation [26]. The samples were diluted 2000 times with ultrapure distilled water, and results were expressed in particle size (nm) and particle concentration.

2.6. *Scanning Electron Microscopy (SEM)*

For the measurement in scanning electron microscopy (SEM), the nanoparticles were deposited on the copper grid. The grids were in contact with the samples for 5 min, and then they were placed in contact with water for 1 min. After this time, it was put in contact with 0.5% phosphotungstic acid for another 1 min, and finally, another 1 min with water. The preparation was performed 24 h before the analysis; the grids were kept in filter paper-lined plates and capped. The measurements were performed using a microscope FEI model Inspect F50 [27].

2.7. *Fourier Transformed Infrared Spectroscopy (FTIR)*

The FT-IR spectral studies were carried on IR-Prestige 21 Shimadzu using the KBr pellets method (hydraulic press Shimadzu, Japan), from 400 to 4000 cm^{-1}. The FTIR spectra were performed for: 4-NC on two different quantities (65 μg and 676 μg), poloxamer 407, polycaprolactone, lyophilized empty nanoparticles and lyophilized 4-NC nanoparticles.

2.8. *In Vitro Evaluation of 4-NC and 4-NCNP Antifungal Activity*

The antifungal activity was evaluated according to M38-A2 guideline with some modifications [28]. The microdilution technique used 96-well plates with RPMI medium, using a clinical isolate of *M. canis*, isolated from a dog. The concentration of 4-NC and nanoparticles with 4-NC (4-NCNP) samples ranged from 250 μg/mL to 0.244 μg/mL and 150 μg/mL to 0.146 μg/mL, respectively. Amphotericin B and terbinafine were used as controls. The inoculum concentration was 5.0×10^4 CFU/mL. The plates were incubated for seven days under constant stirring at 28 °C. Minimal inhibitory concentration (MIC) was defined as the lowest concentration where growth inhibition occurred. Plates were read using 0.1% resazurin (30 μL), and minimal fungicidal activity (MFC) was performed using a sample of each well plated in PDA (potato dextrose agar) before the addition of resazurin. The plates were incubated for seven days at 28 °C. The minimal fungicidal concentration (MFC) was defined as the lowest concentration at which no growth occurred.

2.9. *Preparation of Gel Formulations for Use in In Vivo Study*

Formulations were developed to facilitate cutaneous application, so the samples were inserted into hydroxyethylcellulose gel. The base gel was prepared at the concentration of 2% in water under heating and stirring, and after cooling the samples were added. The concentration of nanoparticles used for the in vivo test was eight times the value obtained in the MIC test (0.072 mg/mL), according to the methodology used by Sharma et al. (2011) [29]. Terbinafine was used as eight times the value obtained in MIC test (0.005 mg/mL).

2.10. *In Vivo Antimycotic Evaluation in SWISS MICE*

The study was approved by the Research Ethics Committee (protocol CEUA/FCF/CAr: 06/2017). Twenty-four adult male Swiss mice weighing between 25 and 35 g were used, kept in individual cages, with feed and water at will. They were divided into four groups of six animals: infected with *M. canis*, treated with gel containing 4-NC nanoparticles, free terbinafine gel (control drug), gel with empty nanoparticle, and the negative control without treatment.

The animals ($n = 6$) were immunosuppressed with 500 μg of estradiol valerate in subcutaneous injection. After three days of immunosuppression, the infection was induced through slots with sterile needles to facilitate infection, where a suspension of 1×10^6 CFU/mL of *M. canis* (clinical isolate) was applied. After the period of infection (about seven days) the treatment was started [29].

Samples treatments were applied using sterile swabs with an amount sufficient to fill the entire infected area (0.3 g). After three days of treatment, three animals from each group were euthanized. After the seven days period, the others were euthanized. Before the sacrifice, blood samples from the animals were collected through the submandibular vein [30] to evaluate the enzymes aspartate aminotransferase (AST) and alanine aminotransferase (ALT) [31]. These enzymes were evaluated to verify if there was liver damage. The areas of the infected and treated skins were collected for microscopic analysis and stored in Karnovisky's solution for 24 h, after which time they were transferred to phosphate buffer (pH 7.4). The experimental model used is due to the greater susceptibility to dermatophytes.

2.11. *Analysis of the Hepatic Profile of the Animals*

Blood samples were centrifuged for 15 min at $1100 \times g$. After separation, the serum was transferred to 1.5 mL Eppendorf tubes and stored at −15 °C. For the analysis, the samples were removed from refrigeration and left at room temperature. Labtest® AST and ALT kits were used, and the tests were performed in triplicate.

2.12. *Grocott-Gomori Silver Methanamine Staining Microscopy*

The analysis of microscopy with Grocott–Gomori staining was carried out in the laboratory of Lauro de Souza Lima Research Institute (Bauru/SP). The skins were stocked in phosphate buffer (pH 7.5) and placed in an OMA DM40 histotechnical model to dehydrate and incorporate into the paraffin. After the skins were embedded, they were cut with a four micron MRP2015 microtome. The dewaxing was started with distilled water and then subjected to chromic acid (4%) for thirty minutes, after which time it was washed with common water. Then, sodium bisulfite (1%) was added for one minute, followed by ordinary water for 10 min and finally in distilled water. Samples were placed in a greenhouse in contact with the silver methenamine solution for 30 min. After this period, the samples were washed again with distilled water six times, followed by gold chloride (1%) for 4 min, and distilled water. Sodium thiosulphate (2%) was placed for 4 min, washed in running water and ending with light green for 45 s. Finally, the samples were dehydrated with 95 °C ethanol, absolute ethanol, and xylol. The samples were observed in an Axioplan 2 microscope, model HBO50.

3. Results

3.1. 4-NC Structural Determination

The results obtained by the ^{1}H and ^{13}C spectra of 4-NC were compared to the literature for structural determination of the substance [32]. NMR spectroscopic data obtained for 4-Nerolidylcatechol at 300 MHz for ^{1}H at 75 MHz for ^{13}C in chloroform-d. Carbons with δ between 110 and 120 ppm are typical of aromatic rings. Thus, the C-3, C-5, and C-6 carbons were assigned to the signals in δ 115.1; 119.2, and 114.3, respectively. Other signals obtained in the ^{13}C spectrum in δ 141.4 and 143.2 were attributed to the substituted carbons of the C-1 and C-2 aromatic ring, respectively, which are characteristic of the catechol group. The C-4 at δ 141.0 indicated that it was bound to the nerolidol group, which was identified by the existence of unsaturated aliphatic grouping signals, in particular by the two signals of two methylene carbons (C-5′ and C-9′) bound to the double bond methyls (δ 23.1 and 26.8, respectively) and three other vinyl methyl (C-12′, C-13′, and C-14′). IR spectroscopy showed high intensity in the absorbing bands with a wave number of 3400 cm-1 relative to the axial deformation of free hydroxyls (OH), also showing bands in 1635 and 1522 cm-1, indicating the presence of axial deformation of alkenes (C=C). In addition to an absorption band, 1283 cm-1 related to phenolic axial deformation (C-O) and the presence of methylene groups due to the presence of absorption bands at 3000 cm^{-1} (axial deformation C-H) (Figure 1) signals corroborated the structure of 4-NC (Figure 2).

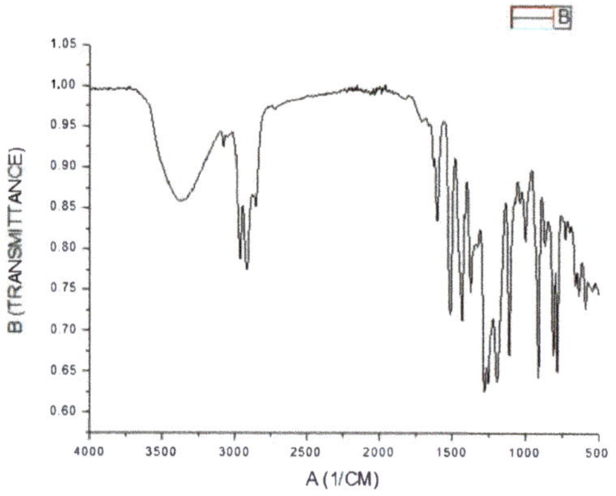

Figure 1. 4-Nerolidylcatechol infrared spectrum.

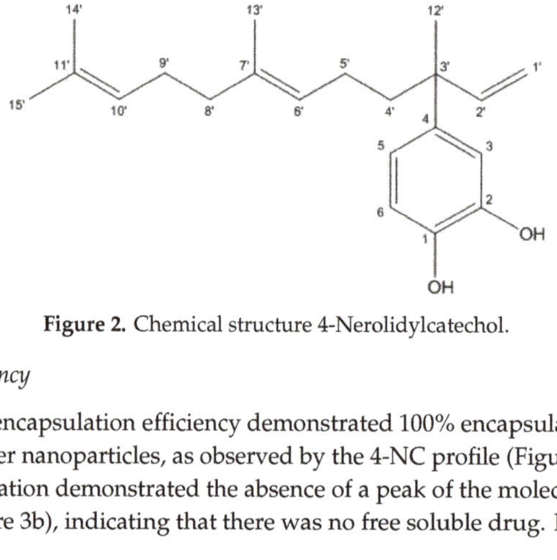

Figure 2. Chemical structure 4-Nerolidylcatechol.

3.2. Encapsulation Efficiency

The evaluation of encapsulation efficiency demonstrated 100% encapsulation efficiency in 4-NC encapsulation in polymer nanoparticles, as observed by the 4-NC profile (Figure 3a). Chromatograms obtained after centrifugation demonstrated the absence of a peak of the molecule at 11.238 min in the Amicom® filtrate (Figure 3b), indicating that there was no free soluble drug. In the chromatogram of material retained in the filter (Figure 3c), the 4-NC peak was observed, attributed to the encapsulated drug. The chromatographic profile of the empty nanoparticles is shown in Figure 4.

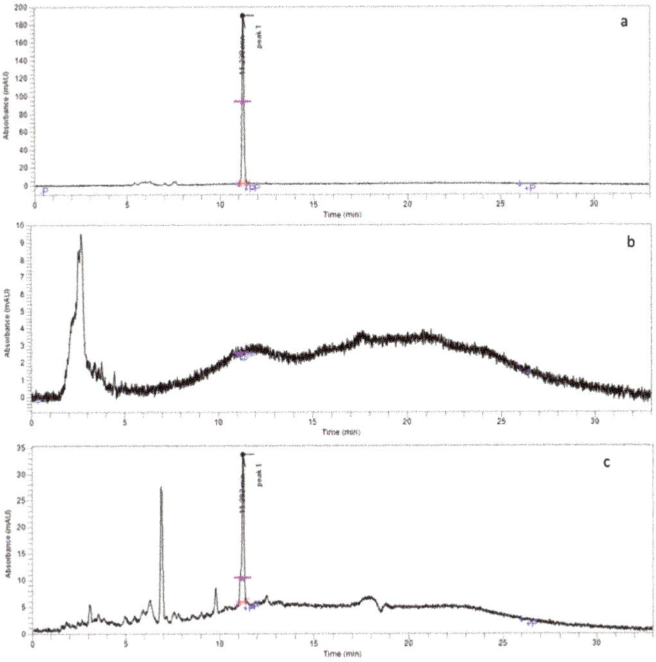

Figure 3. 4-NC Encapsulation efficiency in nanoparticles. (**a**) 4-NC Chromatographic profile. (**b**) Chromatographic profile of 4-NC Nanoparticles filtered in Amicon® tube. (**c**) Chromatographic profile of 4-NC nanoparticles retained in the Amicon® tube.

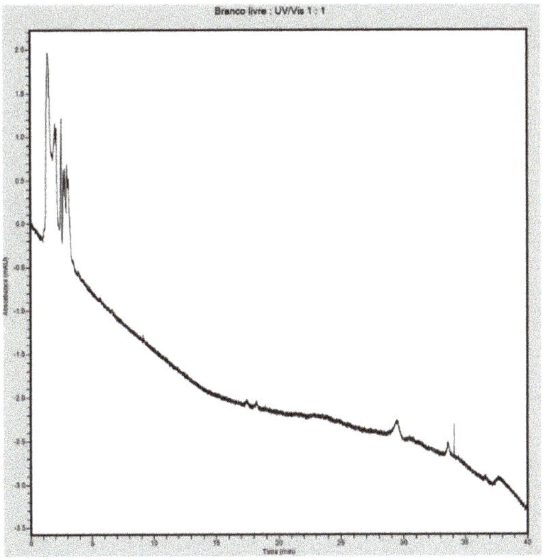

Figure 4. Chromatographic profile of empty nanoparticles.

3.3. DLS, Zeta Potential and NTA Characterization

The polymeric nanoparticle's (NPs) size was 148.1 ± 1.12 nm for empty nanoparticles and 143.5 ± 1.36 nm for nanoparticles with 4-NC. The poly dispersive index (pdi) was 0.149 ± 0.01, with zeta potential (zeta) of −7.15 ± 0.16 mV for empty NPs, while nanoparticles with 4-NC showed polydispersity index of 0.232 ± 0.00 and zeta potential of −9.30 ± 0.17 mV (Table 1).

Table 1. Zeta potential, polydispersion index, and size of nanoparticles.

	Zeta Potential (mV)	pdi	Size (nm)
Empty NP	−7.15 ± 0.16	0.149 ± 0.01	148.1 ± 1.12
4-NC NP	−9.30 ± 0.17	0.232 ± 0.00	143.5 ± 1.36

Empty NP: nanoparticles without 4-NC; 4-NCNP: nanoparticles with 4-NC.

The nanoparticles were also characterized by nano tracking analysis (NTA), showing a concentration of empty nanoparticles of 6.14×10^{11} $\pm 7.74 \times 10^{9}$ particles/mL, and nanoparticles with 4-NC demonstrated a concentration of $3.38 \times 10^{9} \pm 2.4 \times 10^{8}$ particles/mL (Figure 5).

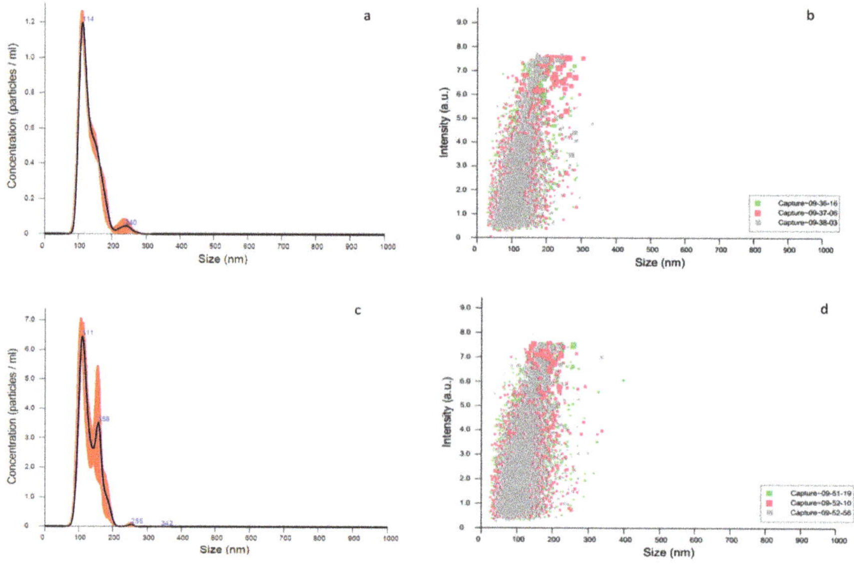

Figure 5. Particle size distribution. (**a**) The concentration of empty nanoparticles. (**b**) The distribution of empty nanoparticles. (**c**) The concentration of 4-NC nanoparticle. (**d**) The distribution of 4-NC.

The photomicrography of nanoparticles obtained for SEM showed a diameter between 35.2 and 162.4 nm (Figure 6).

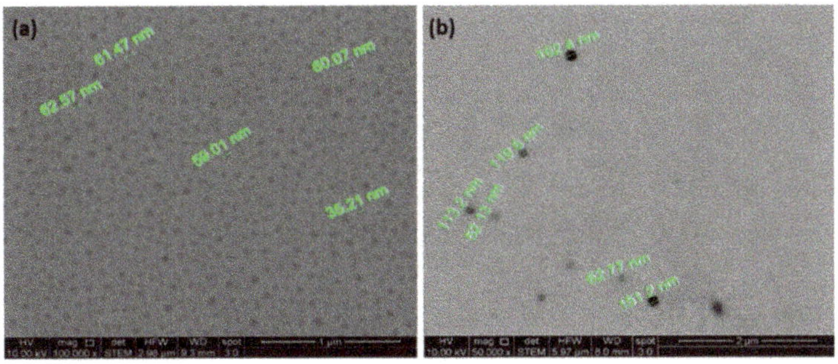

Figure 6. Scanning Electron Microscopy. (**a**) Empty NPs without dilution. (**b**) 4-NC NPs with 10x dilution.

3.4. FT-IR Spectral of Nanoparticles and Compounds

The FT-IR for 4-NC 65 μg did not show any stretching spectra, which could be due to the FT-IR sensibility equipment (Figure 7).

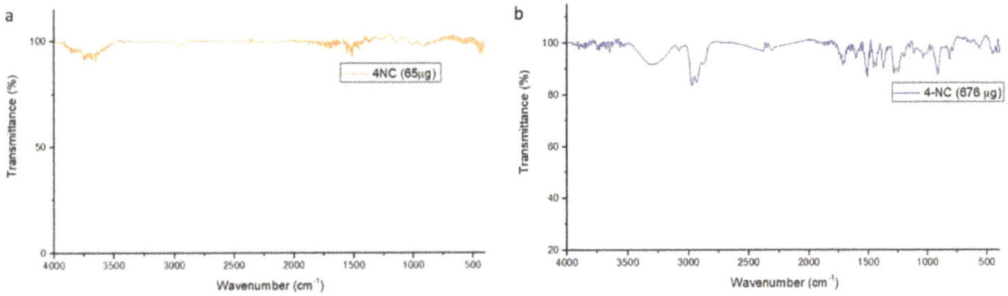

Figure 7. FT-IR spectra of 4-NC (**a**) 65 μg (**b**) 676 μg.

The FT-IR for the 4-NC 676 μg shows high-intensity bands on 3300 cm^{-1} associated to free –OH groups stretching vibrations and strong and broad signal. Other signals were shown on 2900 cm^{-1} related to C-H alkane vibrations. Besides, the 4-NC have more characteristics on 1700 and 1600 cm^{-1} related to alkenes C=C oleafinic and C-C bonds on aromatics, 1200 cm^{-1} the C-O phenolic stretch, and 900 cm^{-1} the C-H alkene oleafinic vibrations.

PCL spectra showed on 3000 cm^{-1} C-H alkane vibrations, 1700 cm^{-1} a strong narrow signal expected from the carbonyls and C-O bonds stretching on 1300–1100 cm^{-1} (Figure 8a). The IR spectrum of poloxamer 407 shows the absorption peaks at 2800 cm^{-1} related to C-H alkane stretch, a signal on 1300–1100 cm^{-1} associated with C-O ether stretch vibration (Figure 8b).

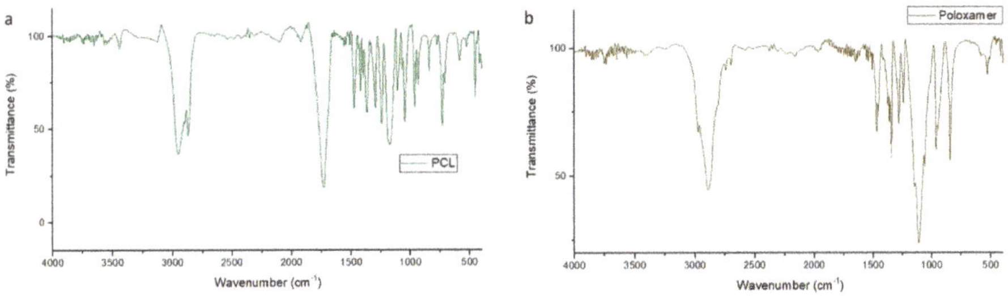

Figure 8. FT-IR spectra. (**a**) PCL, (**b**) poloxamer.

The empty nanoparticles showed a residual water signal at 3500 cm^{-1}, a signal at 2800 cm^{-1} related to the C-H alkane bonds to PCL and Poloxamer 407, a strong narrow signal at 1700 cm^{-1} associated to the carbonyl vibrations of the PCL, and a shorter signal on the 1100 cm^{-1} that corresponded to the C-O ether bond of the Poloxamer 407, indicating an interaction with the PCL (Figure 9).

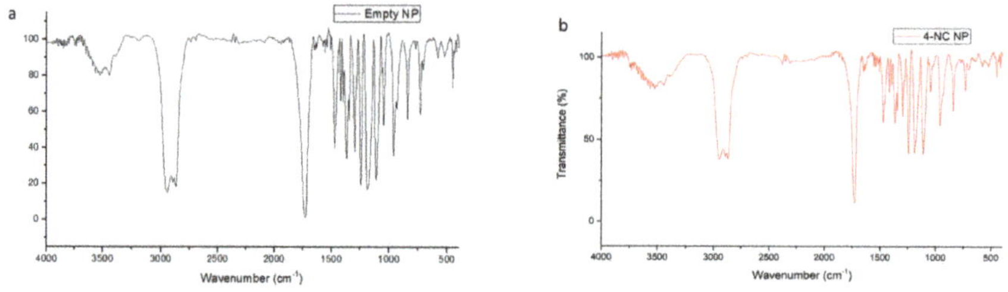

Figure 9. FT-IR spectra for NP. (**a**) Empty, (**b**) with 4-NC loaded.

The incorporated nanoparticles with 4-NC also showed a band assigned to the vibrational mode νOH at 3500 cm^{-1}, characteristic of the presence of water, the C-H alkane bonds at 2800 cm^{-1} due to the PCL and poloxamer characteristics, the carbonyls vibration bond at 1700 cm^{-1} for the PCL molecule, and a reduced signal at 1100 cm^{-1} for the C-O ether bond. The comparison of the FTIR spectral of the 4-NC incorporated and empty nanoparticules showed that the profile of the spectra were similar, showing the water signal at 3500 cm^{-1}, the C-H aliphatic bond vibrations at 2800 cm^{-1}, the strong narrow band at 1700 cm^{-1} due to the carbonyl of PCL, and a reduction of the signal from 1500–900 cm^{-1} on the 4-NC-NP (Figure 10).

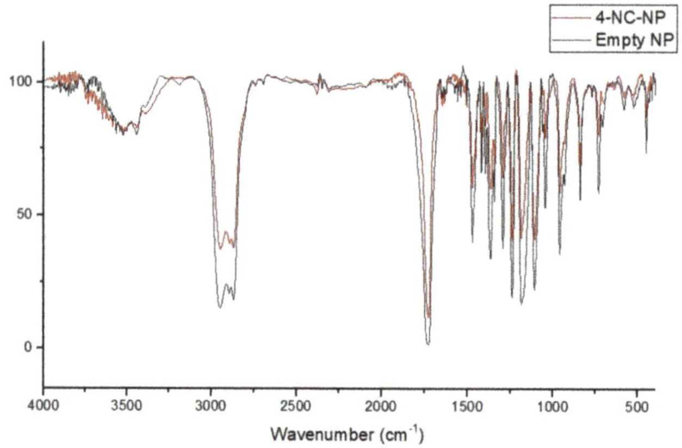

Figure 10. Comparison of 4-NC NP and empty NP FT-IR spectrum.

The spectra results showed that the equipment sensibility could show any 4-NC signal in a 65 μg concentration, and the 4-NC NP were made with 45 μg. Therefore, the 4-NC molecule did not demonstrate a different profile on nanoparticle's signal due to the low concentration, however, the 4-NC NP showed a strong, distinct biologic activity when compared with the empty NP.

3.5. Nanoparticles Antifungal Activity

Table 2 shows the in vitro antifungal activity, evidencing that when the drug was nanoencapsulated, there was an increase of 9.61 times in the MIC and 19.23 times for the MFC. Terbinafine and amphotericin B, control drugs, were evaluated only in free form, without nanoencapsulation.

Table 2. Minimal inhibitory concentration (MIC) and minimal fungicide concentration (MFC) of 4-NC, nanoparticles, and controls (μg/mL).

Samples *	MIC	MFC
4-NC	7.8	7.8
NP	-	-
4-NCNP	75	150
Amphotericin B	0.5	0.5
Terbinafine	0.625	0.625

*: 4-NC, 4-Nerolidylcatechol; NP, nanoparticles; 4-NCNP, nanoparticles with 4-NC. Data are representative of three independent experiments.

3.6. *In Vivo Analysis*

The results showed that there were no changes in liver enzymes resulting from the treatments (Figure 11).

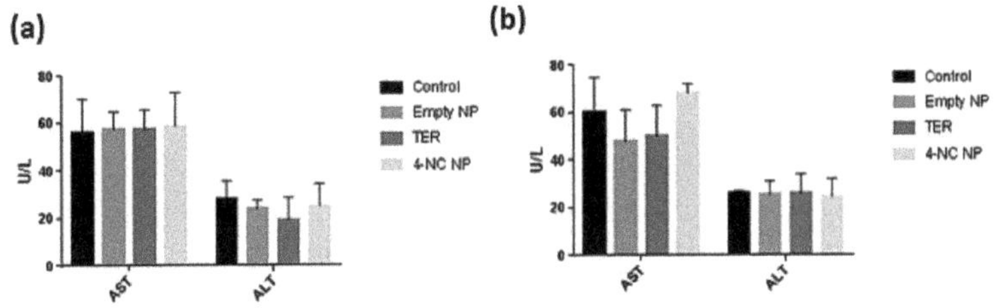

Figure 11. Analysis of the alanine aminotransferase (ALT) and aspartate aminotransferase (AST) enzymes from treated and untreated animals. (**a**) Control, no treatment; TER, free terbinafine; 4-NC NP, Nanoparticles with 4-NC; Empty NP, empty nanoparticles, with 3 days treatment. (**b**) Control, no treatment; TER, free terbinafine; 4-NC NP, nanoparticles with 4-NC; Empty NP, empty nanoparticles, with 7 days treatment. The statistical analysis was performed by Graph Pad Prism Version 7.0 software, through analysis of variance (ANOVA) and Dunnett's test, establishing $p < 0.05$ as the significance level.

In assessing the potential damage to the liver, the levels of transaminases were checked in the plasma, and no significant variation in liver enzymes was observed during the period of 3 and 7 days of treatment. There were evaluated using analysis of variance (ANOVA) and Dunnett's test, establishing a p-value <0.05 as the significant level. No statistically significant difference was observed between the drug-treated and control groups.

The silver methenamine staining of Grocott–Gomori, widely used in fungal detection histology, showed *M. canis* hyphae around the hair follicles indicated by the arrows (Figure 12a), when the skin of an infected with *M. canis* and untreated animal, euthanized three days post-infection was observed. The euthanized animals with 7 days of treatment did not present any more infections, suggesting a recomposition of their immunity. Free terbinafine, after three days of treatment, showed no evidence of *M. canis* infection.

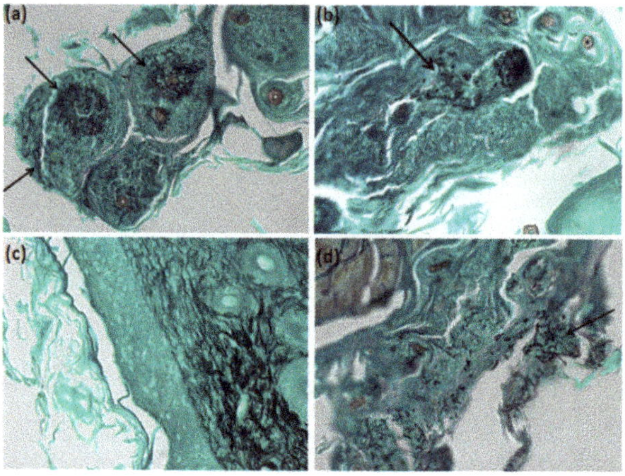

Figure 12. Grocott–Gomori microscopy of the skins of the euthanized animals with three days of treatment. (**a**) The skin of an animal infected with *M. canis* and without treatment. (**b**) The skin of an animal treated with 4-NC nanoparticles. (**c**) The skin of an animal treated with terbinafine. (**d**) The skin of an animal treated with empty nanoparticles.

4. Discussion

The identification of 4-NC was carried out by nuclear magnetic resonance of hydrogens and carbons. 4-NC shows characteristic signs of aromatic and aliphatic hydrogens. Signals in the region between δ 5 and 6 (ppm) are usually attributed to olefins, whereby the signals in δ 5.02 and 5.98 were respectively assigned to the hydrogens bound to the C-1′ and C-2′, and the hydrogens connected to the C-6′ and C-10′ carbons. Signals in the region between δ 1 and 2 (ppm) correspond to methyl, so we can see in δ 1.33 (3H), δ 1.68 (3H), 1.51 (3H), and δ 1.59 (3H), with a chemical shift in the last three signals confirming the presence of double bond, these signals are attributed to the hydrogens connected to the C-12′, C-14′, C-15′, and C-13′ carbons, respectively. The signals corresponding to the aromatic hydrogens presented chemical displacement at δ 6.84, δ 6.74, and at δ 6.79, confirming the catechol grouping. The signals obtained from carbons at δ 141.4 and δ 143.2 are characteristic of the catechol system, corresponding to carbons C-1 and C-2. The ^{1}H NMR and ^{13}C NMR signals are in agreement with data obtained in the literature. The molecular weight of the 4-NC obtained was 314.46 g, the chemical formula being $C_{12}H_{30}O_2$. These results are similar to the results found by Iwamoto et al. (2014) [7], Bergamo (2003) [32], Almeida (2011) [33], and Freitas (2015) [34].

In this study, it was possible to observe that the 4-NC showed total encapsulation (100%), corroborating that the antimicrobial activity demonstrated was of the nanoparticles containing 4-NC. The results obtained showed encapsulation of incorporation superior to those found by Abriata et al. (2017) [25], who used the same polymer and surfactant to incorporate ursolic acid, obtaining results 36.44% lower when using in the same concentrations of compound and polymer. Using the nanoprecipitation technique for amphotericin B incorporation, the results of the encapsulation efficiency were 60 to 80% in the formulations prepared [35].

Analysis of zeta potential demonstrated that poly-ε-caprolactone nanoparticles have a negative potential. In the study by Shao et al. [36], the nanoparticles with negative zeta potential caused little damage to the cell membranes, and the authors justified this result due to the weak interactions with the cells. This low interaction with the biomembranes favors low cytotoxicity.

The characterization analysis of the nanoparticles by DLS, showed an approximate size of 143.5 to 148.1 nm, a much smaller size when compared to the nanoparticles obtained by Souza et al. (2012) [37], which incorporated the herbicide atrazine through the nanoprecipitation technique, but using the surfactant polysorbate 80 (Tween® 80). They obtained diameters up to 341 nm using the same polymer (PCL), and the same technique, i.e., nanoprecipitation.

Comparing the size data obtained by DLS and NTA, it was observed that NTA presented results of smaller nanoparticles. This type of result was also observed by other authors [19,38]. NTA analysis is a complementary technique for the characterization of nanoparticles. The difference between NTA and DLS is that the first provides the concentration of the suspended nanoparticles, and is possible to visualize the sample through videos and obtaining the presented peaks with better resolution [19].

Scanning electron microscopy showed that the nanoparticles have a lower size than that determined by analysis performed in solution and through light or laser beams. This is because, in the microscopic analysis, the samples are dried on a copper grid, and in this way, the reading does not take into account loads that could be around the particle, as in the tests that are carried out in solution, such as DLS and NTA.

Perecin et al. (2016) [39] encapsulated magnetite on a PCL and poloxamer system on a 1:5 ratio magnetite and PCL. The FT-IR spectrum of the nanoparticles does not demonstrate the interaction of the incorporated nanoparticle made of PCL and poloxamer, because the magnetite spectra showed only one strong signal at 600 cm^{-1} and that signal did not appear on the incorporated nanoparticle.

Soares et al. (2009) [40] studied a 4-Nerolidylcathecol system with 2-hydroxypropyl-β-cyclodextrin on a 1:1 molar ratio and the FT-IR spectrum of the 4-NC shows similar signals to out spectra. The 4-NC incorporated into the 2-hidroxypropyl-β-ciclodextrin was not capable of a strong, significant and different signal modification even on a 1:1 molar ratio. The incorporated signal on 3400 cm^{-1} is related to O-H aromatic bond of the sugars and the 1100–1000 cm^{-1} signal due to the ether bond vibration present on the cyclodextrin.

There is a need for further studies of release kinetics in order to improve the formulation and accelerate the release process of the 4-NC of the nanoparticles so that in the free form, they can exert the expected activity in a controlled manner and guarantee the stability of 4-NC-loaded nanoparticle.

The polymeric nanoparticle without 4-NC incorporation did not demonstrate antimicrobial activity; the antifungal activity resulted from the compound incorporated. Nanoparticles with 4-NC compared to the 4-NC isolated demonstrate a higher MIC of 4-NC nanoparticles. The antifungal activity was not potentiated by the incorporation, but neither was inhibited, which could be a consequence of slow-release from nanoparticles. However, the slow release could be an advantage for long-term use of treatment, which could be further investigated in future studies.

It has already been demonstrated in the literature that 4-NC shows certain cytotoxicity for some cell strains [7], besides possessing an antioxidant characteristic [19], is an unstable compound31, and exhibits low polarity, making difficult its incorporation into aqueous formulations. Due to these difficulties, nanostructured systems are an alternative to the use of this molecule for different biological applications.

The in vivo test of liver enzyme profiles of the animals was shown to have the same standard dosage of the ALT enzyme for the treated groups compared to the untreated group, indicating the absence of toxicity. In the present study, the results for AST were significantly lower when compared to the results of the untreated group studied by Nogueira-Neto et al. (2012) [41], which obtained results of 49.67 U/L. Similar data were found by Araujo (2012) [42] comparing Swiss mice with two different breeding strains, where they observed alterations in the values of the animals without any treatment for both ALT and AST. Studies of AST performed by Branco et al. (2011) [43] showed mean values 277.0 ± 18 U/L, whereas values of the present study were significantly lower in all groups. The evaluation of liver enzymes brings promising data since they demonstrate that there was no hepatic damage resulting from the treatment, which is a concern when using 4-NC.

The mouse skins stained with silver methenamine by Grocott–Gomori staining technique showed that groups infected with *M. canis* and treated with nanoparticles, after three days of treatment, still present some infection, however in less extension than the untreated group. The terbinafine group, which was constituted of free drug, no longer had fungi in the analyzed skin areas. Although it is a qualitative analysis, it was shown that nanoparticles are promising for the treatment of filamentous fungi infection.

This study showed that 4-Nerolidylcatechol had high encapsulation efficiency when associated with the nanoprecipitation technique with poly- ε -caprolactone, allowing a more stable formulation, since the evaluation of encapsulation demonstrated that there was no degradation of the compound. The encapsulation allows a possible controlled release for antifungal treatment that is long and difficult. Adjustments to the formulation are required in order to allow the antifungal activity of the compound to be maintained at lower levels even after encapsulation.

Author Contributions: V.R.G. and R.C.L.R.P. conceived and designed the experiments: V.R.G. performed the synthesis of nanoparticles, in vitro and in vivo experiments; V.R.G., F.O., R.S., B.R.K., and C.M.S. performed biological experiments; M.C., P.B.D.S., and J.O.E. were responsible for the nanoparticles study; M.J.K. and J.O.M. were responsible for encapsulation evaluation; A.C.V.B.W. was responsible for microscopy analysis; V.R.G. and R.C.L.R.P. analyzed the data; V.R.G. and R.C.L.R.P. prepared the manuscript; R.C.L.R.P. supervised the study. All authors have read and agreed to the published version of the manuscript.

Funding: This study was supported by Fundação de Amparo à Pesquisa do Estado de São Paulo (FAPESP, Brazil), Process 2016/02107-5, Fondo de Financiamiento de Centros de Investigación en Áreas Prioritarias, Chile (Fondap 15130011).and in part by the Coordenação de Aperfeiçoamento de Pessoal de Nível Superior—Brasil (CAPES)—Finance Code 001.

Acknowledgments: The authors thank the Brazilian Agencies: Coordenação de Aperfeiçoamento de Pessoal de Ensino Superior (CAPES) and Fundação de Amparo à Pesquisa do Estado de São Paulo (FAPESP). We are very grateful to M.Sc. Aline Renata Pavan and Jean Leandro dos Santos with the assistance in carrying out FTIR experiments.

Conflicts of Interest: The authors declare no conflict of interest.

References

1. Maraki, S.; Mavromanolaki, V.E. Epidemiology of Dermatophytoses in Crete, Greece: A 5-year Survey. *Med. Mycol. J.* **2016**, *57e*, 69–75. [CrossRef]
2. Vineetha, M.; Sheeja, S.; Celine, M.I.; Sadeep, M.S.; Palackal, S.; Shanimole, E.; Das, S.S. Profile of Dermatophytosis in a Tertiary Care Center. *Indian J. Dermatol.* **2018**, *63*, 490–495. [PubMed]
3. Lima, E.; Pinto, A.; Nogueira, K.; Silva, L.; Almeida, P.; Vasconcellos, M.; Chaves, F.; Tadei, W.; Pohlit, A. Stability and Antioxidant Activity of Semi-synthetic Derivatives of 4-Nerolidylcatechol. *Molecules* **2012**, *18*, 178–189. [CrossRef] [PubMed]
4. Dorigoni, P.A.; Ghedini, P.C.; Fróes, L.F.; Baptista, K.C.; Ethur, A.B.M.; Baldisserotto, B.; Bürger, M.E.; Almeida, C.E.; Lopes, A.M.V.; Záchia, R.A. Survey of data on medicinal plants of popular use in the municipality of São João do Polêsine, RS, Brazil. i—Relationship between diseases and species used. *Braz. J. Med. Plants* **2001**, *4*, 69–79.
5. Lopes, A.P.; Bagatela, B.S.; Rosa, P.C.P.; Nanayakkara, N.P.; Carvalho, J.C.T.; Mainstro, E.L.; Bastos, J.K.; Perazzo, F.F. Antioxidant and cytotoxic effects of crude extract, fractions and 4-nerolidylcathecol from aerial parts of *Pothomorphe umbellata* L. (Piperaceae). *Biomed. Res. Int.* **2013**, *1*, 1–5. [CrossRef] [PubMed]
6. Bagatela, B.S.; Lopes, A.P.; Fonseca, F.L.A.; Andreo, M.A.; Nanayakkara, D.N.P.; Bastos, J.K.; Perazzo, F.F. Evaluation of antimicrobial and antimalarial activities of crude extract, fractions and 4- nerolidylcathecol from the aerial parts of *Piper umbellata* L. (Piperaceae). *Nat. Prod. Res.* **2013**, *27*, 2202–2209. [CrossRef]
7. Iwamoto, L.H.; Costa, D.B.V.; Monteiro, P.A.; Ruiz, A.L.T.G.; Sousa, I.M.O.; Foglio, M.A.; de Carvalho, J.E.; Rodrigues, R.A. Anticancer and Anti-Inflammatory Activities of a Standardized Dichloromethane Extract from *Piper umbellatum* L. Leaves. *Evid. Based Complement. Alternat. Med. eCAM* **2015**, 1–8. [CrossRef]
8. Roersch, C.M.F.B. *Piper umbellatum* L. A comparative cross-cultural analysis of its medicinal uses and an ethnopharmacological evaluation. *J. Ethnopharmacol.* **2010**, *131*, 522–537. [CrossRef]
9. Rodrigues, E.R.; Nogueira, N.G.P.; Zocolo, J.G.; Leite, F.S.; Januario, A.H.; Fusco-Almeida, A.M.; Fachin, A.L.; de Marchi, M.R.; dos Santos, A.G.; Pietro, R.C. *Pothomorphe umbellata*: Antifungal activity against strains of *Trichophyton rubrum*. *J. Mycol. Med.* **2012**, *22*, 265–269. [CrossRef]
10. PubChem. Available online: https://pubchem.ncbi.nlm.nih.gov/compound/4-Nerolidylcatechol (accessed on 28 October 2020).

11. Rocha e Silva, L.F.; Nogueira, K.L.; Pinto, A.C.S.; Katzin, A.M.; Sussmann, R.A.C.; Muniz, M.P.; Andrade Neto, V.F.; Chaves, F.C.M.; Coutinho, J.P.; Lima, E.S.; et al. In Vivo Antimalarial Activity and Mechanisms of Action of 4-Nerolidylcatechol Derivatives. *Antimicrob. Agents Chemother.* **2015**, *59*, 3271–3280. [CrossRef]
12. Alves-Fernandes, D.K.; Oliveira, E.A.; Hastreiter, A.A.; Faião-Flores, F.; Felipe-Silva, A.S.; Turato, W.; Fock, R.A.; Maria-Engler, S.S.; Barros, S.B. In vivo antitumoral effect of 4-nerolidylcatechol (4-NC) in NRAS-mutant human melanoma. *Food Chem. Toxicol.* **2020**, *141*, 1–12. [CrossRef] [PubMed]
13. Severino, P.; Andreani, T.; Macedo, A.S.; Fangueiro, J.F.; Santana, M.H.A.; Silva, A.M.; Souto, E.B. Current state of art and new trends on lipid nanoparticles (SLN and NLC) for oral drug delivery. *J. Drug Deliv.* **2012**, *2012*, 750891. [CrossRef] [PubMed]
14. Joseph, S.; Bunjes, H. Solid Lipid Nanoparticles for Drug Delivery. In *Drug Delivery Strategies for Poorly Water-Soluble Drugs*; Douroumis, D., Fahr, A., Eds.; John Wiley & Sons Ltd.: Chichester, UK, 2013; pp. 103–149. ISBN 9780470711972.
15. Zhang, W.; Saliba, M.; Stranks, S.D.; Sun, Y.; Shi, X.; Wiesner, U.; Snaith, H.J. Enhancement of Perovskite-Based Solar Cells Employing Core–Shell Metal Nanoparticles. *Nano Lett.* **2013**, *13*, 4505–4510. [CrossRef] [PubMed]
16. Dash, T.K.; Konkimalla, V.B. Poly- -caprolactone based formulations for drug delivery and tissue engineering: A review. *J. Control. Release* **2012**, *158*, 15–33. [CrossRef] [PubMed]
17. Silva, L.G. Chemical Physical Characterization and Evaluation of the In Vitro Release of Poly (ε-Caprolactone)/Tetracycline Conjugates and Poly (ε-Caprolactone)/Ethylsalicylic Acid Conjugates. Master's Thesis, Federal University of Itajubá, Itajubá, Brazil, 2012.
18. Valeriano, V.S.; Leal, A.F.V.B.; Soares, L.A.; Rezende, K.R.; Resck, I.S.; Kato, M.J. Inclusion complex of 4-Nerolidylcatechol in hydroxypropyl-β-cyclodextrin. *Rev. Eletrônica Farmácia* **2005**, *2*, 224–227.
19. Elsabahy, M.; Wooley, K.L. Design of polymeric nanoparticles for biomedical delivery applications. *Chem. Soc. Rev.* **2012**, *41*, 2545–2561. [CrossRef] [PubMed]
20. Souza, A.C.O.; Amaral, A.C. Antifungal Therapy for Systemic Mycosis and the Nanobiotechnology Era: Improving Efficacy, Biodistribution and Toxicity. *Front. Microbiol.* **2017**, *8*, 1–13. [CrossRef]
21. Gaeti, M.P.N.; Benfica, P.L.; Mendes, L.P.; Vieira, M.S.; Anjos, J.L.V.; Alonso, A.; Rezende, K.R.; Valadares, M.C.; Lima, E.M. Liposomal entrapment of 4-nerolidylcatechol: Impact on phospholipid dynamics, drug stability and bioactivity. *J. Nanosci. Nanotech.* **2015**, *15*, 838–847. [CrossRef]
22. Mondal, D.; Griffth, M.; Venkatraman, S.S. Polycaprolactone-based biomaterials for tissue engineering and drug delivery: Current scenario and challenges. *Int. J. Polym. Mater. Polym. Biomater.* **2016**, *65*, 255–265. [CrossRef]
23. Tammaro, R.; Saturnino, C.; D'Aniello, S.; Vigliotta, G.; Vittoria, V. Polymorphic solidification of Linezolid confined in electrospun PCL fibers for controlled release in topical applications. *Int. J. Pharm.* **2015**, *490*, 32–38. [CrossRef]
24. Wang, H.; Xia, Y.; Liu, J.; Ma, Z.; Shi, Q.; Yin, J. Programmable release of 2-O-D-glucopyranosyl-L-ascorbic acid and heparin from PCL-based nanofiber scaffold for reduction of inflammation and thrombosis. *Mater. Today Chem.* **2020**, *17*, 100303. [CrossRef]
25. Abriata, J.P.; Eloy, J.O.; Riul, T.B.; Campos, P.M.; Baruffi, M.D.; Marchetti, J.M. Poly-epsilon-caprolactone nanoparticles enhance ursolic acid in vivo efficacy against *Trypanosoma cruzi* infection. *Mat. Sci. Eng. C-Mater.* **2017**, *77*, 1196–1203. [CrossRef] [PubMed]
26. Filipe, V.; Hawe, A.; Jiskoot, W. Critical Evaluation of Nanoparticle Tracking Analysis (NTA) by NanoSight for the Measurement of Nanoparticles and Protein Aggregates. *Pharm. Res.* **2010**, *27*, 796–810. [CrossRef] [PubMed]
27. Adura, C.; Grerrero, S.; Salas, E.; Medel, L.; Riveros, A.; Mena, J.; Arbiol, J.; Albericio, F.; Giralt, E.; Kogan, M.J. Stable conjugates of peptides with gold nanorods for biomedical applications with reduced effects on cell viability. *ACS Appl. Mater. Inter.* **2013**, *5*, 4076–4085. [CrossRef] [PubMed]
28. Clinical and Laboratory Standards Institute (CLSI). *Reference Method for Broth Dilution Antifungal Susceptibility Testing of Filamentous Fungi; Approved Standard*, 2nd ed.; CLSI document M38-A2; CLSI: Wayne, PA, USA, 2008.
29. Sharma, B.; Kumar, P.; Joshi, S. Topical Treatment of Dermatophytic Lesion on Mice (*Mus musculus*) Model. *Indian J. Microbiol.* **2011**, *51*, 217–222. [CrossRef]
30. Golde, W.T.; Gollobin, P.; Rodriguez, L.L. A rapid, simple, and humane method for submandibular bleeding of mice using a lancet. *Lab. Anim.* **2005**, *34*, 39–43. [CrossRef]

31. Ozer, J.; Ratner, M.; Shaw, M.; Bailey, W.; Schomaker, S. The current state of serum biomarkers of hepatotoxicity. *Toxicology* **2008**, *245*, 194–205. [CrossRef]
32. Bergamo, D.C.B. Chemical Evaluation of Nonvolatile and Volatile Components and Biosynthetic Study of 4-Nerolidylcatecol in *Potomorphe umbellata*. Ph.D. Thesis, Institute of Chemistry, UNESP, Araraquara, Brazil, 2003.
33. Almeida, R.L. Participation of Fractions of 4-Nerolidylcatecol-Free Hydroalcoholic Root Extract of *Pothomorphe umbellata* Root on the Antioxidant and Inhibitory Activity of Metalloproteinases 2 and 9 on Skin. Ph.D. Thesis, School of Pharmaceutical Sciences, UNESP, São Paulo, Brazil, 2011.
34. Freitas, J.A. Investigation of Antifungal Activity, Mechanisms of Action and Protein Profile Analysis against *Pothomorphe umbellata* Extracts. Master´s Thesis, School of Pharmaceutical Sciences, UNESP, Araraquara, Brazil, 2015.
35. Das, S.; Suresh, P.K.; Desmukh, R. Design of Eudragit RL 100 nanoparticles by nanoprecipitation method for ocular drug delivery. *Nanomedicine* **2010**, *6*, 318–323. [CrossRef]
36. Shao, X.R.; Wei, X.Q.; Song, X.; Hao, L.Y.; Cai, X.X.; Zhang, Z.R. Independent effect of polymeric nanoparticle zeta potential/surface charge, on their cytotoxicity and affinity to cells. *Cell Proliferat.* **2015**, *48*, 465–474. [CrossRef]
37. Souza, P.M.S.; Lobo, F.A.; Rosa, A.H.; Fraceto, L.F. Development of poly-caprolactone nanocapsules containing the atrazine herbicide. *Quim. Nova* **2012**, *35*, 132–137. [CrossRef]
38. James, A.E.; Driskell, J.D. Monitoring gold nanoparticle conjugation and analysis of biomolecular binding with nanoparticle tracking analysis (NTA) and dynamic light scattering (DLS). *Analyst* **2013**, *138*, 1212–1218. [CrossRef] [PubMed]
39. Perecin, C.; Cerize, N.; Chitta, V.; Gratens, X.; Léo, P.; de Oliveira, A.; Yoshioka, S. Magnetite Nanoparticles Encapsulated with PCL and Poloxamer by Nano Spray Drying Technology. *Nanosci. Nanotechnol.* **2016**, *6*, 68–73. [CrossRef]
40. Soares, L.A.; Leal, A.F.V.B.; Fraceto, L.F.; Maia, E.R.; Resck, I.S.; Kato, M.J.; Gil, E.S.; de Sousa, A.R.; Cunha, L.C.; Rezende, K.R. Host-guest system of 4-nerolidylcatechol in 2-hydroxypropyl-β-cliclodextrin: Preparation, characterization and molecular modeling. *J. Incl. Phenom. Macrocycl. Chem.* **2009**, *64*, 23–35. [CrossRef]
41. Nogueira-Neto, J.D.; Almeida, A.A.C.; Silva, A.O.; Carvalho, R.B.F.; de Sousa, D.P.; Freitas, R.M. Evaluation of acute toxicity and anxiolytic properties of nerolidol in mice. *BioFar* **2012**, *8*, 42–56.
42. Araujo, F.T.M. Establishment of Reference Values for Hematological and Biochemical Parameters and Evaluation of the Immunological Profile of Strains of Mice Produced in the Research Center René Rachou/FIOCRUZ—Minas and of Laboratory Breeding Center/FIOCRUZ. Ph.D. Thesis, Fundação Oswaldo Cruz Research Center René Rachou, Belo Horizonte, Brazil, 2012.
43. Branco, A.C.S.C.; Diniz, M.F.F.M.; Almeida, R.N.; Santos, H.B.; Oliveira, K.M.; Ramalho, J.A.; Dantas, J.G.; Diniz, M.F.F.M.; Almeida, R.N.; Santos, H.B.; et al. Biochemical and Hematological Parameters of *Wistar* Rats and *Swiss* Mice in the Professor Thomas George Animal Laboratory. *Rev. Bras. Ciênc. Saúde* **2011**, *15*, 209–214. [CrossRef]

MDPI
St. Alban-Anlage 66
4052 Basel
Switzerland
Tel. +41 61 683 77 34
Fax +41 61 302 89 18
www.mdpi.com

Antibiotics Editorial Office
E-mail: antibiotics@mdpi.com
www.mdpi.com/journal/antibiotics

www.ingramcontent.com/pod-product-compliance
Lightning Source LLC
LaVergne TN
LVHW070422100526
838202LV00014B/1504